So you want to be a doctor?

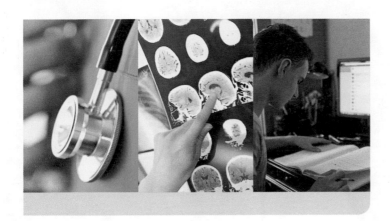

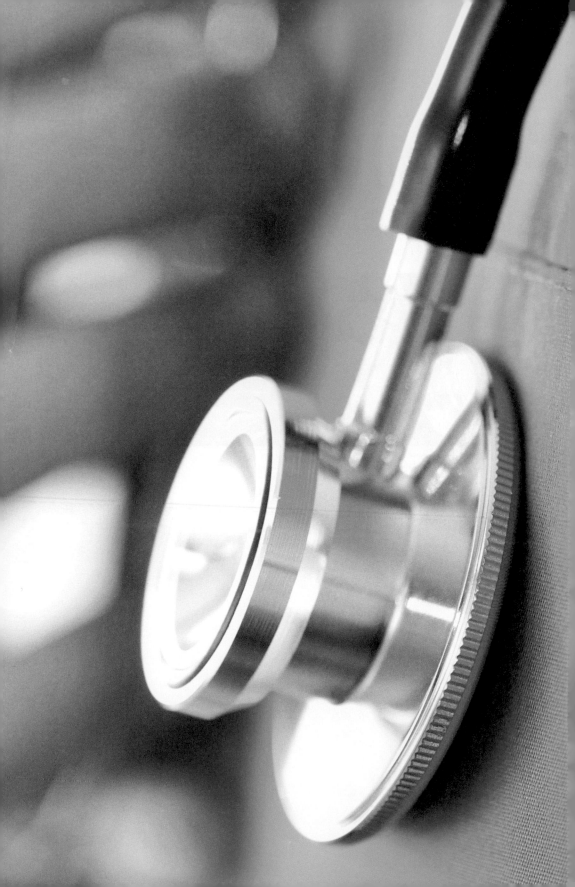

So you want to be a doctor?

The ultimate guide to getting into medical school

Third edition

Edited by

David Metcalfe

Harveer Dev

Michael Moazami

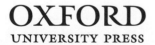

OXFORD

UNIVERSITY PRESS

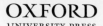

OXFORD
UNIVERSITY PRESS

Great Clarendon Street, Oxford, OX2 6DP,
United Kingdom

Oxford University Press is a department of the University of Oxford.
It furthers the University's objective of excellence in research, scholarship,
and education by publishing worldwide. Oxford is a registered trade mark of
Oxford University Press in the UK and in certain other countries

First Edition published in 2011
Second Edition published in 2014
Third Edition published in 2021

Impression: 1

Published in the United States of America by Oxford University Press
198 Madison Avenue, New York, NY 10016, United States of America

British Library Cataloguing in Publication Data
Data available

Library of Congress Control Number: 2021930034

ISBN 978–0–19–883630–8

DOI: 10.1093/med/9780198836308.001.0001

Printed in Great Britain by
Bell & Bain Ltd., Glasgow

To Mina, my beautiful wife (DM)

To Kiran and Dilan, for making it all worthwhile (HD)

To my family, for their love, and my friends,
for their support and kindness (MM)

Foreword

There has never been a more exciting time to be a doctor. Advances in medical science are allowing doctors to understand human biology, diagnose disease, and ultimately treat patients in ways that would have been unimaginable a few years ago.

There are many reasons why medicine continues to attract the most talented university applicants. The profession offers the respect and trust of the public, a team-based work environment, intellectually challenging cases, and great job security. However, the best reward remains using your abilities to alleviate the suffering of those in the greatest need and witnessing the results.

Winning a place at medical school is the first step to joining this fascinating profession. The selection process is long, complicated, and intensely competitive, so that only the most capable become doctors and care for patients. Earning your place at medical school requires a lot more than just passing exams; at each stage you need to prove that you have the qualities and aptitude required to be a good doctor. This book will take you through the application process and show you how to reach your full potential every step of the way. It will steer you in choosing the medical schools that suit your personality and sending them a clear message that you are the right applicant for their course.

If you work hard and use this book as a guide, you could be strolling the wards wearing your new stethoscope before you know it! Best of luck!

Professor the Lord Darzi of Denham KBE
Hon FREng, FMedSci, FRCS

Preface

Who has the potential to be an excellent doctor?

Medical schools across the UK wrestle with this question as they confront the thousands of applicants every year. A student's life, skills, and personality are reduced to a handful of grades and a single page of writing that will determine their fate. When sorting through these applications, medical schools use fixed criteria to discern 'strong' from 'weak' applications. While this ensures the process is 'fair', these criteria can miss excellent applicants who simply don't know how the system works.

In writing this book, we hope to level the playing field. Regardless of your background or familiarity with the medical profession, this book will help you put together the best possible application.

This book represents the distilled wisdom of over 100 medical students, admissions specialists, and faculty members covering every medical school in the UK. It will guide you through every stage of the application process—from getting work experience, to writing your UCAS form, to preparing for an interview—and with coping with the first term at medical school. It will also help you choose the medical schools that best suit your personality, meaning you have the best possible chance of being accepted.

Getting into medical school is difficult; we hope this guide helps you show that you have the potential to be an excellent doctor.

Good luck!

David Metcalfe
Harveer Dev
Michael Moazami

Acknowledgements

It would not have been possible to produce this book without the help of many kind individuals and institutions who gave their time and energy for our benefit. In particular:

All the contributors for their informative and insightful descriptions of life on each medical course.

The members of medical school faculty and admissions teams who submitted the text for the 'Insider's Views'.

The members of admissions teams who collected the data on admissions statistics that we have quoted in each of the medical school profiles.

The superb information provided by the GMC, UCAT, and BMAT, which made researching this book substantially easier.

Professor Ara Darzi for contributing the Foreword.

Kaplan Test Prep and Admissions (www.kaptest.com) for the material they contributed to Chapter 6 and Appendix 1.

All the contributors to the first and second editions of *So you want to be a doctor?*

Kate Dry for her contributions to Chapter 1.

Jas Toor, Mina Aletrari, and Adina Seaton for their constant support, exceptional proof-reading skills, and wonderful company.

Sarinder, Bobby, and Hardeep for their heroic support throughout the years.

George and Nicholas for putting up with their father disappearing into his office (again) when he should have been pushing them on the swings.

Our excellent editorial team at Oxford University Press, in particular Fiona Sutherland, Geraldine Jeffers, Hannah Lloyd, Abigail Stanley, and Claire Steele. Thank you for your continued support throughout.

▮ Contents

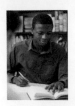

6 Preparing for admission tests 73

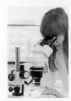

7 Choosing a medical school 89

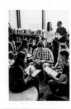

8 Undergraduate medical schools 123

9 Perfecting the UCAS form 215

10 Getting into Oxbridge 237

11 Graduate-entry medicine 251

12 Graduate-entry medical schools 265

13 Non-traditional applications...............................293

14 How to succeed at interview 303

15 If things don't work out...321

16 Making the most of medical school 331

Appendix 1: UCAT and BMAT questions...............347

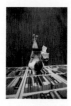

Appendix 2: Useful resources 379

■ Contributors

England

Aston
Keith Leung
Birmingham
Syed Husain
Beth Selwyn
Brighton and Sussex
Emily Mills
Bristol
Keng Siang Lee
Lelyn Osei Atiemo
Cambridge
Laith Alexander
Safia Samah Siddiqui
Central Lancashire
Roham Karimi
Exeter
Rebecca Randall
Harry Theron
Hull and York
Alice Fort–Schaale
Keele
Chantelle Umadia
Lancaster
Sukhbir Khosah
Leeds
Kelsey Loveday
Leicester
Binay Gurung
Liverpool
Biyyam Meghna Rao
Pippa Caine
London—Barts and The London
Joseph Sanders
Eden Seager
London—Imperial College
Dimitrios Karponis
Aleksander Dawidziuk

London—King's College
Anna Harvey
Lisa Hambley
Nathan Hayes
London—St George's
Sandy Ayoub
Vitasta Raina
London—University College (UCL)
Oliver Devine
Manchester
Tonia Forjoe
Newcastle
Shiv Kolhe
Callum McMahon
Nottingham
Afra Akmal
Nanin Rai
Oxford
Emma Flint
Annie Collins
Peninsula
Jonathan Murphy
Sheffield
Lesley Tinkler
Andrew Cinnamond
Southampton
Lizzie Little
Simon Bor
University of East Anglia
Ben McCartney
Warwick
Ollie Burton

Northern Ireland

Queen's, Belfast
Jennifer Tempany
Adam Gallacher

Scotland

Aberdeen
Rekha Gurung
Dylan McClurg
Dundee
Rachel Logan
Edinburgh
William Cambridge
Glasgow
Luai Kawar
St Andrews
Jeremy Samuel
ScotGEM
Callum George

Wales

Cardiff
Emma Rengasamy
Swansea
Christopher Norbury

Overseas

Pleven University, Bulgaria
Ayesha Arora
Charles University, Czech Republic
Taranpreet K. Bhoday

Chapter 1 (Tips for parents)

Kate Dry

▌Becoming a doctor

There are few careers that offer as vast an array of human experience as that of a doctor. It includes the privilege of being present at the birth of a child, relieving pain, taking actions that save the lives of others, and comforting patients and families in times of distress. It is a noble and exciting profession that attracts the most intelligent and caring individuals of each generation.

Getting into medical school

This book is written to help you face the biggest hurdle on the route to becoming a doctor: getting into medical school. Drawing on the experience of over 100 medical students and doctors, it will guide you through every stage of the process, helping you make the best possible decisions for the perfect application.

Medical school applications are amongst the most competitive of any at university. Having top grades is essential, but this is not enough. Medical schools are looking for well-rounded individuals who will make good doctors and who know what the job entails. To ensure that you are the right type of person, they expect to see a range of extracurricular activities (see p. 46), medical work experience (see p. 54), and high marks on your admission tests (see p. 74).

Timeline

A successful application to medical school requires almost three years of planning, from deciding which A levels or Highers to study right up to starting medical school (see Figure 1). The busiest time is Year 12 (England, Wales, and Northern Ireland) or S6 (Scotland), during which you must obtain suitable work experience and engage in extracurricular activities, choose which universities to apply to, sit admission tests, and complete the UCAS application—all whilst studying full-time.

The stages of getting into medical school

To help plan your application, the process has been broken down into five stages (Figure 2).

Deciding

The first step on the road to being a doctor is deciding that you want to be one. Chapter 1 discusses some vital factors to consider, including what being a doctor is like and how much medical school will cost. It is also important to consider which A levels or Scottish Highers to take, as this influences which medical schools you can apply to (Chapter 2). Finally, you must decide if you want to apply for deferred entry and take a gap year (Chapter 3).

Preparing

Once you have chosen to apply to medical school you need to start gathering experience for your application. Extracurricular activities such as volunteer work, sport, and music are an essential part of this process, and Chapter 4 describes how to make the most of these opportunities. Many students find getting the necessary medical work experience to be

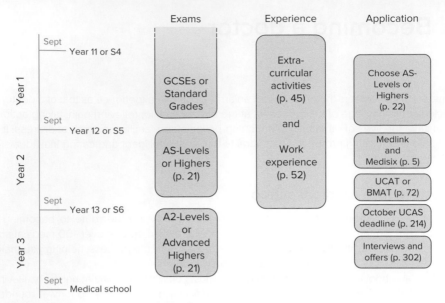

Figure 1 Timeline for applying to medical school.

one of the hardest parts of the application process. Chapter 5 discusses how to arrange this experience and what to expect. The final step of preparation is taking the necessary medical school application exams (e.g. UCAT, BMAT, and GAMSAT). These are discussed in Chapter 6, including which are necessary for each medical school.

Choosing a medical school

Chapter 7 covers how to decide which medical schools to apply to, with an overview describing the different types. This chapter is followed by a detailed description of every UK medical course, written by medical students currently studying there (Chapter 8). There is also a separate description of each graduate-entry medical school (Chapter 12).

Applications and interviews

Once you know where you want to apply, you can start the UCAS form. This process is described in Chapter 9, including how to write a personal statement that makes the most of your experience. Some applications are sufficiently different that they are described separately: applying to Oxbridge (Chapter 10), applying as a graduate to standard courses and graduate-entry courses (Chapter 11), and non-traditional routes including access and foundation courses (Chapter 13). Finally, interview technique is discussed in Chapter 14.

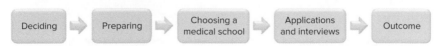

Figure 2 The application process.

Outcome

Hopefully, after all this work, you will gain a medical school offer and achieve the necessary grades. If not, Chapter 15 describes what options are available to you. If you are successful, then Chapter 16 outlines what to expect when starting medical school and how to make the most of the experience.

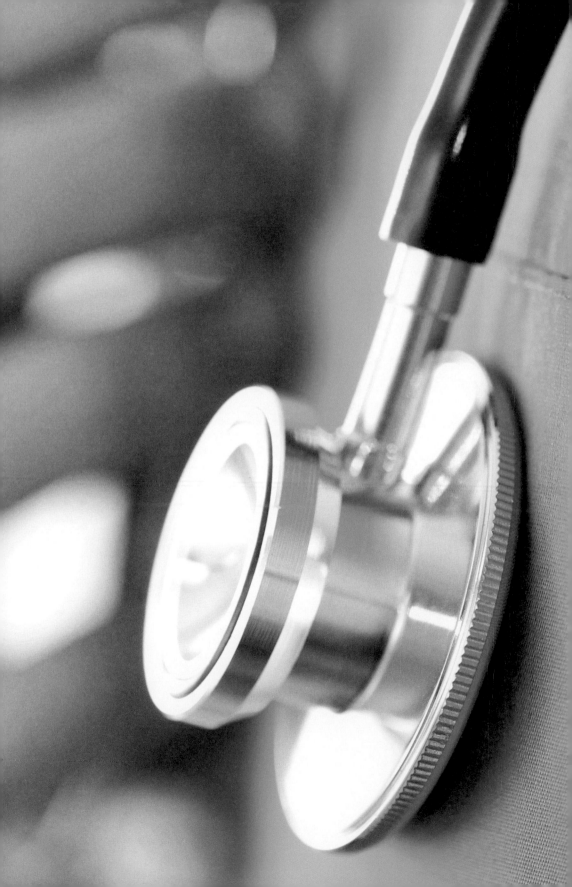

1

Making the decision

▌Do you want to be a doctor?

Applying to medical school is like asking someone to marry you. This might seem like an exaggeration; however, over your life you will spend more hours working than you will spend awake with your life partner. Like marriage, being a doctor will change who you are, influence where you live and affect what you can do with your life. For the right person this can be a wonderful, life-affirming experience. Otherwise, divorce from a medical career can be messy, painful and upsetting.

Would you make a good doctor?

Medicine includes a huge number of specialties (see p. 12), which attract many different personalities. A few qualities are common to all good doctors:

- **Academic ability** While you don't need to be a rocket scientist, you need to be clever to get into medical school and learn medicine.
- **Communication skills** These are the core of medicine; without them you will be unable to diagnose or reassure patients.
- **Caring** This is essential; it is what keeps doctors going when they are busy, tired, hungry, and stressed.
- **Common sense** A lot of medicine involves discerning the key facts and making sensible, rational decisions based on them.

A student's experience ...

I had wanted to be a doctor from an early age and, the older I got, the more determined I became. After the competitive application process I was delighted to get in and the first two years were everything I had dreamed of: fascinating science lectures, great friends, and a stellar social life. However, as the clinical phase began, the magic seemed to fade. I found the work unrewarding and disliked the imprecision and unanswered questions of medical life. I stuck at it (I don't do failure well) and graduated with good marks to start the Foundation Programme, which only intensified my dissatisfaction.

Two years later, aged 25, I took the decision to leave clinical medicine and spent a year travelling with the money I'd saved. On my return I was surprised by the number of interesting job options available to 'ex-doctors' and settled on a pharmaceutical company. While I don't regret doing medicine, I wish I'd thought about it more at the time. I guess I got lost in the challenge of applying to medical school without thinking about what being a doctor was really like.

Why do you want to be a doctor?

This is a question that will keep coming up throughout the application process, particularly when writing the UCAS personal statement (see p. 216) and at interviews (see p. 305). It is important to have thought about the answer very carefully if you want to really convince the reader or interviewer (see pp. 221, 224, and 306).

There is one other person you need to convince: yourself. It is vital that you are honest with yourself about your true motives—not just the positive and noble ones that you'll tell other people, but the less honourable and selfish ones too. There is nothing wrong with liking the fact that doctors are quite well paid or being excited about being called 'Doctor'. By admitting these reasons to yourself, you can then decide whether medicine is the best way of fulfilling your ambitions or whether it does not fit your aspirations as well as an alternative career might.

'I want to help people …' This is a phrase that many applicants volunteer when asked why they want to be doctors. However, if this is the *only* reason you have for wanting to be a doctor, then medicine may not be the best career. This might seem surprising, since the entire point of doctors is to help people, but consider:

- If your only desire is to help people, there are better ways of achieving this goal. Bringing clean water to people in developing countries will save far more lives than being a doctor. Even in the UK, the biggest life-saving effects have been policy changes (e.g. seat belts, sanitation, widespread vaccination).
- Doctors try to help people in the long term, which often leads to short-term suffering, including medication side effects, painful needles, telling them not to do the things they enjoy (e.g. smoking, drinking), or giving bad news.

While all doctors should want to help people, there need to be other motives that keep them going when patients don't get better or the job is difficult.

The importance of being selfish

It is your life. What will make you happy? There is no point becoming a doctor to please parents, impress friends, or satisfy teachers' expectations. Lots of people apply to medical school, so patients will have doctors even if you do not apply. The only sensible reason to become a doctor is because in your heart (and mind) you know that medicine is the career most likely to provide a happy and fulfilling life.

A student's experience …

I was unsure if I was the right sort of person to train as a doctor, so my parents suggested that I try work experience at a local hospital. It was difficult to arrange and it took a lot of attempts, but eventually I managed to get three days on a respiratory ward. I was surprised by how old most of the patients were and at the amount of time the doctors spent writing and filling in forms (very different from TV!), but overall I loved it. One of the younger doctors tried to explain what was going on with each patient and how they were treating them, which was fascinating. She also told me about some of the exams and job applications that she was doing. I'd never considered that there would be more exams after medical school—it made me realize how much doctors have to learn.

I thought long and hard about whether I would enjoy being a doctor and eventually decided it looked better than any other career I had seen. I'm pleased to say that I got into medical school and am now working as a junior doctor, which, despite the anti-social hours, hard work, and responsibility, I am thoroughly enjoying.

Deciding to be a doctor

This is not a decision that comes to you in a flash of inspiration; it is one that you make carefully over several months or years, having considered alternatives and researched what a medical career entails.

How to make the decision

The more you know about the lifestyle of being a doctor, the more likely you are to make the right decision about going to medical school. To find out more about this:

- Consider going on a medical school preparatory course (see p. 5).
- Read 'Being a doctor' on p. 9, which includes a description of the average day for doctors at different stages in their careers.
- Do work experience (see p. 54) with as many doctors in as many settings as possible. If you do not find your work experience fascinating, this is a bad sign.
- Talk to anyone with health-care experience about what it is like to be a doctor.

Medicine on TV

The practice of medicine includes emergencies, ethical dilemmas, life and death decisions, bodily fluids, and rare diseases—a great recipe for dramatic TV. While many TV shows work hard to create realistic scenarios, the vast majority do not reflect the day-to-day life of a doctor very well. Many aspects of a real doctor's job are far less exciting: partially conscious patients unable to communicate; ordering investigations over the phone; taking blood from people with poor veins; and writing a summary of your examination in the notes. While the rare moments of drama can be exciting, you need to be sure that the day-to-day work will satisfy you.

Medical school preparatory courses

There are numerous preparatory courses that can help you to decide if you want to be a doctor and give you advice on getting into medical school. The majority of successful applicants attend at least one such course. There are numerous benefits:

- **Meet other applicants** The value of this cannot be overstated. It allows you to share ideas, get a feel for the quality and enthusiasm of other applicants, and make friends with others going through a similar experience.
- **Learn about medicine** Most courses have doctors sharing details of their job and lifestyle. This is extremely useful for deciding whether medicine is a career that you want to follow and also for getting a feel for how the NHS works (very useful for UCAS applications and interviews).
- **Learn about the application process** Learning from books and websites is no substitute for meeting doctors and admissions experts in the flesh.

Key points

Medical school preparatory courses are not essential to getting into medical school and much of the information they impart can be gleaned elsewhere (e.g. websites, meeting doctors through work experience). However, they do offer a great opportunity to learn, in a short time with minimal effort, the essential facts about medical school applications and the realities of being a doctor.

My biology teacher knew that I was thinking about applying to study medicine and suggested a course for potential medical students. I went with a couple of friends who were also considering medical school. The course was great fun; I had never been in a room with so many like-minded people my age.

The lectures were great too. I learned so much about being a doctor and the different roles they play. A couple of lectures really stuck in my mind—one about emergency medicine that included some horrible pictures of injuries (someone even fainted!) and another one about ways to make sure you get a place at medical school, which was really motivating.

By the end of the course I was convinced that I wanted to apply to medical school. Surprisingly, the two friends I had gone with were convinced that they did not want to apply; however, I made some friends at the course who I've kept in touch with, so I still know other people applying.

Examples of medical school preparatory courses

- **Medlink** (https://medlink-uk.net/) This is the most widely attended medical school entry course in the UK, with events delivered in Nottingham and Dublin. Students attend lectures and practical sessions led by doctors from a range of different medical specialties.
- **The Medic Portal** (www.themedicportal.com/event/medical-school-interview-courses/) The Medic Portal are a reasonably new player in the medical applications arena, organizing this course as well as UCAT and BMAT questions, an interview course, personal statement review service, and application guide. The course is one day long, available in London, Birmingham, and Manchester at a cost of £175 for the day. In addition to the day's teaching, participants also receive an application guide book as well as the chance to practice in a mock interview.
- **Biograd** (www.biograd.co.uk/medical-school-preparation-course-biograd.php) Biograd, partnered with Kaplan, offer this five-day residency course in Liverpool. The course covers specific interview topics as well as tips and tricks for the UCAT examination. Additional past papers, learning materials, and access by email to a tutor is provided in the £780 course fee (excluding accommodation costs).
- **Oxford Summer School** (www.oxford-royale.co.uk/summer-schools/oxford/medical-school-preparation-16-18) Available in Oxford, Cambridge, and St Andrews, these Oxford summer courses are two weeks in duration and include residence in colleges at the university in which they are held. The course purports to cover every aspect of the application process while also giving students some idea of the real-life experience of being a medical student, albeit at the hefty cost of £4,500. Despite the name and images used in advertising, the Oxford Summer School is not affiliated with any of the institutes in which it hosts its courses.

Key points

Many applicants attend medical preparatory courses. They can be useful and provide a lot of value within a short space of time. However, they are also expensive and most of the information they provide can be found elsewhere. As long as you are preparing carefully, you are unlikely to be disadvantaged because you didn't attend one.

Training to be a doctor

Medical school is just the first step in training to be a doctor and getting in is just the first hurdle. Further training after medical school lasts between six and ten years, depending on the specialty, and includes several rounds of competitive interviews and exams (see Figure 1.1).

Foundation Programme In the last year of medical school, students apply for two-year Foundation Programme jobs. Applicants are ranked according to their medical school performance, other achievements, and score on an invigilated test of professional judgement. Students are allocated to the jobs they choose in order of the ranking. Although the vast majority of UK graduates are appointed, the recent expansion of medical school numbers and influx of doctors qualified overseas could see this change in future.

Core training and specialist training In the second year of the Foundation Programme, doctors apply for core training jobs in a specialty (e.g. surgery) and region (e.g. East Midlands) of their choice. Jobs are allocated according to each doctor's CV, application form, and performance at interview. There is a similar selection process for specialist training two or three years later. Both stages can be highly competitive, depending on the specialty and region selected; applicants may need to have passed part of the professional membership exams (see p. 10).

Final career Doctors who complete their membership exams and specialist training can apply for a job as a consultant (see p. 10) or general practitioner (see p. 11). Applications can be very competitive in some regions and specialties. Doctors who do not want the accompanying level of responsibility or who have been unsuccessful in their exams or applications become Staff and Associate Specialists (SAS), doing similar hospital work as consultants but without some managerial responsibilities.

> ⓘ **More information** See *So you want to be a brain surgeon*? by Oxford University Press for details on medical careers, exams, and the different types of medical specialties.

Assessments and exams

Medical school Medical school exams are challenging and stressful, but the majority of students pass. Those who fail usually get a chance to resit and, because there are so many exams, a lot of students resit at least one during their time at medical school. Failing the resits is more serious and a few students have to retake the year or leave medical school (about 1–5% per year). The details of exams vary widely between medical schools, although they often follow this pattern:

- **Pre-clinical years** Exams in multiple subjects occur at the end of each semester (twice a year) with some continuous assessment throughout the year.
- **Clinical years** Exams in specialties recently studied occur once or twice a year with some continuous assessment throughout. Finals are taken in the last year and encompass a mixture of specialties. The exams are usually multiple choice or true/false, and most medical schools also include a practical exam.

Foundation Programme After medical school there is a brief break from exams. Doctors are assessed continually throughout these two years; however, these assessments are rarely failed. For some specialties, doctors must take the first part of the relevant membership exam (see below) in the second year.

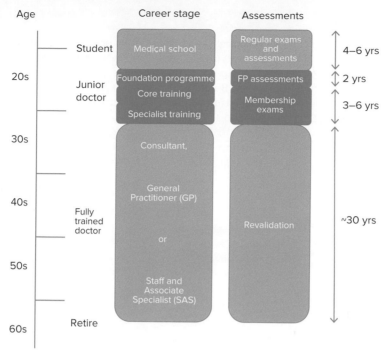

Figure 1.1 Career and assessment timeline.

Core and specialist training (membership exams) The exact format and timing of exams varies between specialties, but almost all have to take membership exams during core training. Membership exams are the hardest that a doctor faces in their career. They are designed so that only the best will pass, with 30–60% of doctors passing at each stage. It is common for doctors to resit at least one part, although each sitting entails two months of intense study alongside a full-time job. They usually follow this format:

- **Part 1 written (science)** A multiple-choice exam testing medical science relevant to that specialty (e.g. anatomy, genetics, physiology) and relevant clinical knowledge.
- **Part 2 written (clinical)** A multiple-choice exam based on diagnosing and managing clinical scenarios. Some specialties also have a viva section where senior doctors grill the doctor being tested.
- **Part 2 practical (clinical)** An exam testing history and examination skills on real patients.

Some specialties also have an 'exit' exam at the end of the junior doctor training. Throughout their training, doctors also need to complete an annual appraisal (e.g. Annual Review of Competency Progression; ARCP), although this is rarely an obstacle.

Consultants, GPs, and SASs Once doctors have reached their final career grade they are regularly assessed by the hospital and the revalidation process organized by the General Medical Council (GMC) every five years to ensure that they remain up to date. Very few doctors have problems at this stage.

Failing exams

There are two main stages in a medical career where exam performance can have very serious implications. The first is A levels (or Highers), where missing your offer can prevent you getting into medical school (see p. 322). The second is membership exams, which must be passed by certain deadlines. Before each deadline it is simply a case of resitting, but after the deadline, doctors may be forced out of the standard career path to work in a Staff and Associate Specialist (SAS) post.

▌ Being a doctor

Unlike most university courses, applying to medicine is a lifelong commitment to one career. It is easy to focus on the choice of medical school (see p. 90), affecting the next five years, instead of whether to become a doctor, which defines the next forty. Many medical students are surprised to find that the job doctors do is different from their expectations. It is essential to learn as much as possible about being a doctor—through work experience (see p. 54) and understanding the different roles that a doctor performs (see p. 12)—before you apply.

Foundation Programme

This is the most junior level for doctors (previously known as the Pre-Registration House Officer or PRHO) and it starts at the end of medical school. The Foundation Programme is two years long and these doctors are responsible for day-to-day management of patients on the wards. This can include a lot of paperwork and organization alongside reviewing patients' progress and simple procedures. These Foundation Year doctors also perform on-calls, where they diagnose and treat patients with new problems.

The Foundation Programme usually comprises six four-month rotations in different hospital specialties or in general practice. A typical job would be:

- **Year 1** Medicine (endocrine), Paediatrics, Surgery (vascular)
- **Year 2** General Practice, Medicine (oncology), Cardiology

A day in the life of a Foundation Year (FY1) doctor ...

07:30 Quick shower and breakfast, then jump on a bus to the hospital.

08:30 Prepare for ward round by writing summaries of new patients on the ward and checking for any new overnight problems or results.

09:00 Ward round led by a registrar; my job is to present each patient, make sure the results are up to date, write the summary of the ward round in the notes, and keep a list of jobs. We cover 14 patients on the main ward and 10 'outliers' on other wards around the hospital. I write requests for investigations (e.g. X-rays) on the way round, to save time.

12:15 Ward round finishes and I divide up the list of jobs with the specialist trainee; most of the jobs are taking blood, referring patients to other teams, or chasing results. Lunch is a sandwich consumed between jobs. The work is often interrupted by bleeps asking me to review patients, rewrite drug cards, and prescribe take-home medications.

16:03 Cardiac arrest call! Elderly patient with no pulse. A specialist trainee leads the team and asks me to take blood from a vein and artery; I manage, but sadly the patient does not survive.

17:15 Frantically write blood request forms for the phlebotomist round tomorrow morning and finish any remaining jobs that must be done today.

17:30 Start on-call for the acute ward where I clerk (perform the initial assessment of) patients admitted from GPs or A&E. I check my management plans with seniors, but otherwise do all the work myself. I get 30 minutes for dinner, which is just long enough to eat at the canteen.

21:30 Hand over my last patient to the night doctor, head home to watch some TV ('The Good Doctor!'), and then collapse into bed.

Core training and specialist training

By the second half of the Foundation Programme, doctors need to have an idea about what type of doctor they want to be (see p. 12) because they must apply for core training in that specialty. The format and length of this phase varies between specialties, with general practice being the shortest (four years) and super-specialists being the longest (may include a research period taking the total to over 10 years). Core training is often quite general (e.g. mixture of medical specialties) while specialist training is more focused (e.g. renal medicine).

As doctors become more experienced, they gain new responsibilities including leading ward rounds, seeing patients in clinic, and learning new procedures or surgery. The on-calls also involve more responsibility and the management of sicker patients.

A day in the life of a Specialist Trainee (ST3) doctor ...

08:00   Drive into work, hoping I'll be able to find a parking space easily.

08:30   Check in with the night registrar about new patients and problems.

09:00   Lead the ward round, checking the progress of each patient and making any necessary changes to medications, nursing instructions, or investigations; there is a consultant-led round the next day so we need to try and get all results ready.

12:00   Leave juniors to handle the ward jobs and check on two patients who have been referred to our team.

12:45   Meet consultant in clinic and discuss the ward patients and reviews over a quick lunch and coffee. There are 32 patients in clinic, that we divide between us; many of them are reviews of known patients, but the handful of new cases can take time.

17:15   Check in with junior staff on the ward and discuss latest developments, then review another patient referred from a different team.

17:30   Handed the on-call bleep; on-call entails discussing referrals from A&E and GPs, supervising the management plans of junior staff, and reviewing the most unwell patients on both the acute ward and the other hospital wards.

21:30   Hand over to the night registrar with a summary of new patients or worryingly ill patients. Drive home to finish an audit presentation.

Consultants

At the end of specialist training, doctors can apply for consultant jobs. Consultants have ultimate responsibility for all the patients on their ward as well as those seen in clinic. While much of the day-to-day work is performed by junior staff, consultants regularly lead ward rounds to supervise the management of patients. This can be a weekly event or happen several times a day, depending on the specialty. Much of their working time is spent in clinic or performing procedures/surgery assisted by the more experienced junior doctors.

Consultants also have a managerial role including supervising the training of their junior doctors, ensuring the smooth operation of their ward, and meeting with hospital management to plan new services and improvements. In teaching hospitals they will also be expected to teach medical students.

The on-call burden varies greatly between specialties, from offering advice from home to being called into the hospital a couple of nights a week.

08:00 Drive into work, making a mental list of emails to send.

08:30 Check in with secretary; quickly read and sign clinic letters.

09:00 Start endoscopy list; five patients in quick succession referred by myself and other members of the team. Phone call to registrar to discuss an acutely deteriorating patient after the third case; offer advice over the phone. List overruns by 30 minutes.

13:00 Review sick patient on the ward with registrar and arrange their admission to the intensive care unit.

13:20 Arrive late to meeting with other consultants and management to discuss methods of reducing hospital-acquired infection rates.

14:00 Afternoon clinic along with registrar; mixture of new patients and familiar faces.

17:30 Check with registrar that there are no urgent problems on the ward, then retreat to office to catch up with paperwork.

19:30 Not my week on-call so no chance of being disturbed; arrive home in time to put the kids to bed and spend the rest of the evening completing a research paper.

General Practitioners (GPs)

Fifty per cent of doctors leave the hospital environment to work in the community. As the name suggests, they see a wide range of medical issues across the complete spectrum of patients (in terms of age, socioeconomic background, etc.). Alongside the medical side of their job, GPs have to run their practice, which operates as a small business; for some this is an exciting opportunity, for others a major hassle.

The GP role generally offers more control and flexibility than medicine in the hospital environment. The training is shorter (two years of Foundation Programme and three years of specialist training) and the pay is similar. The job can be busy and stressful, since the average appointment lasts less than 10 minutes, which is not a lot of time to distinguish a cold from early meningitis.

A day in the life of a GP ...

07:30 Drive to the practice, with time to make a coffee before clinic.

08:00 Clinic begins; patients seen in nine-minute blocks starting with two emergency cases. Cases vary between common problems, chronic care, psychiatric illness, contraceptive pill checks, and the occasional mystery or acutely ill patient that requires hospital admission.

11:30 End of morning clinic, after which I have a coffee break with other GPs to discuss the morning's cases.

12:00 Meet with practice manager and accountant to discuss practice finances.

13:00 Lunch break; once a week I have to visit the patients unable to get to the practice, but today I use the time to update the text for the practice website.

15:00 Afternoon clinic begins; similar pattern to morning clinic except with one long appointment set aside to discuss the medical and social options for an elderly lady who is not coping well on her own. Her son and daughter attend the appointment with her.

18:30 End of evening clinic; out-of-hours care is managed by an on-call service, so no chance of being disturbed. Spend the evening with kids and partner.

▍Types of doctor

The role and lifestyle of a doctor varies greatly according to the specialty they choose. The following covers some of the most common specialties.

Anaesthetics/intensive care

- **Patients** The sickest in the hospital and those undergoing surgery.
- **Work** Almost entirely based in the intensive care unit or operating theatre.
- **Lifestyle** Work is intense, both day and night, but predictable hours.

Surgery

- **Patients** Variable, but average patient younger than other specialties.
- **Work** A mixture of ward rounds, clinics, and time in the operating theatre.
- **Lifestyle** Early starts and late finishes; can be unpredictable.

Medicine

- **Patients** Often elderly with multiple problems; can be admitted for months.
- **Work** Mostly ward rounds and clinics; some specialties do procedures (e.g. endoscopy, bronchoscopy).
- **Lifestyle** Usually a bit more relaxed than surgery, but not always.

Paediatrics (children)

- **Patients** From premature babies to teenagers, though usually under five years.
- **Work** Mostly ward rounds and clinics.
- **Lifestyle** Hours are usually better than those in medicine and surgery.

Psychiatry (mental illness)

- **Patients** Wide range of ages; patients often admitted for long periods.
- **Work** Mostly clinic-based, but some ward-based medicine.
- **Lifestyle** More predictable 9–5 hours than many other specialties.

Obstetrics and gynaecology (pregnancy and women)

- **Patients** Women—obviously! Young in obstetrics, often older in gynaecology.
- **Work** Mixture of ward rounds, clinics, and time in the operating theatre or birth unit.
- **Lifestyle** Childbirth is unpredictable. Busy on-calls.

Pathology (laboratory-based diagnosis)

- **Patients** Mostly looking at samples from patients, but some see patients in the flesh too.
- **Work** Laboratory-based techniques, e.g. microscopes, chemical tests.
- **Lifestyle** Predictable 9–5 hours and light on-calls (if any).

Radiology (imaging)

- **Patients** Complete age range of patients.
- **Work** Mixture of performing procedures and looking at images.
- **Lifestyle** Relatively predictable hours, though on-calls can be busy.

Emergency medicine (A&E)

- **Patients** Complete mixture of patients and problems.
- **Work** Ranges from twisted ankles to heart attacks.
- **Lifestyle** Predictable hours (as shift pattern), but intense and busy whilst at work.

The cost of medical school

The average medical student debt is around £40,000 (slightly higher in London). Many students are worried by these costs, although it is important to understand them fully before letting them affect your decision making.

Where the money goes

The cost of medical school varies depending on type of accommodation, year of study, and location (the pages on each medical school (see pp. 124–290) give an estimate of this cost). The cost also varies widely between frugal and extravagant students. Tables 1.1 and 1.2 give an estimate of the costs of a year at medical school:

Tuition fees These are fees charged by the university towards the cost of teaching. The fees are typically £9,250 per year for all UK students (subject to a yearly increase in line with inflation) except: students from Scotland studying in Scotland (~£1,820 per year); students from Wales studying anywhere (~£9,250 per year); and students from Northern Ireland studying in Northern Ireland (£4,030 per year).

Accommodation Most medical students spend the first year in university accommodation, then move to private accommodation from the second year. Sixteen per cent live at home (27% in London). Mean monthly expenditure on accommodation is ~£535 (~£640 in London).

Transport About 50% of medical students have a car (only 18% in London), which is often necessary at some medical schools during the clinical years. Car ownership costs ~£3,000 per year, though it can result in unexpected large bills when things go wrong. Medical students report spending ~£500 per year on travel to clinical placements.

Where the money comes from

There are several sources of funds to support medical students, although the system is complex, which makes it difficult to calculate what to expect. It helps to know the main organizations/schemes involved:

- **Student Finance England** A non-profit organization that administers student loans and grants on behalf of the UK government to students normally resident in England.

Table 1.1 Typical first-year English medical student costs (30 weeks' term time)

Costs	Per week of term	Per month of term	Per year
Tuition fees	£308	£1,234	£9,250
Campus accommodation	£78–£175	£312–£700	£2,340–£5,250
Living costs	£80–£140	£320–£560	£2,400–£4,200
Expenditure (excluding deferred fees)	**£158–£315**	**£632–£1,260**	**£4,740–£9,450**
Total (including deferred fees)*	**£458–£615**	**£1,832–£2,460**	**£13,740–£18,450**

*Paid through salary after qualification

Table 1.2 Typical clinical-year English medical student costs (48 weeks' term time)

Costs	Per week of term	Per month of term	Per year
Tuition fees	£193	£775	£9,250
Rent	£70–£150	£280–£600	£3,360–£7,200
Living costs	£100–£180	£400–£720	£4,800–£8,640
Expenditure (excluding deferred fees)	**£170–£330**	**£680–£1,320**	**£8,160–£15,840**
Total (including deferred fees)*	**£358–£518**	**£1,430–£2,070**	**£17,160–£24,840**

*Paid through salary after qualification

- **NHS Bursary Scheme** Offered to students on graduate courses (GEM, see p. 252) from the second year, or undergraduate courses from the fifth year onwards.
- **SAAS** (Students Award Agency for Scotland) pays the entire tuition fee for Scottish students studying in Scotland. (Student Finance Wales and Student Finance Northern Ireland are the equivalent agencies in those parts of the UK.)

Student Finance England All undergraduates resident in England and starting university (anywhere in the UK) for the first time should be eligible for a student loan to cover tuition fees and to contribute towards other costs. Check out the student loan calculator under 'education and learning' on the www.gov.uk website.

Student loans Loans obtained through Student Finance England need to be repaid over several years once you start earning over £494 per week (£2,143 per month) and payments are usually taken directly from your salary, like tax and national insurance. You end up paying 9% of what you earn *beyond the threshold* for as long as you're earning. The loan has a rate of interest calculated from the retail price index (RPI—currently 3.3%): 3.3% + 3% interest while you're studying and then RPI only if you earn less than £25,725 per year, RPI + up to 3% if you are paid between £25,725 and £46,305 per year, and RPI + 3% if you earn over £46,305 per year. Tuition fee loans are always set at the level charged by your institution and are paid directly to the medical school. Maintenance loans are partially means-tested and paid directly to you for living expenses (Table 1.3).

The absolute amount of loan available changes year on year and noticeably reduces as the NHS bursary becomes available to you.

NHS Bursary Scheme Students in their fifth or later year on undergraduate medical courses and second-, third-, and fourth-year students on graduate-entry courses receive an NHS bursary in addition to the student loan (which is commensurately reduced).

If you are an undergraduate medical student, the non-repayable NHS bursary covers tuition fees as well as provides some money as a maintenance grant (see Table 1.4).

Table 1.3 Student Finance England maintenance loans

Full-time student	2020–2021 academic year
Living at home	Up to £7,747
Living away from home, not London	Up to £9,203
Living away from home, in London	Up to £12,010

Table 1.4 **Undergraduate** NHS Bursary Scheme (only available in specific years—see p. 15)

Type	Rest of UK	London
Tuition fees paid*	Up to £9,250	Up to £9,250
Student finance loan (income-assessed)	About £2,324	About £3,263
NHS grant	£1,000	£1,000
NHS bursary (income-based, assuming a 48- week academic year)	Up to £4,155	Up to £5,135
Income (excluding tuition bursary)	**Up to £7,479**	**Up to £9,398**
Total assistance (including tuition bursary)	**Up to £16,729**	**Up to £18,648**

*Paid directly to medical school

If you are a graduate-entry student, the non-repayable NHS bursary contributes to tuition fees and provides some money as a maintenance grant (see Table 1.5). The grant is composed of £1,000 for all eligible students, plus an additional means-tested award. It may also cover mileage and parking expenses incurred in travelling to clinical placements (see www.nhsbsa.nhs.uk).

The shortfall ...

Any shortfall between income and expenditure is made up through parental contributions (66% of students), part-time jobs, and professional trainee loans of up to £25,000 (20% of students). Around 25% of students work part-time during term and a similar proportion work during vacations, earning an average of just over £2,700 per year. Over 50% of those with part-time jobs believe paid employment has a detrimental effect on their academic performance. There are also scholarships, hardship funds, and other bursaries available (see www.money4medstudents.org).

University bursaries and grants Some universities offer money to students to help cover the shortfall. Notably, Oxford and Cambridge offer a grant of up to £3,500 per year depending on the financial status of the student's family. Additionally, Oxbridge colleges have many specific grants and bursaries available for students. Most medical schools will have similar funds, although the eligibility criteria and sums available will vary considerably.

Table 1.5 **Graduate** NHS Bursary Scheme (only available in specific years—see p. 15)

Type	Rest of UK	London
Tuition fees paid*	Up to £3,715	Up to £3,715
Student finance loan (income-assessed)	About £2,324	About £3,263
NHS grant	£1,000	£1,000
NHS bursary (income-based, assuming a 48-week academic year)	Up to £4,155	Up to £5,135
Income (excluding tuition bursary)	**Up to £7,479**	**Up to £9,398**
Total assistance (including tuition bursary)	**Up to £11,194**	**Up to £13,113**

*Paid directly to medical school, remainder covered by Student Finance England/Wales/Northern Ireland or SAAS

Medicine as a graduate

If you are applying to study medicine as a graduate student, the finances can quickly become complicated, especially if you have already received a student loan. Generally, if you are a UK citizen and have been resident in the UK for three years preceding the start date of your course, you are eligible for funding as already described.

Stay up to date

Undergraduate student finance will remain a controversial issue for years to come. Medical student finance is even more complicated and most applicants will need to keep up to date for their particular year of entry. Places to look for current information include:

- **BMA Medical Student Finance Guide** www.bma.org.uk/advice/work-life-support/your-finances-and-protection/medical-student-finance
- **Royal Medical Benevolent Fund** https://rmbf.org and www.money4medstudents.org
- **UK Government** www.gov.uk

Tips for parents

Doctors often find the process of being a parent to a medical school applicant even more stressful than their own experiences. Meanwhile non-medical parents confront the dual challenge of navigating the university application process and understanding career advisors to a jargonistic profession which is alien to most.

What to expect as a parent The demands on medical school applicants are ever increasing, and this will be a stressful experience for your child and, by extension, yourself. On top of maintaining their studies, your child will have increasing demands taking on work experience, preparing their application and personal statement, and balancing this with important extra-curricular activities. It may feel like too much, but the ability to balance this now will be important preparation for the competing demands of medical school, and seeing if they can deal with this pace and volume of work. No matter how stressful you find it, it is useful to remember they are going through it, not you. As always, be supportive, and also, be prepared to pay out. There are costs for exams (UCAT, BMAT—see p. 74), attending courses (see p. 76), as well as getting to open days, interviews, and post-offer holder days, which can all add up. You may be eligible for some reimbursements if you meet widening participation requirements (see UCAT Consortium and Cambridge Assessment Admissions Testing websites).

What to do as a parent Parental involvement can vary between avoiding the subject matter in an effort to minimize stress (and conflict!), to setting timetables and micro-managing next steps. There is probably a healthy balance that you will have developed regarding your child's studies; do not feel obliged to mirror any particular approach you may have overheard. There is no one right answer. The key is to focus on where they have succeeded and have faith! Do help them contact anyone you know who may be able to offer work experience or interview practice—suggest rather than push! Keep a lookout for medical school open days. Not all medical schools will offer them, and it is worth attending at least one yourself to get an overview of what is required, how to apply, and how the environment 'feels'.

Try not to bombard your child with health-related news stories. Repeating stories of how applications were 'back in the day' or what so-and-so says you should/should not do are (perhaps not surprisingly) counterproductive, as is 'helpful' advice on what to say or do in the interview. Fly-on-the-wall documentaries set in hospitals are a double-edged sword, so be careful about basing too much advice on these carefully selected vignettes.

Exams, stress, and expectation management In and amongst preparing for what are career- and life-defining events, there will still be mock exams, admissions tests, and coursework deadlines. It is important you look out for signs of stress, especially so around the time of applications. Encourage your child to take regular breaks and, if possible, to work in a different room to their bedroom. Have lots of snacks available during exam time, and while you might want to try to make these healthy, when it comes to the crunch you may quickly learn to give them whatever gets them through! Try to limit screen time if possible (best of luck with that one!). Perhaps find something you can do together that doesn't involve screens and gets them out of their bedroom. A walk or cycle ride might be enough to get some perspective and fresh air.

Do not expect four interviews and four offers. Your child is likely to have been a star performer at school, but so are nearly all other applicants. Even getting one offer is a big achievement, and some very good candidates still don't.

Be sure to talk through their options well in advance. Do they have a plan B? What would the practical next steps be if they do not get any interviews or any offers? See p. 322 and discuss this with them beforehand.

The Medic Portal has a parents' guide to the process of applying, which offers some other perspectives on what to look out for and how to help: www.themedicportal.com/application-guide/parents-guide.

A parent's perspective …

So, your child has just announced that they want to study medicine! If this has always been a lifelong ambition, then you are probably ahead of the game BUT if, like in my son's case, it is a slow realization as they start A levels and start to think about 'what next', then your child will need to 'hit the ground running'. Knowing nothing about the UCAS application process, the work experience, the extra exams that are required before you can even apply to medical school—it all seemed pretty daunting.

Step 1: Work experience We were very lucky, living near a large local teaching hospital that ran a Young Person Volunteer scheme. We were also able to arrange one-week medical shadowing. They will need to have done some work experience in Year 12 for their UCAS application in the autumn term of Year 13.

Step 2: Choosing a medical school Some medical schools hold specific open days. Look out for these early on, as another student at his school waited till the autumn term of year 13 and it was too late to visit before the UCAS closing date. Check out online resources and those available at school or college. Be realistic. It's not necessarily just about where they/you would like to go but where they are most likely to get an offer. Draw up a short list grouped by UCAT or BMAT—unless they really, really want to take two exams. Next, look at entry requirements. Some medical schools pride themselves on being the 'best of the best', so the entry requirements are even higher. My child felt he did not need the added pressure of requiring several A*s when other medical schools will accept As.

We also thought about the environment where he will be happy. There is currently a high dropout rate amongst young doctors. They may be less likely to drop out if they can see themselves living in the same area for 5 to 10 years.

Step 3 Admissions test The UCAT score will determine which medical school they can apply to. There are lots of free resources online but attending a two-day course proved invaluable and gave him access to additional resources (which did not come cheap!). If your child requires extra time in exams, then there are not as many exam centres/time slots, so don't leave it too late to enter for the exam.

Once the application is in, hope for at least one interview. Some medical schools use personal statement, predicted grades, and UCAT score to select solely for interview. Getting an offer is decided on the interview performance. My son was worried this might be a weak point, so we selected at least one medical school that doesn't interview (but needed a very strong application) and one where how you perform on the day wasn't make or break.

Step 4: Interviews Again, preparation is everything. Encourage your child to talk to tutors, colleagues, current medical students who have been through it. Make sure they understand the interview process. Many now use MMI (multi mini-interviews)—a bit like speed dating for medics! Get them to practise, and to read the medical news stories themselves. Each interview we attended was a very different experience. Be confident! You've got an interview—you absolutely deserve to be there.

Step 6: Offers They only need one. If they get more, then amazing! Best of luck.

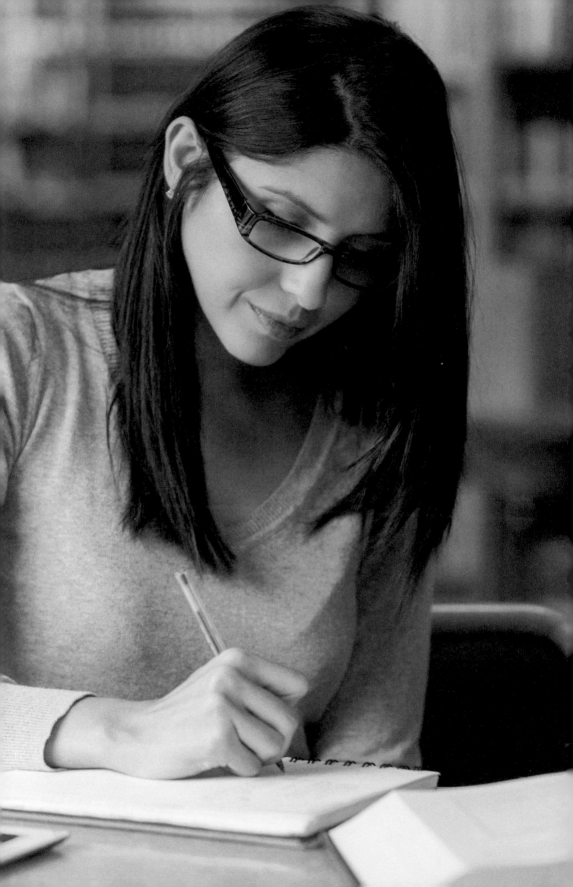

2

Succeeding at A level

Choosing subjects

Medical careers are plagued by exams. School exams are just a first step that will determine whether you win a place at medical school. Most applicants sit a combination of AS and A levels, although the International Baccalaureate and Scottish Highers are often acceptable alternatives.

The transition from GCSE to AS and A2 is a significant one; whilst the number of subjects you study is reduced, your knowledge of each must be far greater. It is this trade-off, from breadth to depth, that requires students to get to grips with the core material in a way quite unlike anything they have done before. This demands time and commitment independent of classroom teaching, so it is essential that you enjoy the subjects you choose.

Which subjects? Admission requirements differ between medical schools. Almost all require A level chemistry and most like to see another science subject at A level as well. Some courses require a third science, at least to AS level. Others prefer breadth and reward candidates taking a non-science subject, such as history. As a general rule, traditional medical schools prefer a spread of science subjects (see p. 92). For many applicants this means chemistry, biology, physics, and maths. Chemistry and biology are particularly helpful, to save having to learn these disciplines from scratch at medical school. However, the 'all sciences' option is by no means the only route to obtaining a place to study medicine.

There are two ways to choose your A level subjects. The first, if you have particular medical schools in mind, is to check their profiles (see pp. 128–290) and look on their websites to find their specific subject requirements and preferences. Most admissions tutors will tell you to use the second method, which is simply to choose subjects you enjoy. This is not just to satisfy a cliché; subject requirements (e.g. chemistry) aside, grades are many times more important than subject options. They are so important that you should be confident of achieving an A or an A* in every subject you choose. As you probably found at GCSE, you are far more likely to score highly in subjects you enjoy.

Choosing AS and A levels: a safe bet

If you follow this strategy, you should be able to apply to almost any medical school:

- Only choose subjects in which you can realistically achieve at least an A.
- Use the medical school profiles (see pp. 128–290) to check admissions requirements.
- Take chemistry and biology, unless you have a particular reason not to.
- Choose two out of physics, maths, and a 'rigorous' non-science.
- Continue chemistry, biology, and one other to A2.

How many? Studying extra A levels can show breadth of interest and impressive academic ability. However, this strategy requires 33% more work and risks a lower set of grades overall. Almost all medical school offers require at least three A2-level grades; some require a minimum grade in a fourth subject at AS level, too. No UK medical schools currently require four A2-level grades.

Many students choose to take four subjects all the way to A2. There are potential benefits to this strategy:

- If you drop a grade in one of the subjects, one of the other ones may allow you to still make your medical school offer.

- Some of the 'academic' medical schools may be slightly more impressed by four A2 subjects than three A2 and one AS.
- If you apply after year 13, once you have received your grades, it may make your application slightly stronger.
- It provides a challenge and fulfils personal interest.

There are also risks to taking additional subjects. AABC looks far worse on a UCAS form than AAB (remember: you have to disclose the grade for all of the subjects you take). If you decide to take additional subjects, you must be prepared to drop one if your overall workload is too high and your results begin to suffer. Nothing should threaten your three core subjects. On balance, it is safer to concentrate on a manageable number of A levels instead of hedging your bets with extra subjects.

What grades? Applicants successful at interview are made an 'offer'. For most candidates this offer is conditional on meeting certain grades. In many cases, applicants are offered AAA, perhaps with additional conditions (e.g. one A must be in chemistry). A few medical schools (such as Oxbridge) usually make an offer of A*AA. Others may offer AAB, perhaps following a strong interview performance, but they are unlikely to go lower. See p. 96 for specific course requirements.

If you are applying before your final A level results, your application is based on predicted grades. These are determined by your school and will be influenced by your performance at AS level. Since there are so many highly qualified applicants applying to medical school, your predicted grades should be at least straight As. This is not an absolute requirement (the minimum required to win an interview at some medical schools is AAB), but the competition is fierce and predictions really do matter. This means working as hard as you can—both to convince teachers to predict good results and, of course, to actually make the grade!

'Good' and 'bad' A levels

Medical schools want to see evidence that you can complete at least three academically rigorous subjects in two years. Some combinations may be considered 'too easy' when taken together, including:

- combinations of maths, further maths, and statistics.
- combinations of biology, human biology, and sports science.

Succeeding throughout the year

Unlike GCSEs, AS and A levels are modular. First-year modules lead to an AS level, which may be taken as a discrete qualification. However, modules taken in the second year will supersede the AS grades and lead to an A level. Together with coursework and assessments, this system means you have to stay committed throughout the second year to achieve the best possible result.

Formulate a plan Whatever you read in the press, achieving A* grades is not easy. Few people rely on talent alone to earn and achieve medical school AAA offers. Instead, you must treat A levels like a military campaign—and every campaign begins with a plan. First, visit the website of the exam board (e.g. AQA, Edexcel) used for your course. Find your specific course (beware of similarly named courses; biology and human biology are not the same!) and download its syllabus (sometimes referred to as a 'course specification'). While you are there, download past papers, mark schemes, and examiners' reports as well.

The syllabus is a list of topics covered by each module. It is what examiners will have in front of them when they write your exam questions. Use this document to guide your studying. If a topic is not in the syllabus, you do not need to know about it. If it is there, you really do. Thorough knowledge of the syllabus is absolutely essential to your success at exam and, while many teachers follow the document closely, you are ultimately responsible for ensuring that you have the required knowledge and skills at exam time.

Coursework Assessed coursework can count for up to 50% of your final A level grade. You cannot afford to be complacent about any piece of assessed work. Even if a piece of coursework is only worth 10%, a D grade (50%) can significantly damage your chances of scoring an A overall. In fact, it would mean needing to average 84% in your exams instead of the normal 80%. To lose a medical school offer for the sake of a few extra hours on a piece of coursework would be heartbreaking.

You should begin coursework as soon as it is assigned. If there is a practical component, go the extra mile to get a reliable set of results. Work hard and redo experiments if they do not run smoothly at the first attempt. Your teacher may be assessing your practical work and, at the very least, will gather an impression of how seriously you are taking the assignment.

Write clearly and ask someone more experienced (e.g. a parent) to proofread what you produce. Aim to write formally but do not get carried away using a thesaurus. Avoid writing in the first person (e.g. using 'I' and 'we') and use course textbooks to see the kind of style you are aiming for. Be sure to follow any instructions you are given; mark schemes rarely award credit for originality.

Very few A level students will use academic references to support their work so, to distinguish yourself, use the internet to find research papers relevant to your assignment (e.g. www.pubmed.gov—look for the 'open access' links for papers that can be read at home). Your school should be able to acquire any papers that you are not able to access directly. Make sure you do not reference Wikipedia as a source, although you can certainly use the references that Wikipedia cites at the bottom of the page (just be sure to read them yourself first). Always reference and never, ever plagiarize—as it will be the quickest way to end your chances of going to medical school (and many other careers in the future).

Don't be afraid to ask your teachers for help and pay careful attention to any advice they offer. They may assess and grade your completed work. If not, they at least have a clear idea of how the mark schemes work. If you finish work early, some teachers will provide comments before you hand it in—this can be very valuable if your teacher is willing. It certainly never hurts to ask politely.

Making the most of your time

- **Be consistent** Throughout your A levels you should be aiming to be at the top of your class. This includes presentations, coursework, and exams. Build an impression of an A* grade student and you're halfway there.
- **Set achievable goals** Be ambitious but remember that you need to be able to achieve your declared goals. You don't get credit for missed targets.
- **Work hard and work effectively** Hard work is certainly rewarded but don't waste effort that could be invested elsewhere; the difference between 96% and 97% is trivial, and the amount of work required to make the distinction may not be worth the net gain. Use the course syllabus and past exam papers to maximum effect.
- **Revision guides** Invest in revision guides early on. It's difficult to make good notes throughout the year and even the best students miss things out. A good revision guide, based on the correct syllabus, fills gaps in your teaching, understanding, and notes.
- **Find a study partner** This doesn't work for everyone but if working alone isn't your thing, find someone to study with. Other potential medical applicants studying similar subjects make ideal study partners.
- **Network with teachers** Always be polite and enthusiastic around teachers. Not only are they a great resource, but they also write your references, make your A level predictions, mark your practical work, and assess your coursework. Your career aspirations will be easier to achieve with others helping you.

Preparing for exams: effective revision

Exam success follows successful revision. Central to this formula are endurance and efficiency. A level revision requires more independence and commitment than GCSEs. You will need to begin reviewing your work early on and develop an effective strategy to maximize the time you spend revising. During this review time you should clarify your understanding of material covered in class and identify knowledge gaps. Your goal is to reach a point where you can answer past-paper questions confidently under exam conditions.

Planning revision There are no fixed rules for revision; to succeed you must be flexible. However, this should not stop you from creating a timetable to organize your revision, ideally a few months before your exams begin. The more time you have to revise, the better. Include key events such as exams and non-academic obligations. Be sure to leave a week or two before the exams to review important topics and to practise past papers. Distribute topics evenly, beginning with those you are least confident about. Remember to be realistic about how much you can achieve in a single day.

- Once you have a schedule, stick to it. Wake at a set time so the morning doesn't just pass you by.
- Experiment with different environments to find where you learn most effectively. You could try working in your bedroom, at the dining table, or in the library, staying in one place or changing location throughout the day.
- Remember to find somewhere away from distractions: the internet, mobile phone, and talkative friends should be saved for scheduled revision breaks.
- Work hard but be careful not to compromise your normal lifestyle. Sleeping, eating, and regular exercise are particularly important. Exercise breaks up the day, keeps the mind alert, reduces stress, and improves quality of sleep.
- Try to ensure revision isn't the last thing you do before sleeping. Reading a novel or talking to your parents will help you think about something other than revision.
- Active recall is more valuable than reading through your notes. Ensure that you incorporate past papers/mock questions/flashcards into your revision schedule.

A student's experience ...

I spent hours 'studying' in my room and everyone seemed very impressed. It wasn't until the exams that I realized how little I knew from all the 'work' I had done. Looking back, 90% of my time was spent on social media. Most of the other 10% was spent rearranging stationery and rewriting my revision timetable. Thirty minutes of studying a day is not enough—even if it is spread across the whole day.

Key points

Don't get too carried away with one topic. The law of diminishing returns states that, beyond a certain level of success, continued effort becomes increasingly wasteful. Learn a topic adequately enough to be able to answer any question you might face in the exam, and then move on.

Making notes There are many different ways of revising and you will need to find the revision strategy that suits you best. The most successful methods require active engagement with your course material.

Making notes helps to reduce masses of information and makes you think about the topic as you express it in your own words. Keep rewriting your notes to condense them even further. The aim is to be left with only a few pages of prompts to review shortly before each exam. Numbered lists and coloured diagrams can also be great to stick around the house. Why shouldn't your family learn about the Kreb's cycle, too? But don't forget that you need to learn, not just create a great set of revision notes. There is only one way to check you have not slipped into the trap of passively copying out words: you have to stop, put your notes away, and challenge yourself. Choose a subject at random and write down everything you know. Then go back and see how well you did. Be ruthless. This is the only way to guarantee you are learning. The exam is not the place to find out!

If you use textbooks, avoid becoming carried away with unnecessary detail. Instead, use textbooks to fill crucial knowledge gaps. Make revision notes from work in class or, even better, invest in a revision guide. This should cover what the course syllabus requires you to know in just the right amount of detail.

Memorizing notes

Three things help with memorizing information:

1. **Concentration**
2. **Repetition**
3. **Emotional response**

Ideally, revision should encourage all of these: for example, copying things out forces repetition and concentration; getting a question wrong (and to a lesser extent right) results in an emotional response. The hippocampus (your memory store) receives strong inputs from the emotion-sensing 'limbic system' of the brain. For this reason, imagining something funny/sad/surprising alongside your notes can help you to remember them. An old adage in medical school is that 'the more ridiculous the memory technique, the better it works'. This holds true outside of medical school, too.

Past papers You wouldn't take a driving test without practising in a car and you should never sit an A level exam without making the most of any available past papers. Past papers are undoubtedly the most effective way to assess your knowledge of the subject matter. A level exams are consistent in terms of difficulty from year to year, so past papers are an opportunity to find out how you will score in the real exam. Clearly it is important to assess this while you still have revision time left!

At regular intervals in your revision, complete a past paper under exam conditions: timed, in a quiet room, away from your notes. Mark it (harshly) afterwards. Do not award extra marks because you know what you meant: examiners are not that forgiving. Try to find the examiners' report for that particular past paper. These offer a great insight into what the examiners were looking for and what they got. When you have marked the exam, appraise your strengths and weaknesses honestly. If you scored an A (usually over 80%), then keep up the hard work. If you didn't quite make the grade, then assess which areas are your weakest and go back to your revision with a vengeance.

Private tuition

Most school teachers are fantastic but they will face obstacles when teaching an A level curriculum. In particular, they have to teach large groups of students, each one of whom has a different set of learning needs. Not every student aspires to straight As and A*s across difficult subjects. This is where private tuition can help. Although it can be expensive, so can dropping a grade and missing a hard-earned medical school offer.

Do you need a tutor? In many cases the answer is 'probably not'. A bright student, supported by good teachers and motivated to work hard for two years, has a very good chance of achieving A* grades. Before hiring a tutor, think hard about whether you are actually using your school resources to maximum effect. Do you concentrate throughout every lesson? Do you look things up if you do not understand them? Do you approach a teacher if you are still stuck? If you already use everything your school has to offer, but still feel you could achieve more, private tuition is certainly an option worth considering.

What does it involve? A tutor is usually a teacher, retired teacher, or graduate providing one-to-one lessons outside of school hours for a fee. They can be self-employed or work for an agency. Fees vary depending on your locality, the tutor's qualifications, and where the lessons take place. Most A level tutors charge between £30 and £40 (up to £95) per hour, including travel expenses.

Who to choose? Finding the right tutor can be difficult. There are no league tables, and although many are highly qualified, this says little about their ability to teach. For this reason, the most reliable way to choose a tutor is by personal recommendation. If you don't know anyone who was tutored, use the internet or a local newspaper to make a list of potential tutors. There are several major online directories of tutors that you can search based on subject and your geographical area.

It's not unusual for a tutor to offer tuition in several different subjects, but be aware of multi-specialists. At A level, it is difficult to keep abreast of so many modules, let alone different exam boards. Medical applicants are already strong candidates and may have more challenging needs than other students. A tutor needs to help push A grades to A*, not simply guarantee reasonable A level grades. Avoid those who have recently finished their own A levels. Undergraduates are unlikely to have the breadth of knowledge and teaching experience needed to keep you on track. If possible, try to find someone currently teaching your subject at A level in a school. They will implicitly understand the level of detail you require as well as the importance of working to a course syllabus. With any luck they will be A level examiners as well!

A student's experience ...

After speaking to a few of my friends, I realized I wasn't alone in wanting a little extra help in one of my subjects. To save on costs, we decided to receive private tuition as a group. The tutor charged extra for teaching more than one student, but it still worked out a lot cheaper than one-to-one lessons. Just make sure that the other students are not included to the detriment of your own work.

Arranging your first lesson Try to speak with potential tutors by telephone before hiring them. It is likely that your parents, if they are picking up the fee, will want to speak with them as well. A telephone call is important to make sure your tutor is familiar with your subject, exam board, and particular needs. It can also provide a preliminary assessment of their suitability. If it is not already clear, use this call to agree the lesson fee and any travel expenses. If travel expenses raise the fee, consider finding someone closer to home, or perhaps meeting your tutor elsewhere.

Many tutors will agree to a free introductory meeting, which is worth taking advantage of. This allows you to get to know each other and discuss how future sessions should be organized. Give your tutor an example question or topic that you would like to go through in the first session; this way you can ascertain how much preparation they have done. Try not to agree on a fixed number of lessons at any stage. This number should depend upon how well you are progressing and the productivity of each session.

Getting the most from your tutor

- Remember these private sessions are an expensive asset: if you feel you would benefit from approaching the sessions in another way, let your tutor know as soon as possible.
- Make a list of topics you need help with. Be as specific as possible and keep a list of questions that crop up when you are studying.
- Most tutors will happily answer questions by email or telephone, but remember they may have a number of students and a full-time job as well.
- Make sure your tutor sticks to the course syllabus as far as possible. They may want to teach outside of the syllabus and, while no education is wasted, this is less likely to boost your exam performance.
- Most students opt for 60–90 minutes of tuition a week. Don't arrange lessons if there is not something in particular that you want to work through.
- To make the most of private tuition, use it sparingly. Ninety-five per cent of your work should take place before the lesson. Always prepare adequately by reading the relevant section in your revision guide and then rereading it after the lesson.
- Never be afraid to hire a different tutor. This might be awkward but private tuition is too expensive a luxury to be wasted. Speak to whoever pays the bill if you think you could achieve more with a different tutor.

Key points

Of course many students cannot afford the luxury of private tuition. This is rarely a problem. Many of the advantages brought by a tutor can be obtained in school. Very few teachers will refuse to see a motivated student at break or lunchtime to discuss a particular learning need. The majority of successful medical school applicants did not have the benefit of a tutor and so they are clearly required to gain a good set of A levels.

Exams

Nobody likes exams, but you will meet them again and again while training to be a doctor. In fact, many doctors are still sitting exams at the age of 40 and beyond. Exams are not only a test of knowledge, they also test technique. After revising hard, avoid making simple mistakes during the exam period itself.

The night before

Make sure you have everything ready for exams the following day. You do not want to rush around in the morning or, worse, forget something. Make sure you have an exam timetable, identification if required, appropriate stationery, and a calculator. Aim to take three good writing pens, just in case.

A student's experience ...

I'd stayed up late revising for a biology module. Even though I had covered most of it already, there were still some gaps and I wanted the opportunity to cover everything again. I couldn't believe my luck when I reached the last question—an essay worth 15 marks. It was the subject I had covered just before going to bed and I could still remember every word on that page of my revision guide. If I don't get every one of those 15 points I shall be disappointed.

Staying up vs. sleeping This is a delicate balance and, to some extent, the answer depends on your body and what you are used to. As a general rule, you are more likely to do well if you feel refreshed: an alert brain will read the questions more accurately, make better decisions, and allow better recall of memories.

Despite this, many students choose to slave away, 'cramming' facts until the early hours of the morning. For some students this can work surprisingly well; the stress allows them to absorb large numbers of facts into their short-term memory (technically, medium-term ...) and they experience only a mild reduction in alertness. For others, the revision is time wasted and they risk sleeping through the exam, missing questions, or putting in an awful performance. It can be extremely difficult to be aware of the effects of tiredness on your own brain; however, if you are finding it hard to make decisions then that is a bad sign.

Critical A level exams are not the time to experiment with new revision strategies; go with what you know works for you.

A student's experience ...

A friend spent ages locked away revising in his room and seemed to think he could keep going while everyone else was sleeping. His valiant efforts came to an end about half way through one of our maths exams. I looked up to see him fast asleep on the desk. Fortunately, an invigilator saw him at the same time and woke him up. But he had lost almost 30 minutes. Needless to say, he stayed awake for the rest of the exam!

During the exam

- **Check the paper** Check you have the correct exam paper (mistakes do happen) and confirm the number of questions you should answer (including the back page). Be sure to follow any specific instructions (e.g. number of answers or pages).
- **Time per question** Divide your time according to the weighting of each question and write down the finish time for each one. This is something you should practise as you revise using past papers.
- **Reading ahead for short-answer questions** If there are multiple parts to a short-answer question, have a quick glance over all of the parts before you begin. This can sometimes give you a clue as to where the examiners want you to go with your answers.
- **Read ahead for long-answer questions** It is worth starting long-answer/essay papers by reading all of the questions that you will have to answer first. This allows your brain to work subconsciously on the later questions whilst you're answering the earlier ones.
- **Understand the question** Be sure you understand the question before attempting an answer. This is more applicable to longer essay-based questions, but it can still be applied to the short-answer type. If necessary, define specialist terms in your question before attempting a response.
- **Anticipate the mark scheme** There are often marks for obvious statements, so write these down before showing off your detailed knowledge. Carefully reading mark schemes from previous papers will help you appreciate that points are often available for things you thought were 'obvious', and that key words or phrases may be required to achieve the marks available.
- **Keep moving** If you find yourself unable to answer a question, then simply move on. If you keep a fast pace throughout the exam there will be time at the end to return to difficult questions. It is best to get full marks for answers you do know rather than waste time getting partial marks for those you don't.
- **Concise essays** Essay questions, particularly in science modules, often have set facts that must be written down to score each mark. You are not publishing a literary masterpiece, so write what you know as clearly and concisely as you can without repetition.
- **Use diagrams** Science answers can often benefit from appropriate use of correctly labelled diagrams, which are faster to produce than text. You do not score double marks for repeating everything in the diagram in text as well.
- **Don't panic!** If you've revised everything, the answer is in there somewhere: reread the question and write your best answer if you are still unsure. You may find the answer is obvious when you come back to the question later on.

After the exam

Having wrangled for hours with an exam paper, it is often tempting to conduct a post-mortem. Most students discuss the exam with friends; others use notes to answer questions they struggled with in the exam room. If you do this, bear in mind that it will create a false impression of your performance. Because memory is so influenced by emotion, you will forget questions you answered with ease and focus on those you were less sure about. For this reason you should try to put aside each exam once you've finished it, at least until the last one is over. Students rarely estimate their exam performance accurately and there are always surprises on results day. You won't know how you did until then!

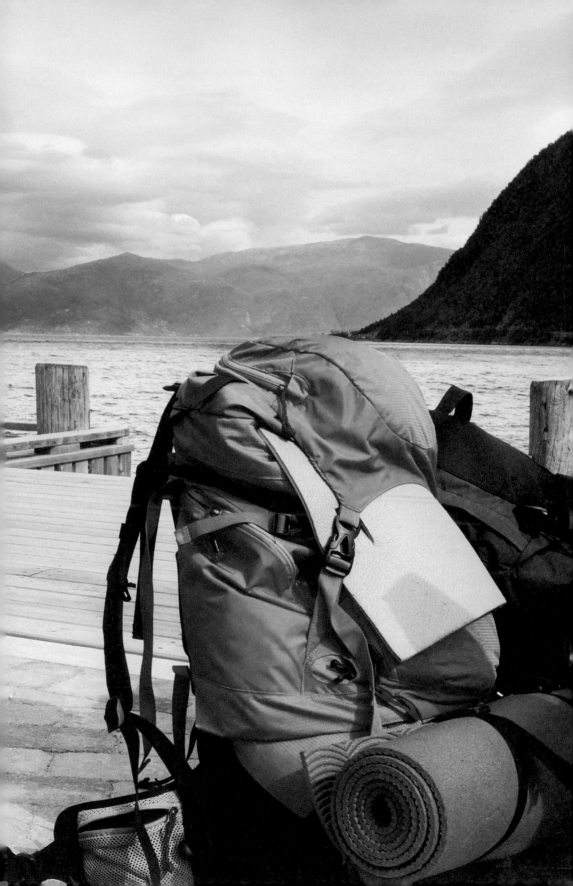

3

Taking a gap year

▌Should you take a gap year?

This might be the last time you can *ever* spend 12 months doing whatever you want. As many as 250,000 young people choose to take 12 months away from full-time work and education every year. You could seize this opportunity to backpack around the world, help a deprived community, or follow your sporting dreams. If you want to try something else before a lifetime of lectures and early morning ward rounds, this chapter will help.

There are good and bad reasons for taking a gap year. The decision could have a massive impact on your life and, like any big decision, needs to be thought through carefully. The list below provides some common reasons for taking a gap year.

- **Life experience** Medicine is a structured career and time out later on is sometimes difficult to arrange. The time between school and university is your own and a great opportunity to pursue your dreams.
- **Maturity** Most medical schools emphasize the importance of early exposure to patients. This means students have to adopt a professional image from their first weeks at medical school. Lots of applicants (and some new doctors!) feel they are not yet ready for this responsibility and would benefit from some personal development time.
- **Skills development** Maturity doesn't come from 12 months of watching daytime television—it's the result of experience. Gap years are an opportunity to develop transferable skills (e.g. professionalism, communication) and practical skills (e.g. a new language).
- **Money** Medical school is an expensive undertaking (see pp. 14–16) and some applicants take a gap year to boost their finances. An applicant living at home in a £15,000 per year job could go some way to funding their tuition before relying on a student loan. However, don't forget that a year of lost earnings over your career could cost in the region of £120,000. So it's worth considering the true 'savings' of working during a gap year before taking one for financial reasons.
- **Work experience** A year away from education means 12 months to collect work experience. This could be long-term employment in the NHS, exotic healthcare placements abroad, or a mixture of UCAS-friendly experiences. However, don't forget that the best experience for being a doctor is a year *working* as a doctor. If clinical experience is your reason for a gap year, remember that those 12 months could be spent as a doctor if you went to medical school straight away.
- **Four medical school rejections** Whether you planned to take a gap year or not, many good applicants find themselves filling time before the next round of UCAS applications. See p. 322 for how to make the most of this time.

Why not take a gap year? While gap years are increasingly common, most students still start higher education straight after school. There are reasons why you should think twice about taking a year out.

- **Time** It's all in the name: a gap year means 12 months out of education. If you include the summer after school ends, it's closer to 15 months. Some people are keen to get started on their career; this might be particularly important to mature applicants (see p. 252) and anyone hoping to be a consultant (see p. 11) by their early 30s.
- **Money** Gap years are an opportunity to boost or break your finances. You can earn a lot of money working (see p. 38) but a whole year travelling costs between £5,000 and £8,000, even if you're frugal.
- **Lack of ideas** Many candidates never think about a gap year. It is always worth considering (if only for a few minutes), so keep reading.

How do medical schools view gap years? Medical schools are broadly in favour of gap years. Admissions tutors understand that they are an opportunity for applicants to develop skills and reflect on their decision to study medicine. However, they will expect a good idea of what you intend to *do* and *gain* from your time off. This doesn't mean that all gap years have to be spent building villages and saving orphans in remote locations. It simply means you have to think hard about your gap year plans and be clear about what you stand to gain from them.

Deferring offers to study medicine There are two routes to taking a gap year. The first is to apply to medical school at the 'normal' time, a year before finishing school, indicating your wish to defer by checking a box on the UCAS form. This will give you the peace of mind of a guaranteed medical school place if you are successful or a second opportunity to apply if you are not. The UCAS reports that between 13,000 and 30,000 higher education applicants (2–7%) choose this option every year.

Although some medical schools (e.g. UCL, Sheffield) explicitly welcome deferred applications from those who can justify their gap year plans, others (e.g. Warwick) are unwilling to defer offers without good reason. They may tightly match offers to places and cannot cope with successful candidates disappearing around the world each year. Others only permit a limited number of deferrals each year. Some medical schools (e.g. Oxford) will offer deferred places but interviewers have to gamble that the candidate requesting deferred entry will be 'better' than those applying the year after. In reality, this means that deferred candidates usually have to be stronger than those asking for traditional direct entry.

If in doubt, ask your preferred institutions about their policy towards deferred applications.

> **Key points**
>
> Twelve months invested wisely can be a huge asset to your application and career but, like any valuable resource, time should be spent devising a clear strategy for achieving a return on your 'investment'.

Applying a year later The alternative is to apply after A levels for admission the following year, so that you already know your A level grades at the time of applying. The obvious disadvantage is that, if your application is unsuccessful, you might be forced into a second year off or into another contingency plan (see p. 322). You also need to consider if being available for interviews will interfere with travel plans.

Of course, there is no rule against doing both. You *could* apply the year before finishing school to see whether or not your deferred application is successful. If so, you could choose to accept or decline the offer. In the event of being rejected, you could start the gap year you were hoping for and submit a better application the following year. This means a year to improve your UCAS application and, potentially, interview experience to learn from. While medical schools may not explicitly express a position on repeat applicants, and it may not weigh heavily in decision making, an experienced panel will still likely recognize someone who has previously applied.

Where to go?

Once you've decided to take a year out, the next stage is to decide where to go. Gap years in the UK are very different from those abroad, and this decision is fundamental to your gap-year plans.

Staying at home

There are advantages to staying in the UK, not least because you're guaranteed three meals a day, flushing toilets, and a hot shower.

- **Money** If your gap year is designed to save money, it's not best spent gallivanting around the world. Round-the-world tickets (four stops) start at £1,000 before factoring in accommodation, food, visa, and activity costs. Staying at home minimizes expense while permitting work in stable employment. However, if your reasons are purely financial, remember that a year out will cost (at least) £120,000 in lost earnings over the course of your career.
- **Work experience** You can arrange healthcare work in any country (see p. 56) but NHS experience is limited to the UK. For this reason, experience at home could provide a better insight into work as an NHS doctor. If you are available for a long period of time (e.g. a year), you could become an experienced healthcare assistant or phlebotomist (see p. 67). However, remember, the best experience for *being a doctor* is being a doctor. Don't spend a year as a phlebotomist in the NHS at the expense of a year working in medicine later on.

The only 'bad' reason for staying at home is the potential lack of new experiences. As a medical student you will be exposed to a huge range of human experience, from helping to assess an acutely psychotic patient to performing chest compressions during a cardiac arrest. If you want to be a doctor you will have to learn how to thrive outside of your comfort zone. A gap year is a good place to begin.

> **Key points**
>
> Try to get away from home for at least part of your gap year. Although you don't have to spend 12 months overseas, making the most of your time means acquiring a broad range of experience. These experiences can be in the UK or abroad; however, a decision to take a year out to stay at home will take some explaining to admissions staff.

Going abroad

Most gap-year students go abroad, at least for part of their time. There are many reasons to go overseas:

- **Opportunity to travel** If you are the typical British medical school applicant, you will have lived in the UK all your life. Experience of the wider world will be limited to television, the internet, and family holidays abroad. A year out is an opportunity to experience just a few of the other 195 countries in the world. Although medical students can travel on their elective, few manage to visit more than one country. After graduation, employment impedes travel opportunities for all but the most adventurous doctors.
- **New experiences** Although experience overseas will undoubtedly be different from the UK, it will depend on *what* you do (see p. 64).

- **Interview ammunition** New and varied experiences mean lots of things to talk about at interview. An interesting gap year will help you stand out and relate questions to your own experiences abroad. Other candidates will be using examples (e.g. grade eight flute and the Duke of Edinburgh Award) that the interviewers will have heard many times before. However, deferring applicants might be interviewed before their gap year begins to bear fruit.
- **Making a difference** Many communities in the developing world are resource-poor and benefit from gap-year volunteers. Volunteering opportunities could include working in a hospital, building a school, teaching English, or disseminating health information to local people. Unfortunately, many small projects are without financial support and rely on volunteers to fund them in return for the opportunity to help.

Where to go abroad? Every country is different but there are similarities (cultural and geographical) within regions. If you want to stay in the English-speaking developed world, where things are broadly similar to the UK, the USA, Canada, Australia, and New Zealand are all possibilities. Travelling through Europe is relatively simple and flights are cheap. Budget airlines fly from London to key European cities for ~£40, less than a train ticket between most British towns. Although flights are cheap, other expenses (e.g. food and accommodation) are less so, and European travel can end up becoming expensive. A further disadvantage is that many people in continental Europe will not speak fluent English. This is, of course, an opportunity to resurrect your rapidly dissipating memories of GCSE French ...

The developing world (much of Africa, South and Central America, and Asia) promises amazing cultural experiences. After visiting these regions, you will be telling stories of your travels (whether or not others want to hear them) for years to come. Backpacking in the developing world is cheap and money lasts a long time—especially if kept safe in a money belt. The disadvantages are largely practical (e.g. booking transport) and related to comfort. If you're willing to forgo flushing toilets for the experience of a lifetime, consider visiting these types of countries.

Other regions promise culture without a need to sacrifice home comforts. These include developed parts of Asia (e.g. Singapore, Japan) and stable countries in the Middle East (e.g. Oman, Jordan, and the United Arab Emirates). Gap-year students rarely visit these destinations and you would be breaking new ground!

Should you stay or should you go? A gap year is probably your longest period of 'freedom' before retirement. With very few limitations, you can choose to do whatever or go wherever you want. For most students, the ideal gap year includes working to earn money then going away to do something interesting. If you *can* afford (and choose) to spend the whole year travelling, you're unlikely to regret the experience. If you're not keen on heading out by yourself, consider taking a friend or don't travel *too* far out of your comfort zone, just far enough to push your own personal boundaries.

If you don't choose a gap year If you remain unconvinced by the value of a gap year, you can still go abroad. There are three months before A level results day and the start of medical school. This is an ideal opportunity to work, relax, travel, or try all three. Think carefully about how to make the most of this time—it might be the last study-free period you have for the next 40 years.

Key points

The potential of your gap year is only limited by your imagination. You can do (or try) almost anything in 12 months. Make the most of your time and you will shine at interview as well as earning memories that will remain with you for life.

▌ What to do?

What to do is at least as important as where to go. These pages set out the benefits, disadvantages, and skills associated with popular gap-year activities.

Working

There are many different ways to work during a year out, either at home or overseas. Most students work for some of their gap year. While health or social care employment is ideal, don't worry if the work you find is less immediately relevant to medicine. Some of the skills you can gain from work include:

- **Teamwork and communication** Most jobs require work with colleagues and/or customers. Some people are not naturally sociable, and human interaction always requires communication skills. Your medical work experience should illustrate how important communication is within the NHS.
- **Working under pressure** Do you become stressed and ineffective when deadlines (or even food orders) are stacking up? If so, gap-year work is an opportunity to learn to work under pressure.
- **Problem solving** Almost everyone is employed to solve problems and initiative will be important at every level of your medical career.

The disadvantage of finding employment is that you have a lifetime of work ahead of you. The trick is to look for a job with added value: either one you really enjoy or one that challenges you to develop new skills. By limiting the time you spend working, you can squeeze other experiences out of your gap year too.

Volunteering

There are many projects needing international volunteers. Many expect a financial contribution to support the project before you start work. You should be wary of projects that resemble commercial tourist activities. If you're travelling to Malawi to build a school, ask yourself why local people (even local builders) can't construct a school themselves. They probably could if they had the necessary resources. Your donation of £1,000 pays for bricks and mortar but, in return, you buy the 'privilege' of building the school yourself. There is nothing wrong with such projects as long as you realize how they work. Projects might include:

- **Health promotion** This could include speaking to local people or visiting schools to disseminate health information (e.g. malaria or HIV prevention).
- **Basic hospital work** Undertaking tasks similar to a healthcare assistant (see p. 67) in the UK. Responsibilities could include basic patient hygiene and monitoring blood pressure, pulse, temperature, and respiratory rate. Do your research before working in countries with a high prevalence of infectious diseases (e.g. HIV). You should always wear some form of personal protective equipment (e.g. gloves) when exposed to bodily fluids.

Be very careful, if volunteering abroad, that you avoid working beyond your competence. Knowing your limitations is vitally important to working as a doctor. Medical school interviewers will not be impressed to hear how you were taught—then practiced—limb amputations in a hospital overseas. As a general rule, if you feel uncomfortable taking on a task then you should politely decline.

As well as seeing the rewards of your labours, volunteering is a way to integrate with a community, as you are not simply there as a tourist. It can also be a good way to gain work experience (see p. 64). (see p. 64) Don't forget that most medical schools provide volunteering projects overseas during university vacations.

Backpacking

Backpacking is a good way to see the world without remortgaging your parents' house. It essentially means travelling with nothing more than a backpack of gear. Backpackers often use local hostels (travel guides are a good place to start, see p. 42) see p. 42 as a base in each new location. As there are thousands of young people backpacking at any one time, you'll almost certainly meet others and end up travelling for a while together. As well as collecting stories for your new (and envious) friends at medical school, think about the kinds of skills you will gain from backpacking.

- **Surviving in a new environment** Junior doctors move jobs every few months to work in a new specialty, team, or hospital. Coping with change will be an important part of your postgraduate training.
- **Meeting new people** You cannot fail to meet new people backpacking. This will mean lots of practice establishing rapport and building relationships with those around you. It won't be long before you notice an improvement in your response to other people, even if you weren't doing badly before. Your ability to 'get along' with new people will be fundamental to your career.
- **Problem solving** You are unlikely to travel without encountering challenges. Cancelled trains, dwindling funds, crime, and disorganization are all possibilities. Meeting these challenges head on is not unlike the work of a doctor, whose role is almost always to solve problems.
- **Perspective** It might be difficult to articulate, but backpacking is great for developing perspective. You will see for yourself how priorities, attitudes, and behaviours differ around the world, and this can lead to a more sophisticated, mature outlook. It has to be an improvement on life spent learning about the world from television and teachers.

A friend and I headed 'down under' to Australia and New Zealand. We had a great time staying in backpacker hostels and making our way slowly through Australasia. We organized work permits and were able to find temporary jobs to fund our most extravagant activities ... and we gained our PADI diving qualification!

How to decide?

Although few students regret their gap-year activities, careful planning will stop you from missing valuable opportunities. There are 15 months between finishing school and starting university; more than enough time for a combination of working at home, volunteering, and travelling overseas.

A student's experience ...

I bought a 'round-the-world' ticket that included five stops. One took me to South Africa and I went to a lion-breeding programme in nearby Zimbabwe. I spent eight weeks feeding and exercising young lions and working in other areas of conservation.

Finding out more

These pages will point you towards informative and reliable sources of information to help in planning your gap year.

Online The most obvious place to look for gap-year information is online. There are many different online resources, including official websites (e.g. the Foreign and Commonwealth Office), charities, commercial gap-year organizations, forums, and travellers' blogs. Before embarking on a project (and certainly before parting with money), find out as much information as possible. If an organization seems well organized, provides lots of information, and is commended by online travel journals, you should be on to a winner. If information is sketchy, think twice, and certainly don't shy away from asking questions. Most reputable companies and charities will put you in contact with previous customers or volunteers for a semi-independent perspective.

Useful websites include:

- **Foreign and Commonwealth Office** Up-to-date travel advice by country. Find out in advance whether your intended destination is considered 'safe' by people in the know: www.gov.uk/fco
- **TrailFinders** Links to all types of travel experience: www.trailfinders.com
- **Madventurer** Useful search engine for healthcare, sports, and educational projects seeking volunteers worldwide: www.madventurer.com
- **Gapwork.com** Connects gap-year travellers to temporary work around the world. Also lists volunteering and adventure activities: www.gapwork.com
- **Responsibletravel.com** Travel 'holidays' from basic to luxurious, including visits to the Arctic and Antarctica for students not short of cash: www.responsibletravel.com

Books If you're someone who likes to see information on the printed page, there are some great travel guides available. Backpacking favourites include:

- *The Lonely Planet* A series of travel guides covering almost every country you could ever hope to visit. These books are beloved and bemoaned by experienced travellers in equal proportions, but if you're going anywhere unusual, add the relevant *Lonely Planet* guide to your kit list.
- *On a Shoestring* Another popular travel series, although from the publishers of *The Lonely Planet*. These guides differ from the latter as they're written with the budget traveller (i.e. gap-year student) firmly in mind. They're also titled by region (e.g. Africa), so you get less detail for your money but don't have to buy a separate guide for every country you visit.
- *Rough Guides* These are the major competition for *The Lonely Planet*. *Rough Guides* tend to include more information but at the expense of glossy pictures. They are often larger than *Lonely Planet* guides.

Take some time in a bookshop or library before committing to one guide or another.

Advice from real people It's a small world and more people travel now than ever before. Perhaps those in the year ahead at school are away on gap years now. Teachers and other students might know how to contact them; email and social networking sites are a good place to start. Those currently travelling will have the best idea of the pros and cons of each individual project or trip.

If you don't know people who are travelling, or even if you do, consider speaking to an experienced travel provider as well. STA Travel has branches around the world (including 53 in the UK) and years of experience negotiating affordable flights for students and other young people. Staff in STA branches often have travel experience themselves and might have an 'insider's view' of your chosen destinations. However, you can often find cheaper arrangements yourself online. Remember to ask whether you can change ticket details later on and, if so, whether this costs extra.

Things to consider

- **Budget** Travel can be cheap, but it can also be very expensive. Flights from London to New York cost as little as £420 return, whereas a 15-day voyage to the North Pole doesn't leave change from £20,000. It's often much cheaper to book accommodation, internal flights, etc. from within a country rather than booking through agents in the UK.
- **Medical school application** If you don't yet have an offer, make a note of the UCAS deadline and potential interview dates.
- **Parents** Parents may be alarmed by your newfound independence. Try to involve them in your planning and negotiate sensitively!
- **Visas** Many countries require visas organized in advance of travel (e.g. from the Embassy or High Commission). Others allow travellers to buy visas when they arrive. Find out so you are not caught out.
- **Vaccinations and disease prevention** Organize vaccinations in good time as some require multiple doses over a period of months. A yellow fever vaccination certificate is required for entry to some countries. Remember that, as a potential medical student, you must take special care to avoid blood-borne viruses that might complicate your career. These include HIV and hepatitis viruses B and C. Identify potential health risks (e.g. from a reliable travel guide) and take care to avoid them.
- **Travel insurance** Insurance might be an unwelcome expense but it is a necessity. Cancelled gap-year plans (e.g. due to bereavement or airline failure) can be financially disruptive as well as disappointing. The average cost of medical repatriation from the USA currently stands at £50,000, without paying for hospital care in that country. Tropical disease and injury are real possibilities for any traveller. Serious injury with multiple operations, a prolonged intensive-care stay, and medical repatriation would be sufficient to bankrupt most parents without adequate insurance coverage.

Key points

Do plenty of research when organizing your gap year, particularly if you intend to travel. This is the best way to stay safe *and* to make the most of your time away.

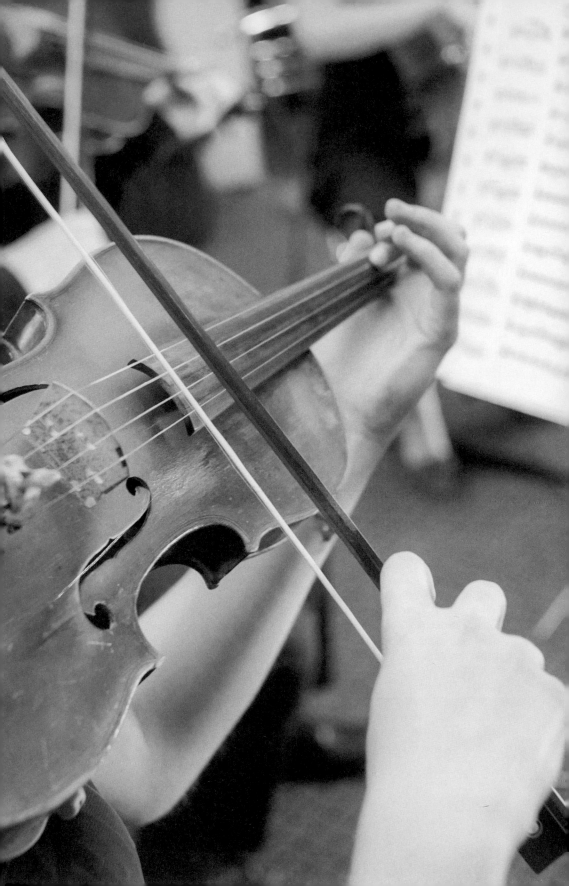

4

Getting a life

Why do extracurricular activities?

Medicine is about science and patients; why does it matter if you play rugby or the violin? An easy answer is that it is one way that medical schools can choose between straight A students, but that's not a complete explanation. Medical schools need candidates who can relate to patients and resist being overwhelmed by the demands of their profession. Having interests outside of medicine is essential to maintaining your mental health and showing you are a well-rounded individual. This chapter will help you think about activities that could help demonstrate these qualities to course selectors.

Discriminating between candidates Extracurricular interests *are* necessary to win a place at medical school, but don't just see them as a 'box to tick'. They are an opportunity to distinguish yourself from other applicants, almost all of whom will boast straight As. In short, you want to stand out. Admissions staff understandably want to select interesting candidates, and one way to be interesting is to have interests. These are best found outside the classroom.

An insider's view ...

One of the ironies of medical school selection is that we pick students with lots of hobbies for a time-intensive course where such activities are difficult to sustain. We know that it's not enough just to accept academically successful applicants. The grades are a minimum requirement. We really want rounded students who will go on to become resilient, insightful, and reflective doctors.

Transferable skills Transferable skills are those that are learned in one environment but which can be applied elsewhere. For example, working with people of different ages and from different backgrounds on a charity project could help you as a doctor working in a multidisciplinary team. You are not expected to have everything you need to be a doctor before getting into medical school. However, admissions tutors expect to see that you have started to develop the qualities necessary for work as a doctor because these cannot be taught in the traditional sense. For this reason, it is important to write about them in your personal statement (see p. 221). It is worth taking a few minutes to consider which qualities are helpful for a doctor. There is no correct answer, but your list could include leadership, effective communication, teamworking, and time management, among many others (see p. 224). With a range of appropriate interests, you should be on your way to developing and demonstrating these skills.

An insider's view ...

It can be tedious shortlisting candidates for medical school interviews. Many are predicted A*A*A*, play a sport to a high level, finished the Duke of Edinburgh Award, and play a musical instrument to grade eight. These things are all very important and many will succeed, but it's the candidate who did something *different* who catches my eye and whom I really want to meet at interview.

Broadening your personality One of the most important transferable skills you can develop is your personality. This is shaped, at least in part, by life experiences and will continue to develop throughout your life. There is no 'right' personality to have as a doctor—good doctors can be shy, scholarly, contemplative, confident, outgoing, or boisterous. However, you can broaden your personality by making the most of extracurricular opportunities.

Adaptability is a vital aspect of any doctor's personality and an important transferable skill. For doctors, no patient, colleague, or working day is ever exactly the same as the last. This is one of the great advantages of a career in medicine—boredom is a rarity—but it can be stressful for people who don't thrive on new experiences. Fortunately, there is a solution. Trying new things will make you more adaptable, achieving will make you more confident, and meeting new people will stretch your communication skills. Almost all experiences will have a positive impact on your personality and, even if you don't realize it at the time, give you a better chance of shining at your interview and beyond.

Relaxation Of course, extracurricular interests should also be fun. Most students work hard to achieve the grades required to win a place at medical school. It is easy to become preoccupied with this aim at the expense of everything else. This can lead to stress and anxiety, which negatively impact on grades, as well as causing health problems. Unfortunately, this is an easy trap to fall into after winning a place at medical school as well. This is one reason why there are such high levels of divorce, addiction, and suicide among doctors. However, stress can be relieved by maintaining a good social circle and a range of hobbies. An hour spent exercising or reading a novel before work can increase your productivity far more than hitting the books straight away.

Key points

Medical schools understandably avoid taking on candidates who cannot strike a balance between work and play. These students might not complete the course or struggle to cope with life as a doctor. This is a key reason why admissions tutors look for evidence of extracurricular interests.

A warning

Extracurricular interests must be considered as part of your overall strategy. They are different from activities that everyone does to relax, such as chatting to friends, watching soaps, or going to the cinema. These alone are unlikely to impress course selectors. Instead, you need to consider more 'interesting' activities. This chapter provides some suggestions but don't forget that extracurricular interests, however important to your application, are also supposed to be fun.

Key points

Extracurricular *achievements* are even better than extracurricular *interests*. This is because most applicants can think up a string of unconvincing hobbies to include on their UCAS application. Examples commonly used include walking, reading, and swimming. If you're going to rely on an example later on you might want to distinguish yourself from the casual swimmer. Strong candidates achieve in their extracurricular life as well as in their academic work.

What can you do?

Choosing extracurricular interests is a personal choice that should be made as early as possible. Of course, your interests should be interesting to *you*. However, a couple of strategic choices can make a difference to the outcome of your application. Applicants often make the mistake of choosing several hobbies that demonstrate similar skill sets (e.g. hiking, climbing, orienteering). Another trap is to accumulate a long list of activities without ever really committing to any of them. The key is to be *selective* in your choice of activities. If you have achieved something amazing—perhaps you are an Olympic athlete or West End actor—one activity may be enough. However, most applicants find they need two or three to impress the admissions team.

There is no single list of extracurricular activities that must appear on every successful application. Although some course selectors award points for playing sport to county level, a musical instrument to grade eight, or the Duke of Edinburgh Award, such an inflexible approach is unusual. The trick is to choose activities you can engage with and gain from. For this reason, it is helpful to pick activities you enjoy. Here are a few ideas to get you on your way.

- **Sports and music** A large number of applicants play a musical instrument or team sport to a reasonable level. These can certainly help show that you are a rounded individual with interests outside of school. However, it is worth noting that *achievement* says more than simply listing an interest. Admissions tutors know 'I enjoy football' could simply mean you once played in PE. Being captain of the school team is far more impressive than simply enjoying the game. Although sport and music are great additions to an application, they are by no means required. Musical success often depends on taking lessons at a young age and no-one expects your medical school strategy to have begun at age seven. Although it doesn't hurt to step out of your comfort zone and pick up a new sport, or even an instrument, there are many other ways to demonstrate a rounded personality.
- **Uniformed youth groups** There are many uniformed youth groups, usually led by volunteers and separated by age range. They are typically well organized and operate at a local level across the country. Groups usually meet on the same evening each week but may require additional time commitments as well. 'Cadets' are associated with different professions (e.g. Police, Army, Navy, Ambulance Service). Although most cadets do not pursue these careers, they learn a lot about themselves and develop many transferable skills. These include an appreciation of hierarchy, command, teamwork, and professionalism. Whilst each group has its own unique qualities (insignia, drills, ceremonies, etc.), these serve as a foundation for community involvement and developing good citizenship.

Key points

Uniformed youth groups include St John Ambulance, Scouts, Boys/Girls Brigade, Police Cadets, and military cadet forces (e.g. Army, RAF, Navy).

- **School activities** Although extracurricular activities are about non-academic achievements, this should not stop you utilizing opportunities at school. Your school is likely to have resources and contacts that are difficult to find elsewhere. A number of schools also permit access to national programmes such as the Duke of Edinburgh Award. Many of these activities occur during or immediately after school, which can reduce travelling time. On the other hand, make sure any hobbies taken up at school do not impact negatively on your lessons. Most schools provide opportunities for student representation. A position as head boy/girl or school president can be taken very seriously by admissions tutors. You will be communicating with senior adults in your school and will have to balance deference with assertiveness. This would undoubtedly improve your confidence and adaptability.

Key points

Don't worry too much if the 'top job' eludes you. Many other committee positions offer the chance to demonstrate these qualities. Examples include joining the school council/committee, working as a prefect, mentoring junior students, and/or helping to organize school clubs. If you don't remember what your school has to offer, your teachers will know. Check notice boards regularly and ask around to ensure you're not missing out!

- **Community involvement** Wherever you live there will be opportunities to help out in the community. This can be distinct from work experience (see p. 54), which is more about finding out what it's like to work in healthcare. Examples of community work include working in an animal shelter, charity fundraising, and volunteering (e.g. in a homeless shelter). Community work can provide opportunities for working with people outside your peer group. It can also provide a great insight into 'real life' as it affects those in your community.

Never forget that hobbies will be interpreted as an outward reflection of your personality. For this reason, you should think twice about developing or describing an interest that could have negative connotations, for example a fringe political perspective. However, this can sometimes work to your advantage, and finding an 'unusual' interest shows sincerity and ingenuity. It can also serve to make your application more memorable, but do be prepared for probing questions at interview.

How many activities?

This depends on the activities and how much time you can squeeze out of your schedule. Your first priority is achieving strong A level grades. However, most good personal statements mention three or four activities, which is enough to demonstrate a range of skills. If you only manage one activity it will need to be exceptional and should speak for itself as to why it is the key focus of your spare time.

A few examples

Applying to medical school is not simply a competition to showcase the most creative hobby. However, it is a distinct advantage to stand out (for the right reasons) from other applicants. The following examples give an idea of what other strong applicants have done in the past and what they believe they gained from their experiences.

World Challenge

I had never travelled further than France on family holidays, so became really excited when someone told me about World Challenge. I raised enough money through working and sponsorship and went on a four-week expedition to Uganda, trekking through the jungle and savannah. I also helped build a classroom for a local primary school. The best thing about travelling through Africa is that I matured and gained a great sense of perspective from seeing how some communities survive with few resources.

Air Cadets

I joined my local Air Cadets when I was 15. As well as learning drill, I made lots of new friends and experienced camping, shooting, abseiling, water sports, flying, and parachuting in just three years. The Air Cadet organization helped me through the Duke of Edinburgh Award as well. Having led other cadets on cold and wet weekends away, I was able to provide lots of examples of having worked as part of a team under pressure.

School visit to Russia

To further my interest in Russian literature, some friends and I organized a visit to a school in St Petersburg with the help of our literature teacher. We stayed with some of the local students, which kept the costs very low, and raised money from sponsored activities to pay for the flights. Along with having a fascinating trip, I learned about a different culture and developed lots of organizational skills.

Bagpipes

Although I have no Scottish ancestry, I decided at the start of my GCSEs to learn the bagpipes. I wrote about this on my UCAS form and my interviewers seemed to think it was really amusing. In fact, they spent most of the time talking about how it's possible to blow into the pipes whilst inhaling at the same time, though they were disappointed to hear that is not how bagpipes work. This really wasn't a topic I'd prepared for!

School photography club

I was very interested in photography and, with two like-minded friends, I set up a photography club. Our school was very supportive and one of the teachers, also a keen photographer, offered to help. In our first year I helped to run a photography competition across the school, which generated lots of interest in photography and earned us quite a few new members as well.

Homeless shelter

During a shadowing placement at a local shelter I met a homeless man who explained some of the difficulties he faced. I spoke to a general practitioner about the problems that homeless people have accessing healthcare and he helped me write a leaflet on this subject that the council has agreed to publish. While working on this I learned about the impact of social circumstances on health and the structure of community healthcare.

Genealogy

I started tracing my family tree and became really interested in population migrations. In fact I became involved with a group of local historians and even co-wrote a chapter for a book about my town that was published. It might sound like a geeky hobby but the admissions tutors seemed impressed that I had an 'academic' interest outside of what was required by the A level curriculum.

Form prefect

As a prefect I was responsible for mentoring younger students. In this role I helped with project ideas, assisted with a class drama production, and tutored students who were struggling. On one occasion, a year eight student approached me to say he was finding maths difficult and felt the teacher picked on him. I arranged a lunchtime meeting at which the teacher explained he believed the student to be very bright but under-motivated. Their relationship improved after this meeting. This taught me that many different problems can be resolved by clear and honest communication.

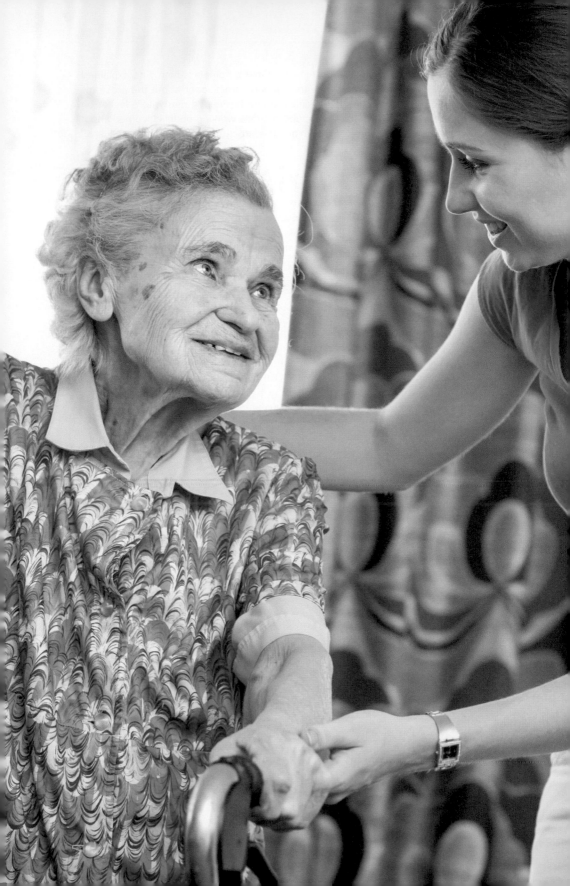

5

Work experience

▎ The value of work experience

Medical school is not just about a university degree; you are choosing a career. Both you and the medical schools you apply to need to know that you understand what it means to be a doctor. This is why work experience is essential.

It is becoming increasingly difficult for school students to find medical work experience. Hospitals and GPs need to protect the personal medical details of their patients from the general public, a principle called patient confidentiality. This can include potential medical students. Although it is difficult, you are unlikely to win a place at medical school without work experience. This chapter will help by suggesting ways to find work experience (see p. 56), to make the most of your work experience time (see p. 62), to volunteer (see p. 64), to find healthcare employment (see p. 66), and to experience research (see p. 68), as well as what to do if all else fails (see p. 70).

How much is enough? The short answer is that you can never have too much work experience. The practical reality is that you have to balance work experience with your work and social life during the school terms and vacations. Although there are no hard and fast rules, the best applicants spend two or three weeks shadowing and several months volunteering or working part-time in a role connected with the caring professions. Many positions only require a few hours a week of commitment, but you will have to begin early to maximize your chance of winning a place at medical school.

It is important to remember why work experience is so valuable; you can't know that you want to enter a career when you have no idea what that actually entails. Work experience will help you distinguish between good and better (there are no 'bad') experiences. Your goal should be to find work experience that helps you to make an informed decision about a career in medicine.

Time frame

The earlier you begin collecting work experience, the stronger your application will be. Applicants often organize their shadowing placements up to a year before submitting their UCAS form. However, it can take a long time to arrange work experience and last-minute panic is best avoided by good planning. Long-term volunteering (e.g. at a hospice or nursing home) shows great commitment to medicine but obviously takes even more time to accrue.

Why work experience is important to medical schools

- Medical schools are choosing doctors, not just students; applicants must show a good understanding of what doctors do.
- Between two and ten applicants apply for each place at medical school. Work experience is a way for course selectors to determine which applicants are genuinely committed to medicine.
- Work experience provides material to discuss with applicants at interview. The importance of this cannot be overstated—questions about your time in work experience are almost certain to arise at interview. It's really important to reflect on what you experience.

Why work experience is important to students

- It provides an insight into what it really means to be a doctor, although bear in mind that doing the job is very different from watching someone else do it.
- It provides an opportunity to talk with doctors about their experiences and lifestyle. This is something that you should endeavour to do as much as possible. Practicing doctors will have personal and unique takes on some of the big issues in medicine— these are valuable opinions and you should take heed of them.
- Students can gain a realistic understanding of the pros and cons of a medical career.
- Students can learn about how hospital and community medical services work.
- It provides plenty of positive (and perhaps negative) experiences to discuss with medical school interviewers.

Problems with work experience

- It can be very difficult to arrange. The next few pages should help.
- Work experience can leave applicants with false or misleading impressions of life as a doctor.
- Medicine is a hugely varied profession. It is impossible to experience every specialty, so it is inevitable that applicants go into medicine without properly appreciating the range of roles available (see p. 12).

A student's experience ...

I remember my work experience like it was yesterday...

'We're losing him, doctor.'

'PADDLES????!'

'Charging, 360 ... CLEAR!'

'Sorry to interrupt your break, doctor, but Mr Wilson in bed four has just been sick again and he's insisting that you look at it.'

We grudgingly switched off the TV. It was a great episode...the sick, on the other hand, was less great. I followed the junior doctor for another four hours, getting in the way and insisting that every patient I saw was having a heart attack (after seeing one earlier that morning).

Of course, being a doctor is not quite as it looks on television. There are considerably fewer crash calls and lots more paperwork! However, this was as useful an insight as any; I learned that if it's hourly crash calls I am after, then perhaps I should have applied to drama school.

Arranging work experience

Finding contacts First, compile a list of everyone you know who works in healthcare. Think laterally. Perhaps a family friend, teacher, or distant relative knows a GP. Maybe a neighbour is a practice nurse or GP receptionist. Any personal connection, however tenuous, could provide a lead. Ideally, try to find contacts working in different healthcare settings (e.g. general practice and hospital). Be thorough and keep returning to the list; at the very least almost everyone has a GP. Ask older relatives if they are, or have recently been, under the care of a hospital specialist.

Using contacts Once you've found a contact, ask for advice. Try to find out which doctors are approachable and likely to help. Ask if your contact would mention you to the health professional before you get in touch. It might seem odd seeking an introduction at this stage but it can reduce the risk of your efforts being 'filed' in the recycle bin. Try to find an email or postal address so you can follow up in person with the doctor (or their secretary). If you are confident, telephoning can be more effective. It is certainly harder to say 'no' to someone in person. Practise what you are going to say before calling and don't be shy about using your contact's name if you have permission to do so.

If contacts don't help If you cannot find a personal contact, drop in to your own GP practice. Ask the receptionist how you could approach the doctors about work experience. They may have a pre-planned scheme for arranging placements. Your own GP might feel a responsibility to help but may worry about confidentiality. If they cannot help, you need to look further afield.

You could have more luck writing to GPs in neighbouring towns where you are less likely to know the patients. You could start by asking each doctor simply to talk with you about medicine. It will be hard for doctors to turn down this humble request. Talking to doctors will be useful in itself but may lead to work shadowing later on. If you have written a letter or email, you should always expect a reply (although be aware this might be hope disappointed, as many medical practices are busy beyond capacity). Many hospitals and GP practices will be unable to help, but it is only polite to say so if you have written to them. You may have to write a second time or follow up with a phone call. Lots of people ask for work experience so you need to be persistent (but not annoying) in order to be 'heard'. Whenever anyone says 'no', don't forget to ask if they can suggest a colleague who can help.

Should your efforts fail, book a normal appointment with your GP. Apologize for taking up their busy schedule and ask if you can discuss their experiences of medicine. Find out whether they could help arrange work experience for you or at least offer advice about who else you could contact.

A more accessible option to work experience in medicine is to utilize the 'Introduction to the NHS' course, a multi-day scheduled work experience that takes place at some hospitals in the UK for the specific purpose of providing a varied work experience. Many hospitals now have specific work experience departments through which you can organize any shadowing experience you want (with age-related exceptions in some trusts). Medify have a work experience map with links to relevant websites that you can use to help you find experience near you: www.medify.co.uk.

> **Key points**
>
> Don't give up. However you approach them, some people will say 'no'. It's not your fault; don't be upset, but simply move on and find someone else to ask. It doesn't matter how many 'no' answers you collect as long as you have one 'yes'.

Special interests If you have an interest in a particular specialty (e.g. paediatrics), phone nearby hospitals to ask for the names of consultants who work in that department. Alternatively, most hospital websites list consultant names and email addresses. Once you have a list, telephone the hospital and ask to speak with the secretary for each consultant. Secretaries will probably pass on your message and call you back to say whether their consultant can help. Call the secretary a second time if you have not heard within a few days. If you have an email address, you could contact the doctor directly. However, it is worth remembering that many senior doctors are not confident with technology. They are also not renowned for strong organizational skills and your message does risk getting lost. This is less of a problem if you have found a good secretary to help you. You should avoid reaching out via social media; less formal means of communication are likely to be rejected, as doctors endeavour to avoid interacting with potential patients via these platforms. There may be exceptions to this general rule, for example online platforms for professional connections.

Most students try to organize placements in specialties such as cardiology, paediatrics, and A&E. However, don't neglect less well-known specialties such as pathology, microbiology, anaesthetics, or ophthalmology.

Key points

If a doctor can't help, ask them to suggest a colleague who may be willing. You will not get anything if you don't ask and asking (politely) will rarely leave you at a disadvantage.

Be creative If you cannot find a contact in healthcare, become one yourself. Lots of healthcare jobs are part-time and require few qualifications. You could volunteer (or find paid work) typing up patient notes in a GP practice, portering in a hospital, or serving tea in a hospice. Many successful applicants find work as a healthcare assistant. Consider working in any job related to healthcare. Ask doctors, nurses, and other healthcare staff about their jobs, the health service, and, of course, about shadowing!

No luck? Don't forget to contact the Royal Colleges or medical schools themselves if you are having trouble arranging work experience. They might also have advice (or contacts) for medical school applicants. You should also remember that shadowing is just one type of work experience. Although it is a very useful thing to organize and to have on your application, it is possible to find out about and show commitment to medicine in other ways. These include volunteering (see p. 64), healthcare work (see p. 66), and research (see p. 68). If after all this you're still short of ideas, see p. 70.

A student's experience ...

I was having difficulties shadowing my doctor because many patients didn't want a student present. One day the hospital porters offered to look after me for an afternoon, and this was the turning point in my work experience. I found out that one of the porters was leaving and I was taken on straight away until a replacement could be found. As a hospital porter I was moving patients around the hospital, preparing surgical kits in theatre, and sitting with patients as they recovered from anaesthetics. I even carried a cardiac arrest bleep! This was great work experience and I got paid to be there; it's definitely worth grasping opportunities in hospital as you never know what might come of them.

▌Preparing for work experience

Before starting your placement, it is useful to have an understanding of how the NHS works (see p. 59 as well).

General practice When a person feels unwell or is worried about their health, they often seek help from their general practitioner (GP). In many cases, the GP is able to give advice or treatment (e.g. a prescription for a medication). If the problem requires specialist skill or knowledge, then the GP refers the patient to another health professional (e.g. hospital consultant, physiotherapist). For this reason, GPs are often described as the 'gatekeepers to the NHS'. GPs have an important role in preventing illness, managing acute health problems, and caring for patients with long-term (chronic) illnesses.

Emergency Department If a patient needs urgent medical attention they can go directly to the Emergency Department or ED (which used to be called Accident and Emergency or A&E—sometimes parodied as 'Anything and Everything'). Most patients are treated directly; however, if further care is required they can be admitted to a Medical or Surgical Admissions Unit (MAU or SAU). GPs can also refer patients directly to the ED, MAU, or SAU. Patients usually stay on a MAU or SAU for less than 24 hours before being discharged or admitted to a specialist ward in the hospital.

Specialists Most specialist doctors (consultants) work in hospitals, where they look after patients who have been admitted for treatment (e.g. surgery, antibiotics). Specialists also see patients from outside the hospital in clinic; these are either patients who were admitted and are now being followed up or patients referred by other doctors such as GPs or other specialists.

A student's experience ...

One of the patients I spoke to had called his GP to say he felt a crushing pain in his chest. His GP thought he might be having a heart attack and called 999. An ambulance went to the man's house and the paramedics brought him straight to A&E. They found out, en route, that he was indeed having a heart attack, and so the A&E doctors were waiting and ready to treat him as soon as the ambulance arrived. He was then moved to the Coronary Care Unit. When he left hospital, he returned for consultations with a cardiologist and later had an operation to improve his heart function. His GP is now managing his blood pressure to prevent a second heart attack. This showed me how every department is vital to patient health. A failure at any step could have been fatal.

Who's who?

- **Foundation doctor** Also known as Foundation Year 1 or 2 (FY1/FY2) doctors, they are involved in the day-to-day care of patients while still learning the skills of medicine. They also ensure that tasks—such as form filling, taking blood samples, and chasing chest X-rays—are completed on the wards. See p. 9.
- **Core/Specialist Training (CT/ST)** After the FY2 year, doctors specialize in a hospital department or general practice. These doctors are training to become either consultants or GPs. See p. 10.
- **General Practitioner** These doctors have overall responsibility for a large number of people in their area. They are usually the first contact for patients and may refer for specialist advice to secondary or tertiary care. See p. 11.

- **Consultant** Consultants are the most senior hospital doctors, with ultimate responsibility for patients. Having trained for over a decade they are very knowledgeable and experienced. Most teach students, research, hold clinics, and lead ward rounds. Some also work privately in their own time. See p. 10.
- **Allied healthcare professionals** Doctors work as part of a multidisciplinary team with nurses, physiotherapists, occupational therapists, speech and language therapists, social workers, midwives, and many others.

How the NHS is structured

The National Health Service (NHS) is the main UK healthcare system; it was launched over 70 years ago, is funded by taxes, and aims to be 'free at the point of use'. It costs the UK taxpayers about £140 billion every year to pay for staff, buildings, equipment, and medications. The NHS is a very complicated organization (1.7 million employees make it the fifth largest employer in the world, just behind McDonald's), but its structure is something you should learn about during the application process. To complicate matters, the way the NHS is run underwent a complete revamp in April 2013 following implementation of the new Health and Social Care Act. See Figure 5.1 for a diagram explaining the structure of the NHS as from April 2013.

The Department of Health and Social Care (DH) The DH has overall responsibility for the NHS and is led by the Secretary of State for Health who is accountable to Parliament and therefore the voting public. However, since April 2013, the DH has delegated day-to-day running of the NHS to a new organization, NHS England. Importantly, responsibility for health elsewhere in the UK has been devolved to the Scottish Government, Welsh Government, and Northern Ireland Executive.

NHS England This organization oversees and allocates resources to around 200 local Clinical Commissioning Groups across England.

Clinical Commissioning Groups (CCGs) These are groups (largely led by GPs) with responsibility for around 60% of the health budget. The role of CCGs is to determine which

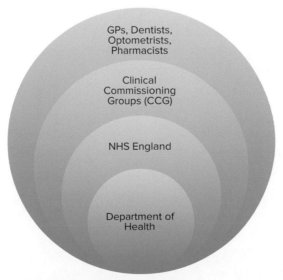

Figure 5.1 Structure of the NHS as from April 2013.

services to 'buy' on behalf of local patients and from which service provider. For example, a CCG might decide to buy all knee replacement services from one local hospital (which is cheapest or has the 'best' outcomes). Or they might decide not to fund a specific treatment altogether, perhaps because it is too expensive or there is little evidence for its effectiveness. The reason for letting CCGs determine regional treatment priorities is that they are thought to be better placed to know what local people want. However, the new structure is controversial (not least because private companies can bid against existing NHS organizations to supply services) and could well come up as a discussion point at interview. Work experience is an opportunity to canvass opinion from NHS employees or to appreciate how few really understand the reforms.

Primary care Primary care describes the 'frontline' services (e.g. GPs, dentists, pharmacists, optometrists) that are the first point of contact for most people.

Secondary care Secondary care describes services that are accessed through a primary care provider. For example, a patient with chest pain may first see their GP (primary care) before meeting a cardiologist (secondary care).

Tertiary care Tertiary care refers to highly specialist services, which are provided in large centres. For example, although knee replacement surgery might happen in most hospitals (secondary care), treatment of a rare bone tumour might be referred to a highly specialized unit in London.

Foundation Trusts Foundation Trusts are NHS hospital trusts that have met specific set criteria and have been rewarded with more autonomy and greater control over their own budget.

▉ Making the most of shadowing

Many students mistakenly try to learn medicine during their placements. This is not what you are there for, as there will be plenty of time for studying later. Instead, try to gain an insight into your future career. Pay attention to what doctors do and how this impacts the doctor, patient, and other members of the healthcare team. For example, if you witness a complicated patient case, use it to appreciate the uncertainty of medicine rather than learning about the disease processes at work. Interviewers expect a realistic understanding of medicine, not someone ready to work as a doctor.

Who to shadow? Doctors are not the only people you will come across in hospital. The truth is that without a team of healthcare professionals to support them, doctors are not a lot of good to their patients. In fact, if you spend all your time with doctors you may never even meet other members of the healthcare team. So branch out; shadow a physiotherapist, speak to a Macmillan nurse, arrange a lunch date with the hospital chaplain. You could even ask to see the laboratories. Gain as broad a perspective as possible and try to appreciate where doctors fit into the wider team.

Reflect To make the most of shadowing, take some time to organize your thoughts. This will help you understand what you are witnessing and learn from the experience. Consider keeping a diary during each placement as this will help organize your thoughts and provide a space to reflect on experiences that made you think. It might also be a useful revision aid on the train to your medical school interview.

- Before starting, ask yourself what you expect, and see if your expectations change throughout the placement.
- What do you hope to get out of shadowing? Obviously, there is a metaphorical 'box to tick' on your UCAS application, but there is much more besides.
- What did you learn? Did anything surprise, please, or disappoint you? Perhaps you saw a distressed relative, an elderly patient being restrained, or a very ill child. You might see a rude or abusive relative, or dislike how a healthcare professional talks to a patient. Make a note of these events and consider how they could have been avoided. If appropriate, talk to the person you are shadowing, who might have a different perspective on the experience.
- Think particularly hard about any ethical dilemmas you come across. Should the GP have prescribed contraception to a 14-year-old? Is it right to sedate an elderly patient with Alzheimer's who shouts on the ward? These questions may well come up at interview and it will be an advantage if you have already thought about them.
- Don't forget the bright side as well; think about how doctors are placed to improve patients' lives. It doesn't always require a crack diagnosis; sometimes a clear explanation or a kind word is all it takes.

The perfect application

Try to shadow each of the following:

- GP
- Hospital specialist (e.g. consultant, registrar)
- Junior doctor
- Another health professional (e.g. nurse, occupational therapist, dietician).

Make sure you also volunteer or work part-time in a hospital (e.g. as a porter, a nursing auxiliary) or in a nursing home. Prepare for interviews by writing down anything that made you think.

Ask questions To really engage with work shadowing you need to ask questions. It is much easier to teach a student who is enthusiastic than one who follows silently behind. Remember to be polite when talking to patients and introduce yourself as a medical school applicant so nobody mistakes you for a doctor.

- Talk to patients—they are important to your future career! Ask what ideas, concerns, and expectations they have about their illness. Don't be afraid to ask questions. 'Does it hurt?' and 'How do you cope at home?' are perfectly valid when asked at appropriate times.
- What do they think makes a good doctor? Most patients will have had a lifetime of good and bad experiences. You will be asked at interview what qualities are important for a doctor, and now is a good time to find out from the people whose opinions matter most.
- Use every opportunity to talk with all types of healthcare professional. Talk to doctors about their work patterns, the NHS, and whether they would choose medicine again. What problems do they face?
- Ask other healthcare workers about their role, the challenges they face, and how they interact with doctors.
- Ask doctors about their lifestyle. What do they like and dislike about their job? How has medicine affected their life's path? How does it impact on their families (if appropriate!)?
- Perhaps most importantly, could you imagine yourself in this job for the rest of your career?

Be proactive You're not just there to ask questions. Offer a pair of helping hands at every appropriate opportunity. This could be as simple as opening the door for patients coming to clinic. You could offer to take wheelchair-bound patients back to the ward to save them waiting for a porter. At the very least you will make a practical contribution to the hospital. At best, the staff will see you are keen and will go out of their way to help you make the most of your time.

A student's experience ...

I spent two afternoons with the nursing staff; the charge nurse was so impressed by my willingness to help that he organized for me to work part-time as a healthcare assistant. This gave me the chance to record patients' blood pressure, complete fluid charts, and distribute meals. It was also an opportunity to meet more doctors and nurses around the hospital.

Volunteering

There is more to work experience than simply shadowing doctors. It is for this reason that medical schools look for students who have undertaken voluntary work, which can demonstrate:

- Understanding of challenges such as working with ill and/or dying patients.
- Long-term commitment to health or social care.
- A genuine interest in people. This is often more valuable than showing you have simply 'ticked the box'. To some extent, demonstrating an interest in people can also be achieved through voluntary work in a non-medical setting (see p. 64).

Where to volunteer?

This depends on what is available locally. The ideal volunteer position will involve contact with people, possibly in a healthcare setting. Remember that long-term commitment to volunteering is much more valuable than just for a shorter time. For this reason, try to choose something you might enjoy and can travel to without too much difficulty. Good places to volunteer include:

- **Hospitals** Volunteering opportunities could include work in the hospital shop or reading to elderly patients on the wards.
- **Residential homes** Elderly people living in residential accommodation can often benefit from help with shopping, tidying, or just someone to talk to.
- **Nursing homes** Individuals in nursing homes often require a lot of care, which can sometimes involve volunteers. Other roles can include befriending and/or taking residents out for a change of scenery.
- **Hospices** These institutions help support people with life-limiting diseases. They are often run by charities and require lots of help from volunteers. There are many lessons to learn in this environment for any potential medical school applicant.
- **Support groups** These groups exist for people with a range of different conditions. They usually hold regular meetings, where you could assist by helping set up and welcoming people to the meeting.
- **Campaigns** Many charities benefit from volunteer fundraisers helping run charity events or appeals. Although you might not be directly exposed to patients, you could still demonstrate an interest and will meet lots of different people in the process.

A student's experience ...

I spent a year working every Saturday afternoon in a nursing home. My work involved feeding patients during meal times, helping the carers to clean immobile patients, and chatting to the residents and their families. I soon found that, most of all, I wanted a career where I could work with so many different people. I'm confident this came across at interview.

How to organize voluntary work?

Compared with work shadowing, volunteering is much easier to organize. This is because many organizations rely on support from volunteers. Nevertheless, as with all your work experience, you should organize opportunities as early as possible. Some organizations require interviews, training, and/or Disclosure and Barring Service (DBS) checks before you can begin working. This can take a lot of time.

Don't forget that telephoning or personally visiting an organization will provoke a quicker response than an email. If you do write first, you may have to call afterwards to encourage a response—don't be shy in doing this but always remember to be respectful. While finding work experience and shadowing is important to you, it is rightfully not the priority of everyone you reach out to. The local newspaper, bulletin boards, and online search engines or telephone directories (e.g. 192.com, thephonebook.bt.com) are useful sources for finding contact details. Wherever possible, try to find the name of an individual to write to. This will make a response more likely and provide someone you can call if an answer is not forthcoming.

There are plenty of voluntary opportunities around, so don't give up at the first hurdle. If you're having trouble, again, think laterally. Maybe you have an elderly next-door neighbour who needs help gardening or a family friend requiring a babysitter. There are opportunities all around you and very few experiences will be wasted. Remember that your ultimate aim is to learn more about a healthcare role and to be able to demonstrate this on a UCAS form or at interview.

Key points

https://do-it.org is an excellent resource for finding local volunteering opportunities. You can search projects based on the group you want to work with (e.g. the homeless, young people) or what you want to do (e.g. build, mentor, counsel). The Royal Voluntary Service also offers a range of volunteering roles in the hospital and community: www.royalvoluntaryservice.org.uk.

Making the most of voluntary work

The same principles of productivity and reflection apply to volunteering as to other types of work experience. You should certainly not dismiss opportunities because there are no doctors present. Great opportunities and insights often arise from a 'less interesting' post, so commit yourself to whatever you sign up for; you never know where it might lead.

Don't forget to ask yourself and others questions about everything around you. What do elderly people who live alone worry about? How did women in a breast cancer support group receive their diagnosis; could their experiences have been improved? You will probably come across some sensitive issues concerning fairly vulnerable people. If it is appropriate to approach these topics you should do so with care and sensitivity. You will learn far more by thinking about your volunteering experiences as much as possible than by simply going through the motions each day.

Needless to say, if you come across a doctor (or other health professional), ask if you can shadow them.

Employment

Many applicants find it hard to set aside time for work experience alongside studies, hobbies, and part-time work. Fortunately, it is possible to combine work experience with employment, essentially getting paid for improving your medical school application.

Advantages

There are many reasons why you might combine employment and work experience:

- **Responsibility** You can often feel as if you are in the way when you do work experience; this is not the case for a paid employee who is an integral part of the team. Doing a job forces you to concentrate more than watching other people at work. That said, when you work as a part of a team, you often only get to see the one aspect that you're responsible for. You can end up in a situation where you miss the forest for the trees.
- **Duration** While work experience might only last a few days, employment will usually continue over a period of months or years. It takes time to become familiar with any new experience and the longer duration will help you feel comfortable in a healthcare setting and around patients. It also demonstrates commitment and interest in working with sick or disadvantaged people.
- **Contacts** Any job in healthcare will be alongside healthcare professionals. These people may respect your initiative and offer further opportunities such as shadowing (see p. 53)—don't be afraid to ask, but expect any shadowing opportunities to be outside of your working hours.
- **Pay** Employers must pay at least the minimum wage to all employees. There are different rates for those aged <18 years, 18–20 years, 21–24 years, and ≥21 years. If there is any doubt, check the minimum wage (www.gov.uk/national-minimum-wage-rates) and contact the Citizens Advice Bureau to clarify if you are unsure.

> **A student's experience ...**
>
> I worked at a GP practice helping summarize paper notes onto a computer system. I was paid £7.50 an hour, more than my friends working in other jobs, and felt I was making a real contribution to the practice. The GPs were keen to talk to me about a career in medicine and sometimes let me spend a few hours with them seeing patients.

Obstacles

As with all work experience, there are obstacles to watch out for:

- **Age** Many healthcare providers require employees to be above a minimum age.
- **Administration** DBS checks often take four weeks to process. It may also be necessary to have immunizations and an occupational health check-up—so apply early.
- **Working hours** Residential homes and hospitals may need evening workers but other employers, such as GP practices, might only open during the day. School holidays are ideal for working.

Types of work

There are thousands of jobs in healthcare but most require specialist qualifications. Work experience applicants often find certain jobs more accessible than others:

- **Healthcare assistant (HCA)** HCAs work alongside nurses and help with washing and dressing patients, bedmaking, and monitoring vital signs (e.g. pulse, temperature). This is an ideal way to experience 'hands-on' care.
- **Clinical support worker** This is a similar role to that of an HCA, although clinical support workers usually assist a therapist (e.g. physiotherapist, audiologist) rather than nursing staff.
- **Carer** Many agencies employ carers to visit elderly or disabled patients in their own homes. Carers will often have a similar role to HCAs, although many posts require a means of transport to visit clients.
- **Phlebotomist** These healthcare workers take blood from patients and ensure it is transported safely to the appropriate laboratory. It is a useful experience as you will meet lots of patients, learn a vital skill, and develop methods of helping patients deal with painful procedures.
- **Hospital porter** Porters move patients and equipment around the hospital. They work everywhere from wards to operating theatres and get to see a wide range of departments, patients, and practices.
- **Domestic services** This includes cleaners, catering, stores, and laundry workers. These roles are easiest to organize and some allow patient contact.

A student's experience ...

As a cleaner on a cardiology ward I got to know many different patients. They often confided in me, so I learned all about their worries, home lives, and thoughts on the hospital staff. In particular, I learned there is more to each patient than a disease.

How to find employment in healthcare?

First choose the organization you want to work for (e.g. hospital, GP practice, residential home). Use the internet or local paper to identify any jobs being advertised.

Small organizations (e.g. GP practices) should be approached directly, whereas hospitals may have their own Human Resources (HR) department. You are more likely to be offered employment if you are available for an extended period of time (e.g. the summer vacation) rather than evenings and weekends.

Large hospitals will often have a website complete with an up-to-date list of vacancies. Many hospitals (and residential homes) take on staff through an employment agency. If you cannot find which agencies place healthcare staff, ask the organization you want to work for which one they use. Most jobs will require you to complete an application form and attend an interview. This will probably be followed by a period of training.

Key points

www.jobs.nhs.uk lists all the NHS jobs available in your area. For non-NHS jobs, use Google to find agencies supplying staff to local care homes.

Research experience

Although it is not a common form of work experience, some applicants organize time in a laboratory helping with research. There is a growing commitment in the NHS towards 'evidence-based medicine' (EBM), which means finding out which treatments actually *work* rather than using them just because they have been used for a long time. Millions of pounds are spent every year on this process. Research is not a substitute for spending time with patients, although it can add a further angle to your application.

Advantages The main advantage of research experience is that you will see another side of modern medicine. Although not all doctors are researchers, many undertake a research project at some point in their career. It would be great if you could show an understanding of this early on. More importantly, seeing research might help you understand the importance of evidence-based medicine and how doctors and scientists learn about disease.

Disadvantages There are three things to consider for any applicant thinking about research work. The first is that it can be very difficult to organize. Laboratories have lots of expensive and potentially dangerous equipment; an electron microscope can cost over £1 million. Laboratories also contain sensitive research work. It is not unusual for a PhD student to work for a year developing a cell line, which could easily be destroyed by an inexperienced work experience student. However, this will depend on the laboratory and most could accommodate showing a student around for an afternoon.

The second point to consider is that you are unlikely to achieve very much with only a short period of time available. This is because it takes a long time to learn laboratory techniques before they can be used to 'discover' anything. It may also be tedious simply watching researchers go about their work. However, going along for a day could be useful in helping to inform your career decisions.

Finally, it may be difficult to explain to interviewers why you chose to find out about research. They will prefer experience with patients and may need convincing that research is a useful addition to your work experience portfolio. This will depend on where you apply and who the interviewers are. However, have an explanation ready in case this unusual part of your application is picked up. Talking intelligently about evidence-based medicine could work very well at this point.

A student's experience ...

I spent a summer working in a laboratory with my neighbour, who is Professor of Physiology at a nearby university. Some of the techniques were hard but I think I was useful to the team in the end. I was given a long time to talk about my project at interview and the interviewers were particularly impressed that I was named on a research paper! I am now a medical student and will be returning to the lab to continue my project as a paid research assistant in my first summer holiday.

Should you try to find research experience?

Research is never a substitute for experience with patients. Admissions tutors want to see evidence of your interest in people above everything else. There are, however, a number of reasons why you might consider looking for research experience:

- You want to learn the importance of research to medicine through first-hand experience. Selling this idea appropriately at interview could show maturity and insight far beyond what the interviewers are expecting.

- You already have a lot of shadowing and volunteering experience. If you are looking to add breadth to your application, research is a possibility.
- You are applying to a medical school with a strong emphasis on basic sciences. These include Oxford (see p. 170), Cambridge (see p. 136), and Imperial College London (see p. 156).
- You are applying to study biomedical science through UCAS, in addition to medicine (see p. 216). Research could fulfil the same role for biomedical science as hospital work does for medicine. Unlike medicine, very few applicants to these courses will have relevant work experience and your chances of acceptance will increase dramatically.
- You are interested in research after graduating as a doctor. Experience now could help confirm this interest or put you off altogether.

Finding research

There are many different types of research. It is unlikely you would be involved in the type of research that goes on in hospitals as this involves patients and may take years to finish. You may, however, hear doctors talk about research projects and/or see patients who are part of clinical trials. Don't forget to ask questions if you do!

You are more likely to find work experience in a laboratory. Although there are research laboratories in some hospitals, most are found in universities. You could try contacting a nearby medical school or Department of Biological Sciences for advice. Most will have websites that list their researchers and current projects. Choose a researcher or project that is relevant to medicine. If you are already interested in a particular field, write to a researcher with similar interests for permission to visit his/her laboratory. Alternatively, don't be shy about exploiting personal contacts. If you or your family know anyone in research—a PhD student, technician, or professor—consider asking them. They may know someone you could approach to supervise you.

The most important thing to remember is that research experience is not a vital part of your medical school application. Very few applicants will have any. If the opportunity arises then seize it; however, it is unlikely to affect your application if you cannot, or do not want to, experience medical research.

Key points

Research experience is not a substitute for work with patients. It should probably only be considered by a small number of applicants such as those applying to very academic courses, those who already have an existing interest in research, and/or those who have already undertaken a wide range of different work experience placements.

If all else fails...

Successful applicants often have a long record of experiences such as shadowing, volunteering, and part-time employment. These are important and often necessary. However, an additional tactic is to find something that makes you stand out from the other applicants. Have a look at some of the following examples for ideas—but don't feel limited by them!

Hospitals abroad

On holiday with my parents, I visited a small clinic in a remote area of Malawi. I had finished two hospital attachments in the UK but was interested to see how things worked abroad. Fortunately, the medical assistant in charge understood my interest and spoke good English. He showed me around his clinic and I was amazed to see how much could be achieved without expensive equipment. This taught me that many conditions can be diagnosed simply by talking and examining patients. These are vital skills anywhere that medicine is practiced.

Occupational therapists

Occupational therapists help people who have restricted activity as a result of their illness. During a shadowing placement I spent a couple of days with the occupational therapy team. I watched them conduct assessments, provide vital equipment, and even visit patients in their own homes. If I am honest, I hadn't really thought about healthcare taking place outside hospitals and GP practices. I was able to see first-hand how much important work goes on in the community and how it is not just doctors and nurses who treat patients.

Pathologist

During a summer vacation I worked as a lab assistant in the histopathology department of a hospital. Although I didn't think this would be useful for medical school, as I didn't see many live patients, I was wrong. At interview I talked about the importance of hospital support services, which often go undervalued because they are hidden away from patients. This seemed to please the pathologist on my interview panel!

I was also invited by one of the consultants to see deceased patients being prepared for post-mortem. This was fascinating, although I was apprehensive at first, and writing about it on my UCAS form led to a discussion at another interview about when and why post-mortems should be carried out. Fortunately, I had asked the consultant very similar questions so found myself in a great position to answer them.

Mountain rescue

As a keen climber, I read an article in a climbing magazine about mountain rescue teams. This seemed like an ideal opportunity to combine work experience with something I already enjoyed. Although I wasn't able to join one of the teams because of my age, I met with the team doctor who gave me a tutorial on the effects of low temperature on the body. This helped me see how basic science, anatomy, physiology, and biochemistry all fit into clinical medicine. It also gave me some ideas about what I might like to do when I finish medical school.

Army doctors

During my time as an Army cadet, I listened to a talk by an Army doctor. He described his journey through medical school and working in NHS hospitals, before touring conflict zones such as Afghanistan. This helped me identify another reason for studying medicine: the skills learned as a doctor can be applied in thousands of different situations. Wherever there are people in need of help, there is an important role for doctors.

A brief warning Finding work experience abroad can be a great way to have fun and set your application apart from the competition. This is much easier to organize during a gap year after school (see p. 33). Always remember to put patient safety and dignity before your own need to gain experience. Do not put yourself in a position (e.g. by doing things you are unqualified to do) whereby patients are put at risk. Any suggestion of this could result in a premature end to your application.

If things still aren't working out Work experience is difficult to arrange. However, successful applicants will almost always have managed to organize something; if you think laterally enough there will always be opportunities available. You could contact local pharmacists, hospital laboratories, travel clinics, hospices, or baby-weighing clinics, all of whom might be able to help.

An insider's view ...

Students often want to know what experience they need to win a place at medical school. There is no simple answer. We want to know that applicants have learned something about being a doctor and are enthusiastic about medicine. At the very least, applicants should have read about healthcare. They should have spoken to doctors (at least their own GP) and patients about the qualities needed to be a good doctor. Students struggling to find work experience should remember that there are many ways to learn about medicine. Even simple things can help persuade interviewers that you want to be a doctor.

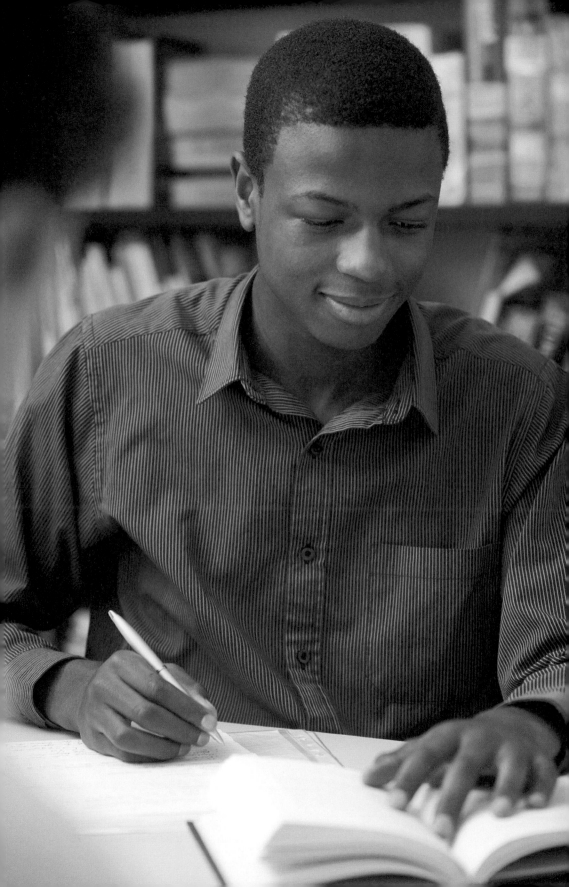

6

Preparing for admission tests

▌The use of admission tests

Most medical schools require an admission test to help identify the best candidates. You only get one chance each year to take each test (admissions cycle), but with careful preparation it is possible to maximize your score.

The tests are very different from A levels and appreciating this difference is the key to doing well. They do not test what you know; rather they test how well you can think under *considerable* time pressure. To succeed, you must focus on answering lots of questions well rather than a few questions perfectly. The test designers claim that preparation does not help since the questions are based on intellect and not knowledge. However, it is the opinion of probably everyone that's ever taken these tests that, in practice, being familiar with the question styles and refining your technique makes all the difference.

This chapter describes the format of these tests, explains how the scores are used by medical schools (see p. 75), offers strategies to get the best marks (see p. 80), and includes an overview of the UCAT (see p. 82) and BMAT (see p. 86). The GAMSAT, a test usually reserved for graduate-entry courses (see p. 251), is described on p. 255. To help explain the format of the different question types we have included sample questions in Appendix 1 (see p. 347); these were contributed by Kaplan (www.kaptest.co.uk) who run preparation courses for these tests.

The admission tests

There are two main tests used by medical schools in the UK: the University Clinical Aptitude Test (UCAT) and the Biomedical Admissions Test (BMAT). They are used by all medical schools except:

- The graduate courses at Cardiff, Liverpool (see p. 272), Nottingham (see p. 277), ScotGEM (see p. 290), St George's University of London (see p. 275), and Swansea (see p. 286), which use the Graduate Medical School Admissions Test (GAMSAT) (see p. 255).
- Keele (see p. 144), which permits the GAMSAT for graduates who don't meet the GCSE/A level requirements.
- Exeter (see p. 140), which requires the GAMSAT for graduates applying to the five-year course, or for those for whom more than two years have elapsed since completion of their A levels.
- Plymouth/Peninsula (see p. 172), which requires the GAMSAT for anyone applying to their five-year course who isn't coming straight from school.
- Buckingham (see p. 201) and University of Central Lancashire (UCLan) (see p. 138), which do not use an admission test.

The UCAT has five sections: 'Verbal reasoning', 'Quantitative reasoning', 'Abstract reasoning', 'Decision analysis', and a 'Situational judgement test' (see p. 82). The BMAT consists of three sections: 'Aptitude and skills', 'Scientific knowledge and applications', and the 'Writing task' (see p. 86).

The purpose of admission tests

Tests have become a necessary part of the admissions process due to the high number of students applying to study medicine. They offer:

- **A way to distinguish between candidates** Most medical school applicants are predicted straight As/A*s. The admission tests offer universities a way to distinguish between them.
- **A fair comparison** Admissions tests allow the medical schools to compare all applicants using a fair and consistent standard. Unlike A levels, where students taking the same subject sit exams set by different exam boards, every candidate answers the same standard of questions.
- **Identical mark schemes** The marking is done to the same standard; in fact the UCAT is marked by computer and the BMAT is multiple choice except for the essay, which has a consistent mark scheme (see p. 87).
- **Teaching independence** Since the tests require limited background knowledge, the benefits or disadvantages of different schools and teachers are minimized.

Key points

The admissions tests are very different from other exams. You need to be willing to skip questions, make quick guesses, and prioritize which questions to go back to. Practising the tests under time pressure will make a big difference to your technique and eventual results.

How are the tests used by medical schools?

This is not an easy question to answer because the use of admission test scores differs between medical schools. Furthermore, many institutions do not describe their selection methods in great detail. As a general principle, the tests are used to filter out the 'best' applicants:

- **Is there a cut-off score?** Some medical schools set an explicit 'cut-off' score: those above the specific score get invited to interview, while those below do not. Often this is determined year on year (for example, some schools set a cut-off above a certain decile for that year). Other medical schools derive a total score by assessing GCSEs and UCAS forms alongside admission tests, and set a cut-off for this value instead.
- **Are the cut-off scores available?** Medical schools used to keep very quiet about their cut-off scores; however, this has not always been the case in recent years. If a specific school does not list their requirements on their website, you can often search for a Freedom of Information Act request for the scores of successful applicants (www.whatdotheyknow.com).
- **What is the estimated cut-off score?** A UCAT score of 2,500 out of 3,600 (i.e. an average of 625 out of 900 in each of the first four sections) appears to be a common cut-off score. There is less information about the BMAT cut-off, but it is generally thought to be 13 out of 23 (i.e. 5 out of 9 in each of the first two sections and 3C out of 5 on the essay—see p. 87).
- **Is it difficult to reach this estimate?** Not for above-average applicants: in 2018, the average scores for the UCAT were 567, 624, 658, and 637 for sections 1–4 respectively. For the BMAT, the mean scores were 4.0 for section 1, a split mean of 4 and 5 for section 2, and 3A for section 3. The cut-off scores are not unreachable, but you need to do better than average.
- **Test scores in context** Admission tests are an important component of your medical school application; however, they are considered alongside GCSEs, AS-level results, predicted A level grades, and your personal statement (see p. 221). For some medical schools, a bad admission test score means no interview; at others it means that the rest of your application must be outstanding.

Preparing for and taking the tests

There are several resources that you may call upon to help you prepare for admission tests:

- **This chapter** These pages should be used to gain tips about how to answer admission test questions. By reading about the format of the UCAT (see p. 82) and BMAT (see p. 86), you will learn more about what is involved in each section. You should then try the sample questions in Appendix 1 (see p. 347).
- **Specimen questions** The UCAT and BMAT websites offer sample question papers for each section. These have the advantage of being identical in format and style to the questions you will receive on the day. However, there are a limited number of questions and you risk becoming overfamiliar with them if you practise too often. This can lead to a false sense of security.
- **Practice books** These usually consist of a bank of questions similar to those in the UCAT and BMAT. Make sure that the book has explanations along with answers, so you can learn where you went wrong and how to improve. Such books have two limitations: a lack of individual feedback and an inability to assess BMAT essay performance (see p. 87). You could try asking your teachers to look at your practice essays, together with a copy of the mark scheme.
- **Websites** Alongside practice books, a number of websites have practice questions for UCAT and BMAT. They range in quality and cost; up-to-date lists and reviews can be found on medical student forums. Some of the most commonly recommended websites are Medify, The Medic Portal, Kaptest, and Passmedicine.
- **Preparatory courses** These offer the opportunity to practise test questions under timed conditions, with experts who can provide tailored feedback and explain the answers to questions you don't understand. Preparatory courses are also invaluable for going through answers to BMAT essays. Kaplan, who provide the test material (see p. 347), offer preparatory courses in the UK and online in real time.
- **Further reading** There are various books available on thinking skills, logic, and critical reasoning that may be used to better understand these areas. These skills are particularly useful for sections 1–4 of the UCAT and section 1 of the BMAT. It is likely also to be worth investing in some GCSE physics, chemistry, biology, and maths revision books for section 2 of the BMAT.

Preparatory courses and websites

Almost all students prepare for their UCAT or BMAT using a combination of the resources just described. The questions in Appendix 1 (see p. 347) were provided by Kaplan Test Prep and Admissions, who offer classroom courses that teach methods and strategies for the test and also provide website resources (www.kaptest.co.uk).

UCAT practicalities

Taking the UCAT The UCAT is taken before completing the UCAS form and choosing the medical schools to which you will apply. The test can only be taken once a year, before the beginning of October (see www.ucat.ac.uk for exact dates) and you need to book a test date, often four to six weeks in advance. It is a computer-based test performed at one of the official Pearson VUE test centres. There are many centres across the UK and internationally; an exemption list of countries without a test centre, in which students do not need to take the test, is available on the UCAT website. An extended version of the test is available for candidates with special educational needs (UCATSEN). In both versions you can mark questions for 'review' and go back to them at the end.

Practical hints Aim to sit the UCAT as soon as possible, allowing you to focus your efforts towards your UCAS application form and preparing for interview. This also allows you to reschedule if you are feeling unwell or unprepared in the days leading up to your test date. Whatever you do, make sure that you don't set your only test date for the last date possible in the cycle. Make sure you have been given your pen and laminated booklet to make notes on before the test begins—with the invigilator still there, check that your pen works before the test starts. Ear plugs might be available, but take your own to ensure your comfort while helping to prevent distractions.

UCAT results Your test answers are marked by computer and the result is available immediately after the test. The test centre then sends your result to UCAS, who will pass it on to the universities to which you send an application.

If your results aren't quite what you expected, don't panic! UCAT results are usually considered alongside other factors such as exam results and your personal statement (see p. 221). If it is obvious that you scored very low, you should consider applying to medical schools that are not strict about cut-offs (although identifying these can be tricky) or do not use the UCAT at all (see p. 74).

BMAT practicalities

Taking the BMAT This test is taken after choosing medical schools and submitting your UCAS form. Applicants must register with the Cambridge Assessment Group before 15 October (the same closing date as UCAS applications); however, there are late booking fees so it is best to register earlier. There are three sittings of the BMAT—in February, September, and November—and some universities have strict requirements as to which sittings are acceptable. You can only sit the exam once a year and so, if you sit an early session that isn't accepted, you might have forfeited a chance at accessing your preferred universities. The BMAT is a written test that must be taken at an official test centre. The majority of candidates will sit the BMAT at their own school or college, around the beginning of November. A soft pencil should be used for sections 1 and 2 (take an eraser as well) and a black ink pen for section 3.

BMAT results Most people leave the BMAT test feeling that it did not go well. Nevertheless, you should avoid trying to anticipate your results until they arrive, as the BMAT is not the type of test that you finish feeling you've nailed it! It's designed so that you feel you could have done better with more time. The BMAT results are usually released online at the end of November.

Key points

The full BMAT specification and additional specimen questions can be found on the Cambridge Assessment Group website (https://www.admissionstesting.org). This is also where you will need to register to sit the BMAT as well as find further details regarding reimbursement. The cost of the BMAT varies depending on the session. UK medical schools almost exclusively specify either the August or October sitting.

Admission test strategy

There are three ways to improve your performance in the admission tests: practise, practise, and practise! You are very unlikely to learn a question that will come up. However, you will learn to manage your time, concentrate on questions you can answer, and become familiar with the format so that you don't waste valuable seconds on instructions on the day.

- **'Revising' will not help (much)** Your strategy for the admission tests needs to be different from that for your A levels. 'Cramming' before the test won't help you since outside knowledge is irrelevant to the UCAT, and is only required to a limited degree in the BMAT. Revision serves to familiarize you with the nature of the exam and style of question you can expect; you aren't revising material at all.
- **Learn the format** Instead, you need to focus your efforts on learning the format of the questions so no time is wasted on the day trying to understand the task (see Appendices).
- **Learn about the mark scheme** You should be familiar with what the sections are examining and, in particular, those taking the BMAT should be aware of what examiners are looking for when marking the essay question (see p. 87).
- **Maximizing your marks** In the multiple-choice sections you can maximize your marks by answering as many questions as you can in the time allowed. On the BMAT essay, marks are maximized by an essay that directly answers the questions and achieves the requirements of the marking criteria (see p. 87).
- **Do not be afraid to skip questions** It is not a realistic aim to answer all of the questions correctly. In order to succeed you must be prepared to leave questions and return to them later on if there is time.
- **Guess** Because there are no negative marks, if you do not know the answer, guess (see p. 80).
- **Practise** You need to practise mock tests under timed conditions in order to maximize your mark on the test day.

Practise your pacing

Many students have their first experience of sitting the UCAT or BMAT under properly timed conditions on the test day. For many this experience is stressful and ultimately disappointing since they find there are far more questions than they can answer in the time available. These test-takers tend to score below average in one or more sections, which means that they miss the cut-off score and fail to qualify for interview. It's a hard lesson to learn and an unpleasant way to learn it. This can, of course, be avoided by adequate preparation.

There are a few things you can do as part of this practice to get yourself in the test-day mindset:

- **Average time per question** Work out the average timing per question for each section of the test. For example, the Quantitative Reasoning section of the UCAT requires you to answer 36 questions in 23 minutes. Be careful here, as the minute to read directions cannot be used to answer questions; so instead of having 23 minutes, there are only 22. With only 22 minutes to answer 36 maths questions, you must answer each question in about 36 seconds, and that's without allowing extra time to look over the charts and tables that accompany the questions. See p. 82 for timing calculations.

- **Triaging the 'stinkers'** This highlights the importance of triage. You may find that with a bit of timed practice you have no trouble answering most maths questions in 30 seconds. Unfortunately, the test designers have thought of this, so they mix in questions that are more complicated. These could be complex because there is more information to read or because the maths required is significantly more elaborate. Instead of taking about 30 seconds, these questions might take three or four minutes. Working even one of these out completely could cost you five or more marks on later, quicker questions. In the UCAT you can guess an answer, mark the question for review, and come back to it. In the BMAT, guess an answer and place a star in the margin reminding you to come back to it if you have time later.
- **Timed practice** You've probably never had a test that required answering so many maths questions so quickly. The good news is that, with timed practice, you can improve your speed and accuracy. However, this practice must be *timed* and it must include questions that are similar in terms of their format, structure, and range of difficulty. Timed practice is a feature available on most of the websites referred to earlier in this chapter.

Key points

By practising your pacing you can learn to triage questions, rather than waste time answering long or complicated ones. You can guess strategically and move on to quicker marks later in the section. Knowing this, and practising for it properly, can make all the difference in qualifying for interview.

An insider's view …

Every year we have many students on our admission test prep courses who sat the UCAT or BMAT in the previous year and failed to qualify for interview. They simply didn't score highly enough, despite having great A levels. Although these students are incredibly bright, they made the mistake of assuming that the UCAT and BMAT are similar to school exams. They had never encountered a test that is designed to be difficult for a bright student to finish. In fact, most of them had never left questions on an exam unanswered until they sat the UCAT or the BMAT. Unfortunately, they had this experience of leaving questions unanswered on the test day, which destroyed their hopes of getting a place to study medicine that year. These students always say the same thing: they wish someone had told them about the benefits of practising beforehand, because then they would have invested time preparing for the test and earned the score required the first time around.

Kaplan Test Prep and Admissions (www.kaptest.co.uk)

The following tips apply specifically to the multiple choice-type questions you will face in the UCAT and BMAT.

Triage

Triage is a French word meaning 'to separate, sort, or select'. Imagine that you are the only medic in the Emergency Department of a rural hospital on a quiet night. Following a car crash, five patients come in at once. Assessing them quickly, you find that one is unconscious, not breathing, and has no pulse, while the other four are bleeding profusely but are conscious. By ignoring the unconscious patient initially, you can save four lives by quickly stopping their bleeding (elevate and compress). Once the 'bleeders' have been stabilized you can see if there is anything you can do for the last patient.

- **Why triage?** When resources are limited, triage is essential. It allows you to achieve the most benefit with the time, equipment, and experience that are available.
- **Triage in admission tests** To maximize your marks on the UCAT and BMAT you must triage each question as it appears. If a question appears to be time-consuming, you do not have time for it. This includes questions with unusually long sections of text or pages of information with them. There are more marks, and quicker marks, in the questions you have yet to encounter. This is a skill you should practise as you actively revise.
- **Returning to the rest** If you have time left over after a first pass through the questions in the section, you can come back to the ones you've skipped. This approach may be unfamiliar, but these tests have been designed to give you a hard time finishing if you answer all the questions in order. Triage is the surest way to maximizing your marks.

This strategy works because virtually all the questions on the UCAT and BMAT are multiple choice; this means there's another strategy you can use as well…

Strategic guessing

- **No negative marking** An essential fact: there is no penalty for incorrect answers on the UCAT or BMAT, so there is no penalty for guessing. Thus, it's essential that you put down an answer for every question. Leaving questions blank means giving up on marks that could have been yours.
- **Strategic guessing** Guessing strategically means doing a quick assessment of a question to eliminate one or more answers before guessing from the remainder. Because a multiple-choice question can only have one correct answer, there must be a reason why all the other answers are wrong. You can either work out the correct answer through straightforward reasoning/maths, or you can work out the correct answer by eliminating all of the wrong answers. Guessing strategically is a variation on this latter option: when you don't have time to eliminate all of the wrong answers, simply eliminate the obvious ones and make your best guess from the answers that remain.

The odds of guessing correctly when guessing blindly, as compared to guessing strategically, are shown in Table 6.1.

When you can eliminate one or more answer choices, guessing strategically gives you a much stronger chance of answering correctly and picking up the mark.

Table 6.1 The odds of strategic guessing

Number of answer choices	Odds of correctly guessing blindly	Odds of correctly guessing strategically after eliminating:	
		1 answer	2 answers
3	33%	67%	100%
4	25%	33%	50%
5	20%	25%	33%

- **Blind guessing** The odds of guessing blindly are not bad, particularly when there are only three answer choices. Still, you should only guess blindly if you are running out of time and at risk of leaving questions unanswered. In that situation guessing blindly gives you some chance of picking up the mark. If you leave a question unanswered, the odds of picking up the mark are nil.
- **BMAT exceptions** Note that the BMAT sometimes includes a few questions in section 1 or section 2 that have write-in answers (e.g. a number or a phrase). These questions are relatively uncommon and not susceptible to strategic guessing. As you triage the BMAT, it's usually best to leave the write-in questions for later, unless of course you find they are quick work and easy marks. Importantly however, this style of question hasn't been used since 2010, so it's highly unlikely that you'll be expected to answer questions with numbers or phrases.

Key points

You must be prepared to guess strategically and maximize your marks with questions you don't have time to work out properly.

▌The UCAT

The Universities Clinical Aptitude Test (UCAT) is currently employed by:

- **England** Anglia Ruskin (see p. 201), Aston (see p. 128), Birmingham (see p. 130), Bristol (see p. 134), East Anglia (see p. 178), Edge Hill (see p. 202), Exeter (see p. 140), Hull/York (see p. 142), Keele (see p. 144), Kent and Medway (see p. 202), Leicester (see p. 150), Liverpool (see p. 152), London—Barts (see p. 154), London—King's (see p. 158), London—St George's (see p. 160), Manchester (see p. 164), Newcastle (see p. 166), Nottingham (see p. 168), Plymouth/Peninsula (see p. 172), Sheffield (see p. 174), Southampton (see p. 176), Sunderland (see p. 203), Warwick (see p. 282).
- **Northern Ireland** Queen's University Belfast (see p. 182).
- **Scotland** Aberdeen (see p. 186), Dundee (see p. 188), Edinburgh (see p. 190), Glasgow (see p. 192), St Andrews (see p. 194).
- **Wales** Cardiff (see p. 198).

The UCAT is produced by the UCAT Consortium to assess a wide range of 'mental abilities and behavioural attributes' that medical schools have identified as being important. The entire test takes two hours and each of the five sections of multiple-choice questions is timed separately.

Section 1: Verbal reasoning

44 questions: 11 reading passages, 4 questions per passage

21 minutes: less than 2 minutes per passage

Section 1: Verbal reasoning

The first section assesses your ability to think logically about written information presented in a passage of text and to reach a reasoned conclusion. For each passage you are given there are four corresponding questions. Your answer must be based *only* on the information you have been given in the passage, not on any personal prior knowledge. This is a hugely important point, as some of the passages will contain information that is false—it's your job to ignore what you know and to treat every passage as though it were true. Some questions ask you to choose 'True', 'False', or 'Can't tell' to describe a statement. Other questions require you to select the most suitable response to a question or incomplete statement. For practice of this section there are four sample questions based on a single passage of text on p. 348, which you should aim to complete within two minutes. The answers are on p. 362.

Section 2: Quantitative reasoning

36 questions: 9 sets of graphs/charts/tables, 4 questions each

24 minutes: ~2½ minutes per graph/chart/table

Each question has five options, one of which is correct

Section 2: Quantitative reasoning

After the verbal reasoning section comes an assessment of your ability to solve numerical problems. You will need to be able to quickly extract relevant information from graphs, charts, and tables. Although good mathematical ability helps, it is less a test of numerical competency and more to do with problem solving, such as manipulating simple ratios, fractions, percentages, and averages. For practice of this section there are four sample questions based on one set of charts on p. 350, which you should aim to complete within two minutes. The answers can be found on p. 362.

Section 3: Abstract reasoning

55 questions associated with sets of shapes

13 minutes: ~1 minute per pair of sets

Section 3: Abstract reasoning

This section assesses your ability to infer relationships from information by convergent and divergent thinking. You are presented with two *sets* of shapes, labelled 'Set A' and 'Set B'. All the shapes in each set are similar to each other, but Set A is not related to Set B. You have to determine whether the test shape belongs to Set A, Set B, or neither set. The items include irrelevant material, so it is important that you remain focused in identifying a rule that relates each item of a set to all the others. Once you are sure you have identified the rule for each set, it should be easy to get the marks for all five test shapes.

You may also be presented with two sets of shapes labelled 'Set A' and 'Set B' and asked to select which of four possible options belongs to each set. Fewer questions will involve showing you the progression of a figure in some logical way and requiring you to suggest which of a selection of options would come next, or, which shape would complete a statement involving a group of shapes.

For practice of this section there are five test shapes based on one pair of sets on p. 354, which you should aim to complete within one minute. The answers can be found on p. 362.

Section 4: Decision making

29 questions

31 minutes: ~2 minutes' reading time to familiarize yourself with the codes and any additional instructions, and ~1 minute per question

Section 4: Decision making

The penultimate section investigates your ability to deal with various forms of information, infer relationships, make informed judgements, and decide on an appropriate response in situations of complexity and ambiguity. Deciphering each code will require a skilful combination of logic and judgement to reach an answer. There are four or five options for each question and in some questions more than one option may be correct. For practice of this section there are five sample questions based on one code on p. 358, which you should aim to complete within seven minutes. The answers can be found on p. 362.

Section 5: Situational judgement test

69 questions associated with 22 scenarios, with up to five questions associated with each scenario, and each offering three or four potential response options

26 minutes

Section 5: Situational judgement test

This section assesses your judgement in healthcare-related scenarios, testing for the interpersonal skills, self-awareness, professionalism, and ethical values necessary for successful medical practice. After reading a hypothetical clinical scenario you will be asked to make judgements about a series of options relating to it, by selecting their appropriateness or importance. Each response option must be considered irrespective of the time frame (i.e. short-term options may be more or less important/appropriate than long-term options) and independently; therefore you may choose the same option multiple times for any given scenario. The list of options is not meant to be exhaustive, and you are asked to make a judgement only about the options presented to you. You may also be asked to rank three options in order from most to least appropriate.

For practice of this section there are eight sample questions based on one scenario on p. 360, which you should aim to complete within three minutes. The commentary to this section can be found on p. 362.

Key points

If you wish to see more examples of situational judgement test-type questions, you could try some (harder!) questions intended for final-year medical students—*Oxford Assess and Progress: Situational Judgement Test*.

The BMAT

Brighton & Sussex (see p. 132), Cambridge (see p. 136), London—Imperial (see p. 156), Keele (see p. 144), Lancaster (see p. 146), Leeds (see p. 148), Oxford (see p. 170), and University College London (UCL) (see p. 162) require applicants to have completed the BMAT. The BMAT is produced by the Cambridge Assessment Group and consists of three sections. The following pages describe the structure and format of each section, the qualities they are testing for, and the approach you should take when answering them.

Section 1: Aptitude and skills

35 questions: multiple choice or short-answer questions

60 minutes: 1 minute 40 seconds per question

Section 1: Aptitude and skills

According to the specification, this section of the BMAT aims to test generic skills that will be used as an undergraduate medical student:

- **Problem solving** This refers to encoding and processing numerical information into simple numerical and algebraic operations in order to solve problems. Around 13 marks are available for your ability to select relevant information, recognize analogous cases, and apply appropriate procedures.
- **Understanding arguments** A series of logical arguments are presented that require the candidate to reason, make assumptions, and form appropriate conclusions. There are 10 marks available for these questions.
- **Data analysis and inference** You will need to interpret and reach appropriate conclusions from verbal, statistical, and graphical information. There are 12 marks available for these questions.

Drawing diagrams can help you to answer these questions and often single letters can be used to represent different names/groups. You must also be able to manipulate integers and fractions easily. You are unlikely to be able to solve all the questions in your head and a single question often needs extensive jottings on scrap paper. There are four sample questions on p. 368 as practice for this section, which you should aim to complete within seven minutes. The answers can be found on p. 374.

Section 2: Scientific knowledge and applications

27 questions: multiple choice or short-answer questions

30 minutes split between biology (7 questions), chemistry (7 questions), physics (7 questions), and maths (6 questions): just over 1 minute per question

---

Section 2: Scientific knowledge and applications

The designers of the BMAT have created this section to test whether candidates have the core biomedical sciences knowledge necessary for studying medicine, as well as the capacity to apply their understanding. The material is restricted to that normally included in non-specialist school science and maths courses (i.e. equivalent to (dual award) science and maths at GCSE).

Many students become obsessed with revising GCSE material for section 2 of the BMAT. While the questions are based on GCSE science and maths, the GCSE content is used as a basis for multiple-choice questions that test the *application* of knowledge and quick thinking. You only have a minute for each question in section 2 so it is important to remember that you will face time pressure.

Drawing diagrams, especially when faced with dense descriptive passages, will often help you towards the correct answer. There are four sample questions on p. 370 for practice of this section, which you should aim to complete within four minutes. The answers can be found on p. 374.

Section 3: Writing task

Answer one question out of three: answer to be handwritten on a single page of A4

30 minutes: including any planning time

No dictionaries or reference books allowed

Section 3: Writing task

For this section you have half an hour to answer one from a choice of three questions. The questions will be based on topics of general, medical, or scientific interest. They are often preceded by a short proposition, such as a famous quote or theoretical hypothesis. You will then be asked to consider the argument that has been proposed, as well as its implications, propose your own counterargument, and/or resolve the conflict raised by the proposition.

You are limited to a single side of A4; therefore selection and organization of your ideas is critical. You should spend at least five minutes planning your essay (up to 20% of marks are given for organization and structure of the essay). That will leave you with 22 minutes to translate this plan into a concise and accurate piece of written work, leaving three minutes spare to read it through and correct any mistakes.

Outside knowledge is necessary to complete the BMAT essay since you will need to provide examples from real life to illustrate the points you make (i.e. historical or current events). It is difficult to prepare, other than by writing practice essays in the proper format (i.e. limiting yourself to 30 minutes and one side of A4, handwritten). You could also try learning about a few common ethical dilemmas (see also p. 312) and the merits and pitfalls of science, law, and the arts. BMAT essay titles almost always require examples from science and/or medicine, so preparation for your medical school application should be sufficient for this essay.

There are three sample questions on p. 372 for practice of this section; you should aim to answer one on a single side of A4 within 30 minutes. Advice can be found on p. 374.

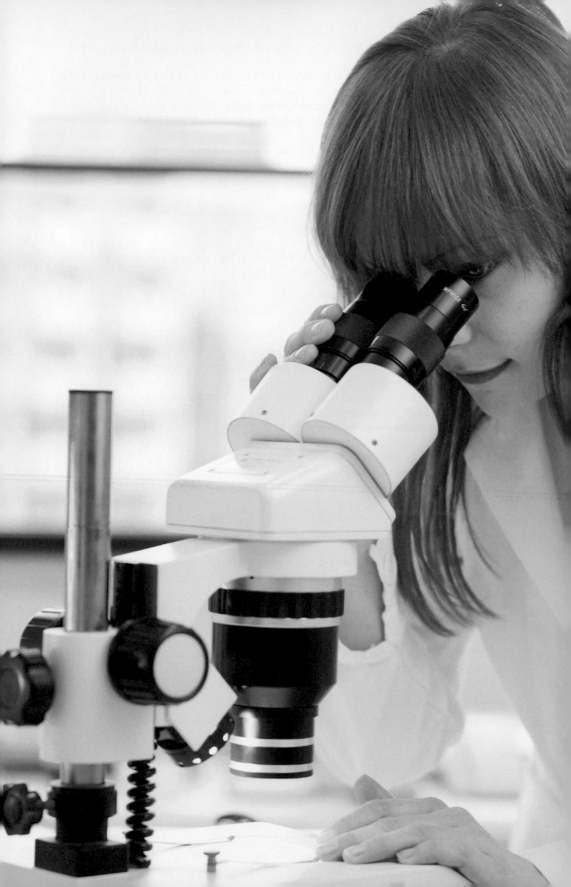

7

Choosing a medical school

Factors to consider about the medical school

Once you have decided to become a doctor, the next big decision you have to make is where to study. The years spent at medical school will be some of the most important of your life as you acquire the necessary skills and knowledge and develop professionally to be a doctor. The choice of medical school also greatly affects your chances of getting an offer to study medicine. You need to select medical schools that match your individual academic and non-academic skills.

This chapter will take you through what you need to consider about the medical school, including course type (see p. 92), university type (see p. 94), how difficult each medical school is to get into (see p. 98), your own personality (see p. 100), teaching styles (see p. 102), medical school league tables (see p. 106), and where to find further information (see p. 120). Chapter 8 gives details of every undergraduate medical school in the UK.

Drawing up a shortlist

If you want to become a doctor, the medical school you choose is unlikely to affect your career path. Your focus should be on finding a medical school that will accept you. Start by making a shortlist based on the following:

- **Basic eligibility criteria** You need to check basic admissions criteria for the university and course for which you are applying. This includes age, nationality, GCSE grades, A level subjects, and health and criminal record checks. If you are in any doubt about whether you meet their criteria, check with the admissions office before applying. See p. 96.
- **Competition** It is hard to know how you compare with the other medical school applicants; however, it is worth considering how competitive the different courses are so that you always include a 'safe bet'. See p. 98.
- **Types of course** These can be divided into problem-based learning (PBL), integrated, and traditional (see Table 7.1). It is worth bearing in mind that elements of PBL are increasingly being incorporated into all types of course. Similarly, don't expect to avoid scientific theory in PBL courses—you will need a minimum amount to become a safe and competent doctor. See p. 102.
- **University** The geography of the university/medical school will either be campus, city-based, or collegiate. See Table 7.2.
- **Intercalated degree** This offers you the chance to obtain an additional degree during your medical studies. See p. 91.
- **Reputation** This is difficult to define and less important for most medical careers than for other careers. Generally, universities with medical schools have strong reputations. All medical schools receive a stamp of approval from the General Medical Council (GMC), which guarantees high standards of education. For the very small minority of high fliers who may benefit from attending an internationally renowned medical school, the league tables on p. 106 are worth considering. Everyone else should concentrate on finding a medical school that fits them, rather than listening to hearsay.

The intercalated degree

In addition to a medical degree, most undergraduate courses offer the chance to complete an additional degree (often a Bachelor of Science or BSc). These courses last an additional year and provide an opportunity for you to research another subject that you are interested in. It is worth considering whether you want to pursue an intercalated degree when making your list of possible medical schools.

Advantages The intercalated degree is a great chance to explore an area in which you might want to specialize later in your career. It also provides an opportunity to become involved in original research and earn CV points, especially if your project leads to a conference presentation or publication. With increasing numbers of medical students taking intercalated degrees, there is an increasing need to have one if you are applying for the more competitive medical specialties. There are also many transferable skills to be gained, such as learning to critically appraise research literature. It also provides a pleasant break from the dictatorial routine of medicine, providing a more self-directed learning experience. One final benefit, a little further down the road, is that if you find yourself applying to a competitive deanery or for an academic foundation programme spot, having an additional degree counts for points to help bolster your application.

Disadvantages It is worth remembering that whatever you spend your time studying, it is unlikely to be relevant to general medical practice. This is because most research projects are very specialized. Even if you attempt a research project, there is no guarantee that you will come away with publishable data during your limited laboratory time. An intercalated degree will also delay you from paid employment by one additional year (as well as adding an additional year of costs—see p. 14).

Choice Intercalated degrees are offered as an option at all UK medical schools (except for graduate students) but the following universities have a compulsory intercalated degree year: Cambridge (see p. 136), Edinburgh (see p. 190), London—Imperial (see p. 156), Oxford (see p. 170), St Andrews (see p. 194), and UCL (see p. 162). Nottingham (see p. 168) includes a BMedSci qualification within their five-year course and without requiring an additional year of study. Other medical schools only permit students to intercalate based on their academic performance during the core medical degree. See individual medical school profiles in Chapter 8 for details.

A student's experience ...

The year I spent studying for a BSc in physiology was divided between lectures and laboratory time. These lectures were different from those in medicine as we were expected to familiarize ourselves with important relevant developments in the scientific literature. In the second half of the year I worked full-time in a lab, using a special type of microscope to assess the structural composition of a protein. The majority of this time was spent on long, repetitive, and often fruitless procedures. However, hours of work were rewarded by publishing in a good biochemistry journal. After passing my exams at the end of the year, I was successfully awarded a BSc.

Key points

www.intercalate.co.uk has good up-to-date information on most of the intercalated degrees offered across the UK. It also specifies whether the courses are available for external candidates, should you wish to consider pursuing an intercalated BSc at a different university (though this is less common).

Types of course

Use Table 7.1 to help you decide which type of course would suit you best.

Table 7.1 Types of course offered by UK medical schools

	Problem-based learning (PBL) course
Description	Students meet their weekly learning objectives by working in teams to solve a clinical scenario (e.g. management of a 72-year-old male with poorly controlled diabetes in the community). Each student's findings are presented to the facilitator and the rest of the group at the end of the week.
Pros	• Large element of teamwork and encourages problem solving, both of which are required daily by doctors. • Develop lifelong skills of self-directed learning. • Engaging and 100% clinically relevant from day one. • Early clinical exposure to supplement the problems presented.
Cons	• A less established technique subject to the criticisms of some older doctors. • Less standardized teaching and the experience is highly dependent on the quality of the non-medical facilitator. • May have large gaps in scientific understanding.
Offered at	Liverpool, Manchester, Glasgow, Queen Mary, Plymouth/Peninsula, Sheffield, Keele, Hull and York, Barts, and UEA.
	Integrated course
Description	Lectures on systems of the body (their normal function and aberrations in disease) are integrated with clinical attachments. There are different learning styles that can form part of the 'integrated' family of courses including problem-based learning, enquiry-based learning, and case-based learning. There is significant overlap between these specific monikers.
Pros	• Good relevant scientific understanding delivered at the appropriate stage. • Early clinical exposure.
Cons	• Early clinical exposure may unnerve those who prefer grasping all the theory before facing patients. • Still receiving lectures in the final years of the course. • Lack of depth in theory may frustrate those favouring scientific detail.
Offered by	Liverpool, Cardiff, Glasgow, and Birmingham as well as, in some contexts, the medical schools given for PBL above.
	Traditional course
Description	Pure sciences are taught in the first (pre-clinical) half of the course, followed by hospital/GP attachments in the clinical half of the course.

Table 7.1 *(Continued)*

	Traditional course
Pros	• Best understanding of the theoretical science underpinning medicine. • Clinical exposure only after a substantial knowledge base has been built.
Cons	• Out of touch with *real* medicine during pre-clinical time. • Less clinical exposure in total. • Hours spent learning unnecessary scientific detail that is often quickly forgotten after exams. • Clinically relevant details can be lost in the ocean of facts.
Offered by	Oxford and Cambridge

▋Types of university

Use Table 7.2 to help you decide which type of university appeals to you.

Table 7.2 Different types of university

	Campus
Description	The students live and work in a fairly self-contained area, separate from the local town/city.
Pros	• Sense of community between students.
	• Very student-orientated services/facilities; cheap and convenient.
Cons	• Students everywhere!
	• Quite artificial and distant from the 'real world'.
	City
Description	The university buildings are dispersed throughout a town/city.
Pros	• The experience of living within a real town/city.
	• The benefits of the local facilities of a town/city.
Cons	• Can be expensive.
	• Living arrangements and travel to work can be impractical.
	• May live far away from other students on your course.
	Collegiate
Description	Independent colleges that are dispersed throughout a town/city providing catering, accommodation, social, and welfare services. Members of different colleges are brought together in laboratories, lecture theatres, and GP practices/hospitals.
Pros	• Close contact with non-medical students.
	• Wealthy institutions that can often provide additional financial support (although very variable).
Cons	• Often provide additional regulations (e.g. mandatory minimum attendance for evening dinner; college fees for international students).
	• Little interaction between colleges—lack of central Students' Union/bar, hence poorer sense of university spirit.

An insider's view ...

It's impossible to appreciate the different types of university until you've spent at least a day exploring each one with someone familiar with the area. Open days are ideal for this and you should avoid making any decisions about which medical schools to apply to until you have had a good look around.

Summary of medical schools

Table 7.3 shows the key details of each undergraduate medical school in the UK for quick comparison. The full details of each medical school are shown in Chapter 8. See also Table 11.2 on p. 261 for graduate-entry courses.

Table 7.3 Summary of undergraduate medical schools in the UK

Medical school	Type[1]	Grade[2]	Qualification	Location	Length (years)
Aberdeen	Stone	AAA	BSc, MSc	Campus	5
Aston	Carbon fibre	AAA	BSc	City/campus	5
London-Barts	Plate glass	A*AA	BMedSci, BSc	City/campus	5
Birmingham	Red brick	AAA	BMedSci	Campus	5
Brighton and Sussex	Plate glass	AAA–AAB	BSc/MSc	Campus	5
Bristol	Red brick	AAB	BSc	Campus	5
Cambridge	Stone	A*A*A	BA[3]	Collegiate	6
Cardiff	Red brick	AAB	BSc	Campus	5
Central Lancashire	Plate glass	AAB	MRes	Campus	5
Charles, Prague	Stone	Admission test	Not available	City	6
Dundee	Red brick	AAA	BMSc	Campus	5
Edinburgh	Stone	AAA	BSc, BMedSci	Campus	6
Exeter	Stone	AAB	BA, BSc, MClinEd	Campus	6
Glasgow	Carbon fibre	AAA	BSc	Campus	5
Hull and York	Carbon fibre	AAA	BSc, MSc	Split campus	5
London-Imperial	Stone	A*AA	BSc[3]	City	6
Keele	Carbon fibre	A*AAb	BSc, MSc, MMedsci	Campus	5
London-King's	Red brick	A*AA	BSc	City/campus	5
Lancaster	Carbon fibre	AAA	BSc, MSc	Collegiate	5
Leeds	Red brick	AAA	BA, BSc	Campus	5
Leicester	Plate glass	AAA	BSc, MSc or PhD	Campus	5
Liverpool	Carbon fibre	AAA	BSc, MSc	Campus	5
Manchester	Carbon fibre	AAA	BSc, MSc, MRes	Campus	5
Newcastle	Plate glass	AAA	BSc	City/campus	5
Nottingham	Red brick	AAA	BMedSci[3]	Campus	5
Oxford	Stone	A*AA	BA[3]	Collegiate	6

Table 7.3 *(Continued)*

Medical school	Type[1]	Grade[2]	Qualification	Location	Length (years)
Plymouth/Peninsula	Carbon fibre	A*AA–AAA	BSc, MSc	Campus	5
Pleven, Bulgaria	Stone	Admission test	No	City	6
Queen's, Belfast	Red brick	AAAa	BSc or MSc	Campus	5
Sheffield	Red brick	AAA	BMedSci	Campus	5
Southampton	Plate glass	AAA	BSc	Campus	5
St Andrews	Stone	AAA	BSc[3]	City	6
London-St George's	Plate glass	AAA–A*AA	BSc	City	5
London-UCL	Red brick	A*AA	BSc[3]	City	6
UEA	Carbon fibre	AAB	BSc, MRes	Campus	5

[1] See p. 102 for descriptions

[2] A2 levels, with AS levels indicated by a lowercase letter

[3] Compulsory intercalated degree

Competitiveness of medical schools

It is important to avoid applying only for the most competitive medical schools. The obvious number to consider is applicants per offer; however, this is not a complete picture. Prestige gives an idea of how sought after each place is; a lower score is more prestigious. The final score is subjective, based on considerations of the quality of applicants, required grades, and applicants per place. Table 7.4 ranks each school in the UK by competitiveness. See also Table 11.1 on p. 261 for graduate-entry courses.

Table 7.4 Competitiveness of undergraduate medical schools in the UK

Medical school	Competition (applicants per offer)	Chance of interview (applicants per interview)	Success after interview (offers per interview)	Prestige (offers per place)	Competitiveness score
Oxford	10.5	4.2	2.5	1.1	5
Cambridge	4.7	1.32	3.5	1.2	5
London—Imperial	4.0	2.9	1.4	1.7	4
Edinburgh	4.8	n/a	n/a	2.5	4
Nottingham	3.5	2.2	1.6	3.0	4
St Andrews	2.9	2.3	1.3	2.8	4
London—UCL	4.1	3.3	1.2	2.1	4
Plymouth/ Peninsula	3.5	1.6	2.2	3.0	2
Glasgow	3.8	2.4	1.6	1.9	3
Cardiff	5.3	2.8	1.9	1.5	3
Bristol	5.2	3.6	1.4	3.3	4
Southampton	8.6	n/a	n/a	1.7	3
Leeds	6.7	2.6	2.5	1.9	3
Manchester	3.5	2.0	1.8	2.1	3
London—St George's	3.8	2.1	1.8	2.2	3
London—King's	3.1	2.6	1.2	2.7	3
Brighton and Sussex	3.0	1.4	2.2	1.2	2
East Anglia	2.3	1.4	1.6	2.9	2
Sheffield	2.5	1.8	1.6	2.6	2
Liverpool	2.2	1.2	1.9	4.3	2
London—Barts	2.2	1.5	1.5	2.4	2
Queen's, Belfast	2.6	1.9	1.4	1.9	2
Aberdeen	3.5	1.9	1.85	2.6	2

Table **7.4** *(Continued)*

Medical school	Competition (applicants per offer)	Chance of interview (applicants per interview)	Success after interview (offers per interview)	Prestige (offers per place)	Competitiveness score
Dundee	4.2	2.5	2.3	2.3	2
Newcastle	3.7	2.3	1.6	2.0	2
Keele	4.0	2.4	1.7	2.2	2
Birmingham	5.0	4.0	1.25	2.2	2
Exeter	3.5	1.8	2.0	1.4	2
Hull and York	2.6	1.8	1.4	3.0	1
Leicester	3.3	2.1	1.6	2.4	1
Lancaster	3.4	1.9	1.8	2.2	1

The applicant

Once you've made your shortlist of possible medical schools, it's time to be intro-spective, to identify the courses that suit your own talents, learning style, personality, and circumstances.

Personal factors to consider

Teaching/learning styles Choose a type of course (see p. 90) that suits your preferences, skills, and CV. If you have a particular penchant for molecular sciences, a traditional course will probably suit you best. If you cannot wait to have your first exposure to clinical medi-cine, an integrated course may be what you're looking for. Or if you would prefer self-directed learning, group work, and seminars over lectures, a PBL course might suit you better.

Equally, look at what you can realistically achieve. If interpersonal skills are your strength, you might be more successful on a modern, clinically focused course. If you're a closet sci-entist or enjoy rote learning, a traditional course might be better suited to your particular talents. There is always a mix of teaching styles at any medical school, so you cannot avoid a particular one in its entirety, but the emphasis does vary between courses. Take the time to find the most suitable mix for you.

Competition Use objective measures (e.g. your grades, practice admission test results) and subjective judgements (e.g. teacher's advice, amount of preparation) to estimate your relative strength as an applicant. Table 7.4 on p. 98 estimates how competitive each med-ical school is; try to apply to those appropriate to your estimation of your abilities, but re-member that it is sensible to choose one of the less competitive schools too.

Assessment methods A variety of assessment strategies are used by most courses, including vivas (oral exams), multiple-choice questions, extended matching questions, short answer papers, and essay papers. Some courses involve exams at the end of every module while others hold them at the end of each year. Again, play to your strengths. Make sure you ask at the open days which methods are used, as this may change from year to year.

University life Do you enjoy the busy city life or would you prefer a more peaceful sub-urban environment? If you are moving away from one extreme, think carefully about this. Stay with a friend or relative for a few days—you never know what will make you love or hate a new place until you've experienced it properly. Birdsong at 6 a.m. or crowded underground trains might make this decision for you.

An insider's view ...

The most successful applicants are usually those who have applied to a medical school that suits them. Anyone who has read a prospectus can describe the layout of first-year accommodation, and a quick Google search will bring up a university's international ranking for that year. What is more persuasive in a medical school application is for the applicant to describe what makes them uniquely suited to that particular medical school.

Hobbies and interests If you have a specific interest outside of medicine (e.g. you play a sport competitively) it may be worth looking at what facilities/opportunities the university can offer. Use the Students' Union website of each university as a starting point for more information.

Distance from home This is important for many people and you should consider the practicalities of travel. You need to strike a balance between living an independent life and having your family near enough for support (and potentially clothes washing or food packets…). A common approach is to draw two circles around your home town, one for too near and one for too far, and consider the regions between the two circles.

Costs Given standardized tuition fees, the cost of education will not vary between medical schools unless you are a Scottish, Welsh, or international student (see p. 14). Other costs can vary greatly depending on where you choose to live. In general, London is very expensive and the further you travel away from London, the cheaper the cost of living is. There are some notable exceptions to this rule, including Edinburgh, Oxford, and Cambridge.

The other key variable is your own frugality. It is easy for a student in Newcastle to spend far more than one in London if they are leading a life of relative extravagance. See p. 14 for estimates of living costs and Chapter 8 for the relative living costs at specific medical schools.

Future career Choosing a medical school for its expertise in a particular specialty requires unrealistic foresight. By the time you have finished medical school it is likely that your career aspirations will have changed dramatically as you discover more about each specialty.

Future life Most qualifying students tend to work close to the medical school at which they qualified. This is especially true for FY1/FY2 doctors (see p. 9). So consider whether you would be happy living in the surroundings of the medical school for the next seven years or more. Although there is nothing to stop you moving away upon qualifying, you are likely to stay put whilst you adjust to your new job.

Key points

Once you graduate from medical school, you are free to move anywhere in the UK for work. The application process makes a point of ensuring that hospitals cannot pick and choose doctors who qualified locally. However, many graduates choose to stay in the same region for personal reasons—they know the hospitals and consultants and have made friends locally.

As the job application process is competitive, graduates of universities in popular locations may find themselves forced to move due to competition. These locations vary from year to year but often include London and Oxford.

A decision-making guide

Armed with facts about medical schools and secure in the knowledge of your own strengths as a medical school applicant, you are ready to narrow down your options. UCAS permits applications to four medical schools each year (see p. 216). The following pages will help you identify the medical schools that suit you best and ease your decision-making process.

The choices

Each medical school has its own character and artificially grouping them inevitably leads to generalizations. For example, Liverpool and Manchester are often described as two of the six 'official' red-brick universities, but both teach a more modern PBL type of course. With this in mind, use the following groupings as a *guide*, to help focus your attention on similar medical schools to the ones you have already shortlisted.

Carbon fibre Ultramodern PBL courses (see p. 92). These are the 'Marmite' of medical schools—you either love them or hate them: *Aston, Exeter, Keele, Glasgow, Lancaster, Liverpool, Manchester, Plymouth*.

Plate glass New, sensible, and made for the city, if somewhat commonplace. Campus- or city-based courses with a mixture of PBL and lectures include: *Barts, Brighton and Sussex, Hull York, Leicester, Newcastle, Southampton, St George's, University of East Anglia (UEA), Warwick*.

Red brick These tried and tested courses are likely to feature in your application. Lecture-based city courses with early clinical exposure and minimal PBL include: *Birmingham, Bristol, Dundee, King's College London, Leeds, Nottingham, Queen's Belfast, Sheffield, UCL*.

Stone Established but a little stuffy; old academic (occasionally collegiate) courses with an emphasis on science: *Aberdeen, Cambridge, Edinburgh, Imperial, Oxford, Charles University Prague, St Andrews*.

Key points

You need to be cautious if your shortlist contains medical schools at opposite ends of the spectrum. If you are completely stuck, use the algorithm (see Figure 7.1) as a starting point to identify the group of medical schools that you should focus your research on.

Key points

Applicants commonly ask: what is the best medical school? The bottom line is that your choice will not make a huge difference to your professional career. Your knowledge, skills, and attitudes will depend much more on the amount of time you invest in the course than the institution you attend. Regardless of your medical school, you will be as free as anyone else to pursue the specialty of your choice. Choose institutions because you would thrive there, instead of perceived indicators of quality or status.

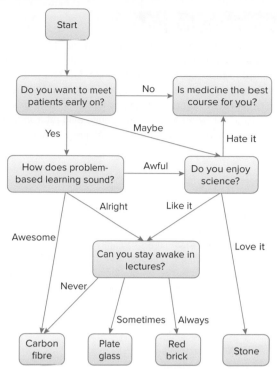

Figure 7.1 An algorithm for choosing a type of medical school.

An algorithm for picking medical schools

While Figure 7.1 grossly simplifies a complex thought process, it should help to highlight some of the most important factors and the types of courses that embrace them. Medical schools have many subtle distinguishing factors, so don't discount them until you have read more (see Chapter 8).

Tailoring your application to the shortlist

The preparation doesn't stop once you have chosen four medical schools. You need to work through the appropriate medical school profiles (see Chapter 8) to identify similarities, and consider writing your personal statement (see p. 221) to fit these specific schools' priorities.

Your four choices should ideally be similar types of course to allow such tailoring of your personal statement. If you've gone for the more traditional science-based teaching, you might want to write about how you've demonstrated an interest in science through learning more about a particular discovery. Alternatively, if you are applying to PBL-based courses, you could describe an example from your work experience where a doctor discussed a management plan with their colleagues and researched additional options. In this way, you could draw parallels between the self-directed group learning of PBL and everyday clinical practice.

At this stage it is worth writing, for interview purposes, some brief notes on the courses to which you are applying. These can be used to refresh your knowledge of the course when it comes to interview day (see p. 304). This will help avoid the risk of discussing the prospect of an intercalated humanities degree at a university where this is not an option.

A student's experience ...

A large proportion of my Cambridge interview was dedicated to discussing the research project I participated in during my summer holidays. Whilst this appeared successful at Cambridge, my attempt to replicate the conversation a few weeks later at Liverpool was less well received. Eventually we went on to talk about my part-time employment as a Health Care Assistant and the insights I had gained into the challenges of healthcare. This seemed to impress the panel far more! It became quite evident from this experience that different medical schools are not looking for identical qualities and experiences.

An insider's view ...

We need to be satisfied that the candidates sitting before us will become safe and competent doctors, and this can be achieved by applicants demonstrating a fairly generic set of skills. However, we also have to consider the suitability of the candidate to the course that we offer. Assessing whether the medical school and the student are a personality fit is a more subjective decision that is based on our limited exposure to the applicant as they discuss their experiences and answer our questions.

Key points

It is possible to write a personal statement (or answer an interview question) that is attractive to all types of medical schools, but having an idea of your target audience is an obvious advantage.

League tables

League tables must be approached with caution. Using medical school and university league tables is often fraught with difficulties because of conflicting results. Even when the popular league tables agree, be careful in the way you use the information. The following pages discuss this oft-cited but poorly understood topic, and include some important tables that you should consider.

How are rankings calculated? League tables use various criteria to reach their final scores. The following criteria are commonly used:

- **UCAS entry score** Average number of student UCAS points.
- **Student satisfaction** Scores based on students' views on teaching.
- **Quality of research** The Research Excellence Framework (REF) score, which rates departments based on academic research.
- **Staff** The expenditure on staff per student or the staff to student ratio.
- **Class of degree** The percentage of 2:1 and first-class degrees conferred.
- **Employability** The likelihood of securing full-time employment after graduation. This is more applicable to university league tables, which include students studying non-medical degrees.

Table 7.5 summarizes the medical school rankings in 2020 from some of the most popular producers of league tables, including: *The Complete University Guide, The Guardian* and *The Times*. Tables 7.6 and 7.7 show a detailed breakdown of the scoring for *The Guardian* and *The Complete University Guide* rankings respectively.

The ranking of universities is discussed more frequently than that of medical schools. University league tables look at all courses offered by a particular university, not just medicine, when assigning scores. Table 7.5 shows the position of medical schools in both UK and international university rankings.

What really matters? While the rankings of medical schools are unlikely to affect the careers of most doctors, the teaching styles may have an impact. Figure 7.6 shows the results of an interesting study that assessed performance in a membership exam taken after medical school (see p. 117), which is required for medical graduates to proceed into a specialist training post. There are many reasons to question the findings, including medical school examination styles giving an unfair advantage, selection bias (i.e. the best applicants choose the more competitive courses), and changes in medical school teaching since the doctors qualified. Nevertheless, this study shows an apparent benefit from studying at Oxford, Cambridge, and Newcastle.

How should rankings be used? Whilst many people (including parents) look at medical schools in relation to league tables, you should not rely too heavily on these. Ask yourself how important a score for staff research is for assessing the quality of your education. Similarly, the number of 2:1/first-class degrees conferred by a university might not relate to high-quality teaching. Whilst weaker applicants may want to avoid higher-ranking universities and stronger applicants may want to consider them, remember that you should use league tables in context, after considering everything else about each medical school.

Medical school rankings, 2020

Table 7.5 shows the rankings of (undergraduate) medical courses according to four of the most respected league tables—three national and one international.

Table 7.5 Rankings of UK medical schools from four sources

University	League table rankings for medicine			
	The Guardian University Guide 2020[1]	The Complete University Guide 2020[2]	The Times Good University Guide 2020	QS world rankings, 2020[4]
Cambridge	4	2	5	3
Oxford	1	1	1	2
Edinburgh	11	5	15	19
UCL	16	13	13	8
Newcastle	13	14	7	51–100
Aberdeen	2	11	10	151–200
Imperial College, London	9	7	4	10
Dundee	6	6	10	151–200
Queen Mary's, London	15	8	8	51–100
Hull and York	31	27	28	401–450
Plymouth/Peninsula	8	20	23	501–550
Leicester	27	30	26	151–200
Leeds	17	19	20	51–100
Sheffield	24	18	19	101–150
Birmingham	20	28	24	51–100
King's College, London	32	17	27	20
St Andrews	21	25	21	301–350
Warwick[3]	33	29	33	101–150
Nottingham	23	24	25	101–150
Manchester	29	26	29	34
Southampton	28	31	30	51–100
Bristol	19	12	14	51–100
Queen's, Belfast	25	23	16	101–150
Brighton and Sussex	10	22	17	301–350
Liverpool	30	32	32	101–150
East Anglia	12	21	18	301–350
Glasgow	7	3	2	51–100
Cardiff	18	15	22	101–150
Keele	3	9	6	351–400
St George's, London	26	33	31	201–250

Table 7.5 *(Continued)*

University	League table rankings for medicine			
	The Guardian University Guide 2020[1]	*The Complete University Guide 2020*[2]	*The Times Good University Guide 2020*	QS world rankings, 2020[4]
Lancaster	22	16	12	351–400
Swansea[3]	4	4	3	351–400
Exeter	14	10	9	251–300

[1] Table 7.6 shows the breakdown from which *The Guardian* ranks were obtained.

[2] Table 7.7 shows the breakdown from which *The Complete University Guide* ranks were obtained.

[3] With the exception of Warwick and Swansea graduate medicine courses, all rankings are for undergraduate courses

[4] After the top 50, the QS World University Rankings by subject list universities in categories rather than specifying individual ranks, e.g. as "top 51-100" rather than "75th".

Data from *The Guardian University Guide 2020, Complete University Guide 2020, The Times Good University Guide 2020,* and QS World University Rankings, 2020

The Guardian University Guide league table for medicine, 2020 The medical school rankings for *The Guardian University Guide* shown in Table 7.6 are based on objective scores; however, the relative weight of each component (e.g. is student satisfaction more important than research quality?) is open to interpretation.

The Complete University Guide rankings for medicine, 2020 The medical school rankings for *The Complete University Guide 2020* are shown in Table 7.7.

Table 7.6 Breakdown of *The Guardian* 2020 ranking of UK medical schools*

University	Guardian score[1] (/100)	Satisfied with course[2] (%)	Satisfied with teaching[3] (%)	Satisfied with feedback[4] (%)	Student:staff ratio[5]	Spend per student[6] (/10)	Average entry tariff[7]	Value-added score[8] (/10)	Career after 6 months[9] (%)
Oxford	100	91.9	94.9	78.0	9.8	10	221	4	95
Aberdeen	96.9	98.0	93.0	75.3	7.6	3	232	4	99
Keele	95.4	99.0	96.7	82.8	6.7	5	188	8	100
Swansea	95.3	92.4	94.0	72.3	6.7	5	n/a	9	100
Cambridge	95.3	70.7	85.7	56.1	6.7	10	232	4	98
Dundee	91.0	91.0	93.0	62.0	8.2	4	239	7	100
Glasgow	88.5	90.1	94.7	69.6	8.4	3	230	6	100
Plymouth/ Peninsula	86.9	95.6	96.0	72.6	6.8	5	189	5	99
Imperial College	86.0	88.0	89.6	70.8	7.2	8	201	4	100
Brighton & Sussex	85.5	98.0	95.3	84.7	8.4	8	174	8	100
Edinburgh	85.4	71.3	84.4	48.9	5.4	8	231	4	99
UEA	84.0	98.0	93.3	70.8	5.7	3	188	6	99
Newcastle	81.8	94.1	96.0	75.5	7.9	6	193	5	100
Exeter	77.0	93.1	93.3	72.2	8.9	4	209	4	99
Queen Mary	76.2	93.1	94.3	77.4	9.8	5	202	7	100

Table 7.6 (Continued)

University	Guardian score[1] (/100)	Satisfied with course[2] (%)	Satisfied with teaching[3] (%)	Satisfied with feedback[4] (%)	Student:staff ratio[5]	Spend per student[6] (/10)	Average entry tariff[7]	Value-added score[8] (/10)	Career after 6 months[9] (%)
UCL	76.1	84.2	87.7	51.7	5.8	5	201	4	99
Leeds	73.5	96.0	94.4	74.3	9.0	4	192	8	100
Cardiff	69.8	83.8	89.3	61.3	9.3	9	203	4	100
Bristol	66.9	89.0	93.3	69.8	9.2	5	196	5	100
Birmingham	66.1	84.2	90.3	63.5	8.0	4	191	7	100
St Andrews	66.0	94.0	94.4	64.0	10.9	3	207	7	99
Lancaster	63.6	88.0	88.3	79.7	9.1	4	176	8	100
Nottingham	60.4	80.0	89.3	52.8	7.3	3	189	7	100
Sheffield	59.4	94.0	94.3	78.2	10.7	3	183	6	100
Queen's, Belfast	59.1	93.0	92.7	80.8	10.4	4	192	1	99
St George's, London	58.5	81.2	84.0	58.5	8.7	5	189	7	100
Leicester	53.4	87.9	92.3	59.0	9.9	5	180	6	100
Southampton	53.3	76.2	86	47.7	7.6	4	186	6	100
Manchester	49.9	75.0	82.1	59.6	8.3	6	184	1	100
Liverpool	48.2	56.4	72.2	52.1	7.6	6	183	7	100
Hull-York	48.1	78.0	87.9	70.6	10.1	3	181	5	100

University	Guardian score[1] (/100)	Satisfied with course[2] (%)	Satisfied with teaching[3] (%)	Satisfied with feedback[4] (%)	Student:staff ratio[5]	Spend per student[6] (/10)	Average entry tariff[7]	Value-added score[8] (/10)	Career after 6 months[9] (%)
King's College, London	42.2	64.0	82.8	44.5	9.0	4	185	6	99
Warwick	36.1	58.0	73.9	50.1	9.7	5	n/a	10	100

[1] The Guardian score (out of 100) is an exclusive rating of excellence based on a combination of all the other factors.

[2] Course satisfaction is the percentage of final-year students satisfied with overall quality, based on the National Student Survey (NSS).

[3] The teaching quality score is the percentage of final-year students satisfied with the teaching they received, based on the NSS.

[4] The feedback score is the percentage of final-year students satisfied with feedback and assessment by lecturers, based on the NSS.

[5] Staff:student ratio is the number of students per member of teaching staff.

[6] Spend is the amount of money spent on each student, given as a rating out of 10.

[7] Average entry tariff means the typical UCAS scores of students currently studying in that department.

[8] The value-added score compares students' individual degree results with their entry qualifications, to show how effective the teaching is, given as a rating out of 10.

[9] The career score is the percentage of graduates who find graduate-level jobs, or are studying further, within six months of graduation.

Table 7.7 Breakdown of *The Complete University Guide 2020* ranking of medical schools*

University	Student satisfaction (/5)	Entry standards (UCAS tariff)	Research assessment (/4)	Graduate prospects (/100)	Overall score (/100)
Oxford	4.42	3.45	0.74	97	100.0
Cambridge	3.77	3.43	0.77	99	99.9
Glasgow	4.23	3.20	0.78	100	99.5
Swansea	4.27	3.49	0.66	100	99.3
Edinburgh	3.65	3.30	0.85	99	99.3
Dundee	4.15	3.04	0.56	100	99.0
Imperial College London	4.11	3.35	0.88	99	98.4
Queen Mary's, University of London	4.34	3.28	0.71	99	98.4
Keele	4.47	3.27	0.92	100	98.1
Exeter	4.32	3.16	0.77	99	98.1
Aberdeen	4.36	2.89	0.52	99	98.0
Bristol	4.06	3.24	0.88	100	97.9
University College London	3.76	3.20	0.96	99	97.8
Newcastle	4.28	3.20	0.84	100	97.8
Cardiff	3.96	3.25	0.63	100	97.6
Lancaster	4.22	3.27	0.99	100	97.2
King's College London	3.58	3.40	0.77	99	97.0
Sheffield	4.35	3.14	0.77	100	96.9
Leeds	4.20	3.10	0.68	100	96.8
Plymouth/Peninsula	4.49	3.16	0.45	99	96.7
East Anglia (UEA)	4.34	3.07	0.68	99	96.7
Brighton & Sussex	4.49	3.24	0.61	100	96.6
Queen's, Belfast	4.30	2.88	0.91	100	96.6
Nottingham	3.80	3.13	0.73	100	96.5
St Andrews	4.29	2.79	0.57	98	96.5
Manchester	3.79	3.19	0.66	100	96.2
Hull–York	3.91	3.20	0.67	100	96.2
Birmingham	3.96	3.04	0.70	100	96.1
Warwick[1]	3.54	3.05	0.61	100	95.9
Leicester	4.01	3.03	0.74	99	95.8

Table 7.7 (Continued)

University	Student satisfaction (/5)	Entry standards (UCAS tariff)	Research assessment (/4)	Graduate prospects (/100)	Overall score (/100)
Southampton	3.70	2.94	0.85	100	95.7
Liverpool	3.63	3.09	0.68	100	95.4
St Georges	3.87	2.95	0.48	100	95.4
Central Lancaster	4.00	2.63	0.31	n/a	90.8

[1] Warwick is a graduate medical school and a UCAS tariff calculated for school leavers was not included.

* Copyright *The Complete University Guide* © 2020, www.thecompleteuniversityguide.co.uk

▌Performance after medical school

After medical school, most new graduates apply to a region ('Foundation School') where they will spend the first two years of their careers. These allocations are competitive and based on a number of factors, such as performance at medical school. Figure 7.2 shows the proportion of new graduates that are allocated their first choice of region when they qualify as doctors. When looking at Figure 7.2, it is important to know that many new graduates choose to stay near their medical school. As some regions (such as London) are more popular than others, this will explain some of the variation in the proportion that are able to stay in their first-choice location.

Medical school should help foster the knowledge and attitudes that graduates can develop throughout their careers. Figure 7.3 shows how many doctors at the end of their first year of working said that they felt 'well prepared' by their medical studies. This data is likely to be highly valid as it is based on a national survey of almost all first-year doctors. However, it is possible that highly theoretical courses would be ranked low in this domain despite providing graduates with a strong knowledge base that may prove more useful as their careers develop.

Postgraduate exams are an important feature of life after medical school. There have been many studies, across a range of different postgraduate exams, showing that

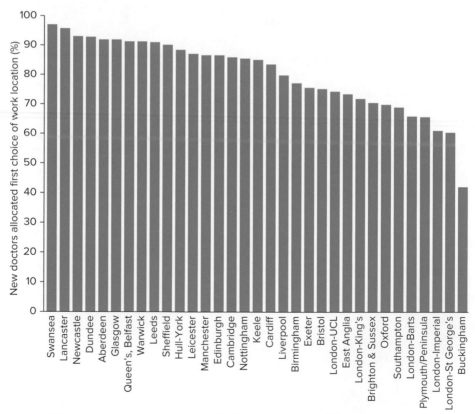

Figure 7.2 Foundation Programme application results by medical school.
Data from UK Foundation Programme. 2019 recruitment stats and facts report: https://foundationprogramme.nhs.uk/resources/reports/

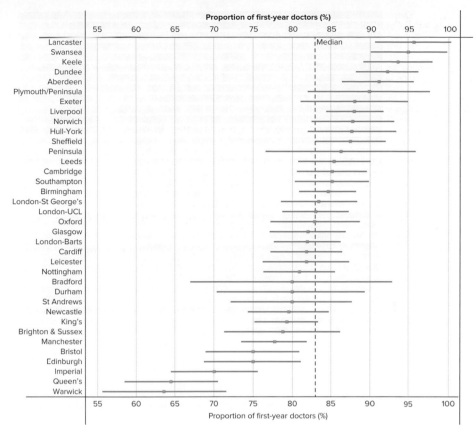

Figure 7.3 Proportion of first-year doctors who felt 'adequately prepared for their first post'.

Data from the General Medical Council. National training surveys reports, 2019: https://www.gmc-uk.org/about/what-we-do-and-why/data-and-research/national-training-surveys-reports

performance varies by the medical school from which each candidate graduated. Figure 7.4 shows, by medical school of qualification, the proportion of doctors that passed their postgraduate exams at the first attempt. Figures 7.5 and 7.6 show scores achieved by doctors sitting exams necessary to complete training in anaesthesia and general practice. Importantly, all postgraduate exams can be attempted on a number of occasions and it is not uncommon (as should be evident from Figure 7.4) for good doctors to pass on the second or third attempt.

Postgraduate exam performance is not the only important indicator of post-qualification career success. As doctors progress through their postgraduate training, they are required to maintain an e-portfolio that shows how they are meeting the objectives of their training programme. Their development is reviewed annually at an Annual Review of Competency Progression (ARCP). Most trainees achieve a 'satisfactory' outcome at each ARCP, but the range of 'unsatisfactory' outcomes extends from trainees having to provide further evidence through spending longer in training to being released from the programme. Table 7.8 shows that graduates from some medical schools are more or less likely to run into trouble later on in their careers. However, it is important to note that these are population

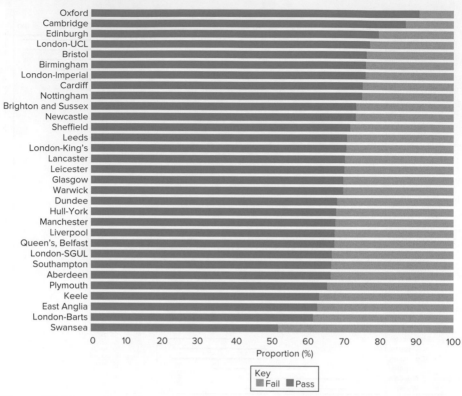

Figure 7.4 Mean pass rate across all postgraduate examinations based on General Medical Council data, 2014–2018.

Horizontal bars indicate 95% confidence intervals.

Data from Richard Wakeford, personal communication.

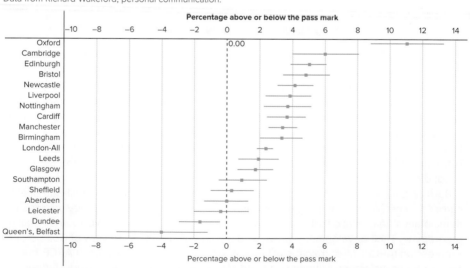

Figure 7.5 Results of the multiple-choice question part of the primary Fellowship of the Royal College of Anaesthetists (FRCA) examination.

Horizontal bars indicate 95% confidence intervals.

Data from Bowhay, A.R., Watmough, S.D. An evaluation of the performance in the UK Royal College of Anaesthetists primary examination by UK medical school and gender. *BMC Med Educ* 9, 38 (2009). https://doi.org/10.1186/1472-6920-9-38

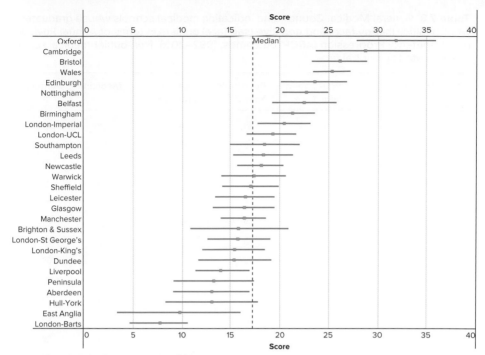

Figure 7.6 Results of the Membership of the Royal College of General Practitioners (MRCGP) applied knowledge test (AKT).

Horizontal bars indicate 95% confidence intervals.

Reproduced with the permission of the Royal College of General Practitioners. Report by Royal College of General Practitioners (RCGP). MRCGP Statistics 2012–2013. Annual report (August 2012–July 2013) on the results of the AKT and CSA Assessments. RCGP, London, UK. https://www.rcgp.org.uk

averages (they do not indicate how *you* would perform) and most doctors from all medical schools progress without difficulty.

Clearly, the data presented in this section should be interpreted with caution. It is uncertain to what extent applicant selection and quality of medical school education contributes to postgraduate performance. Such 'rankings' of graduate performance are also likely to vary between years and to lag some time behind any changes made to each institution's admissions and teaching processes. There are also relatively small differences in some of the comparisons. They are interesting nevertheless.

Figure 7.7 shows that medical schools also vary by the career destination of their graduates. Some medical schools are more or less likely to produce doctors who go on to work in general practice than in hospital specialties. There are many possible reasons for these differences, including exposure to general practice and career mentorship at medical school. Importantly, all postgraduate career destinations are accessible to graduates of all medical schools

Table 7.8 General Medical Council data indicating medical schools whose graduates were positive (happy face) and negative (sad face) outliers in terms of Annual Review of Competency Progression (ARCP) outcomes, 1992–2016. Non-outlier medical schools are indicated by neutral face

Medical school	Foundation Year 1	Foundation Year 2	General practice	Medicine[1]	Surgery[1]
Aberdeen	😐	😐	😐	🙁	😐
Birmingham	😊	😐	😐	🙁	😐
Brighton & Sussex	😐	😐	😐	😊	😐
Bristol	😊	😐	😊	😊	😐
Cambridge	😐	😐	😐	😊	😊
Cardiff	😐	😐	😊	🙁	😐
Dundee	😐	😐	😐	😊	😐
East Anglia	😐	😐	🙁	🙁	🙁
Edinburgh	😐	😐	😐	😊	😐
Glasgow	😐	😐	😐	😊	😐
Hull–York	😐	😐	😐	🙁	😐
Keele	😐	😐	😐	🙁	🙁
Lancaster	😐	😐	😐	😊	😐
Leeds	😐	😐	😐	😐	😐
Leicester	😐	😐	😐	😐	😐
Liverpool	😐	😐	😐	🙁	😐
London–Barts	😐	😐	🙁	🙁	🙁
London–Imperial	🙁	😐	😊	😊	😐
London–King's	😐	😐	😐	😐	😐
London–St George's	😐	😐	😐	😐	🙁
London–UCL	😐	😐	😊	😊	😐
Manchester	😐	😐	😐	🙁	😐
Newcastle	😐	😐	😐	😊	😊
Nottingham	😐	😐	😐	😐	😐
Oxford	😐	😐	😊	😊	😊
Plymouth/Peninsula	😐	😐	😐	🙁	🙁
Queen's, Belfast	😐	😐	😊	🙁	😐
Sheffield	😐	😐	😐	😐	😐
Southampton	😐	😐	😐	😊	😐
Swansea	😐	😐	😊	😐	😐
Warwick	😐	😐	😐	🙁	😐

[1] Data refer to those in 'core' medical or surgical training.

Data from the General Medical Council national training surveys reports: https://www.gmc-uk.org/about/what-we-do-and-why/data-and-research/national-training-surveys-reports

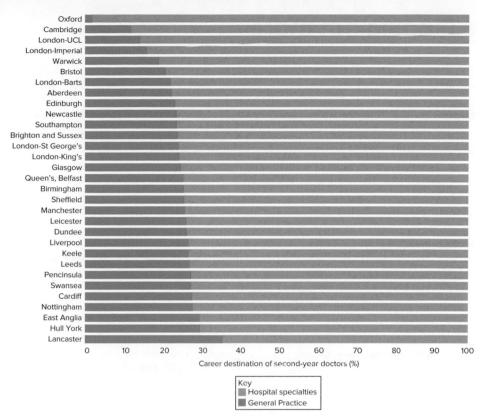

Figure 7.7 Next career destination for doctors in the second year of the Foundation Programme.

These data do not include doctors choosing to take a break from training in the UK.

Data from the UK Foundation Programme Office (UKFPO). F2 Career Destinations Report 2018. https://foundationprogramme.nhs.uk/resources/reports/

Finding out more

There are many factors that determine whether a particular medical school makes your shortlist. Some of these are easy questions with easy answers, such as basic eligibility criteria. However, a lot of what you are looking for is more subjective—you are, after all, searching for the ideal medical school *for you*. Making this decision requires good resources and the right questions.

Visiting Unless distance makes travelling impractical, there is no excuse for not visiting the university at least once before you apply. Otherwise it is difficult to make an informed decision as to whether each university justifies a space on your UCAS form.

It is worth contacting university admissions offices or checking their websites in advance to find out practical details such as when the medical school is open and parking arrangements. If you are travelling by public transport, plan the route in advance to avoid wasting time on the wrong bus out of town. Note that some medical schools may not be where you expect them to be (e.g. Warwick is in Coventry), so it is well worth checking exactly where they are to be found before setting off. Occasionally universities provide guest rooms that you can book if you decide to stop overnight.

Some medical schools restrict access, which is why you are best visiting on an open day. If you've missed it, ask a friend who studied there or get a contact from your sixth-form college. A friendly medical student might be willing to give you a guided tour if you ask nicely.

Gauging the atmosphere Visiting the medical school and attending the open day is the best way to appreciate the character of the medical school. Is it a team-spirited environment or a constant battle of wits? Were the staff open and approachable or cold and distant? There are more similarities than differences between medical schools but you will often develop a 'feeling' for each institution's ethos when visiting. Speak to as many different students as possible to judge for yourself whether you would fit in. Remember that medical schools like to impress candidates at open days, and so if you have reservations on the day, things may be even worse in reality.

The open day Open days are organized by medical schools and provide an opportunity to talk to students, tutors, course organizers, and other applicants. Your first priority should be finding the date of the next open day for medical schools you are interested in. Telephone the admissions office to verify the date and time of the open day and to confirm your place. Book early as there is often a limited number of spaces available.

Remember to dress and act appropriately whilst visiting the medical school. Open days are not interviews but potential interviewers may be in attendance and you don't want to be remembered for the wrong reasons.

Key points

Try not to be influenced by the weather. The campus might look green and beautiful in the middle of June but it will rain there sometimes as well. Environment is important but try not to fall into the trap of 'sunny = good, raining = bad'.

What to ask? The open day is your golden opportunity to clarify discrepancies between information sources and reassure yourself about admissions criteria. Speak to as many people as possible and, if you get on especially well with someone, ask for their email address. Fellow applicants are a good source of support and might be your medical student colleagues in 12 months' time. Questions you may wish to consider asking current medical students include:

- What's a typical day like for you? (Note though that this will differ between years.)
- How much contact do you have with your tutors?
- What is the pastoral support like for students?
- How much clinical exposure do you get in the first two years?
- What are the facilities like for…?
- How expensive is it to live in this area?
- How many students passed/failed their exams in your year?
- Where do people live in different years?
- Is it a safe, student-friendly area?
- What was your interview process like?
- Would you apply here again? Why/why not?

Other sources There is very little that a successful open day or friendly telephone call will not be able to answer. However, should you experience any difficulties, try the following:

- Obtain a copy of the prospectus from a careers fair, open day, admissions office, or via the university website (see Chapter 8).
- Use the Students' Union/JCR websites for 'unofficial' prospectuses that are often written by students and offer a more informal perspective.
- Utilize contacts acquired from the open day/personal visit.
- Ask your high school for details of successful applicants from previous years and contact them. Social networking sites are a good place to begin.
- Compare notes with colleagues at school who are considering applying for the same course.
- Search the internet for the MedSoc student committee and drop them an email asking for advice, or try online forums. However, take everything you read with an extra large pinch of salt.

Key points

If all else fails, pay another visit to the university and approach a friendly student in the library or cafeteria. If they can't help, they should be able to point you in the direction of someone who can.

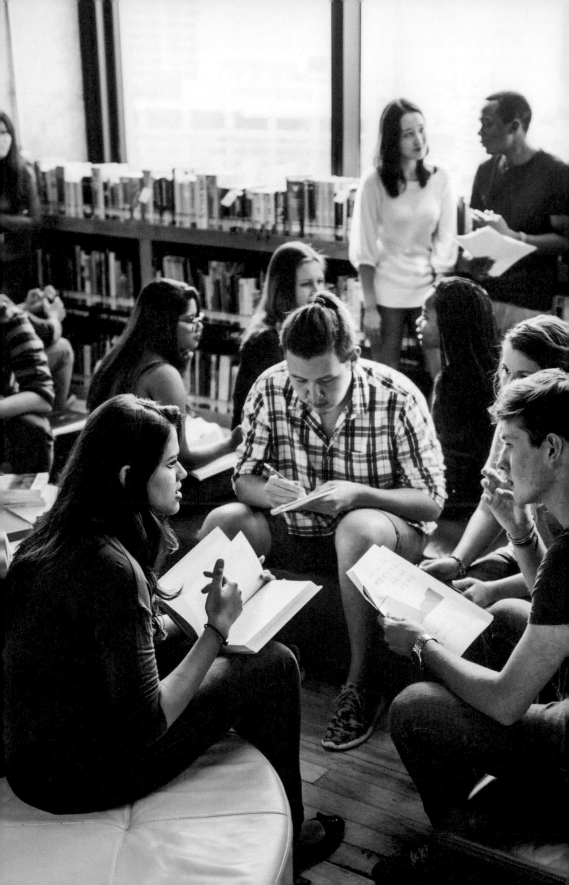

8

Undergraduate medical schools

∎ Understanding the profiles

Since choosing the right medical school is so important to winning a place (see p. 90), this chapter gives detailed descriptions of every medical school in the UK. Separate profiles are available for graduate-entry courses (see p. 252); graduates on standard courses may face different entry requirements (including admission tests). Foundation and access courses follow the same pattern after the first year as described here, although entrance requirements will be different.

The writers To ensure the most accurate information, the profiles have been written in collaboration with one or two medical student representatives from each medical school (see p. xiv). A senior member of the admissions team or medical school faculty was also asked to describe what makes their medical school unique and what types of students they are looking for in the admissions process.

Warning!

While every possible step has been taken to ensure the accuracy of this information (including multiple reviews by the admissions team at each medical school), errors may persist. Furthermore, medical schools are continually striving to improve their courses and methods of picking the best students, so the details may change from year to year. Before you make an important decision based on this information, check the medical school website or contact its admissions team. Double-checking is a good principle to follow when working in the NHS too!

Key to the profiles

To make it simple to compare medical schools, the profiles have been written in a consistent format (see also Table 8.1):

University This section gives a broad overview of the structure of the university and how it relates to the medical school, and describes some of the facilities available to medical students.

Course Teaching and clinical exposure vary widely between different courses (see p. 92). This section outlines the structure of each course, how different stages are taught, and some of the options that students can select.

Lifestyle There is far more to medical school than studying, so this section describes some of the options available for life outside the classroom.

Factoid An interesting snippet or little-known fact about the city, university, or course.

Entrance requirements

There is no point in applying to a medical school when you do not meet basic requirements; always check these before submitting your UCAS form. Also bear in mind that:

- Medical school websites offer extensive details on alternative entrance requirements such as Scottish Highers and the International Baccalaureate.
- Not all A levels are created equal; some combinations will not be accepted (see p. 22).

Table 8.1 Sample profile explaining the criteria collated for each medical school

Myth	A popular myth about each medical school …
Reality	… and the reality according to the locals
Personality	Personality traits commonly found at each medical school
Best aspects	Why studying there is better than sliced bread
Worst aspects	Why studying there can make your blood boil
Requirements	Admission test, A level and GCSE requirements (please take the warning on p. 124 into account)

Course length	Total length of course	Structure	Campus, City, or Collegiate (see p. 94)
Type of course	Carbon fibre, Plate glass, Red brick, or Stone (see p. 92)	Year size	Medical students per year group
Typical offer	Required A level grades (AS levels indicated by lowercase)	Intercalated degree	Extra degrees available (see p. 91)
Applicants	Number of applicants	Student mix:	Proportion of mature (>21 years old) and international students in a year group
Interviews	Number interviewed	% Mature	
Offers	Number given offers (see p. 98)	% International	

Competition	All medical courses are highly competitive; this subjective scale aims to highlight how they compare to other medical schools
Living costs	A subjective rating of living costs
Work	All medical courses have packed timetables and intense workloads (expect at least 40 hours per week); this subjective scale aims to highlight how much additional free time you might get compared to other medical schools

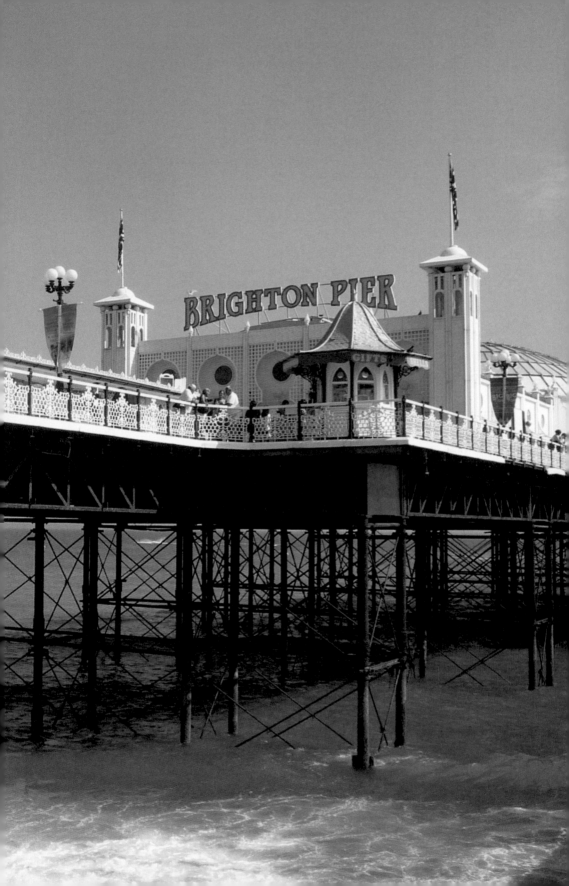

England

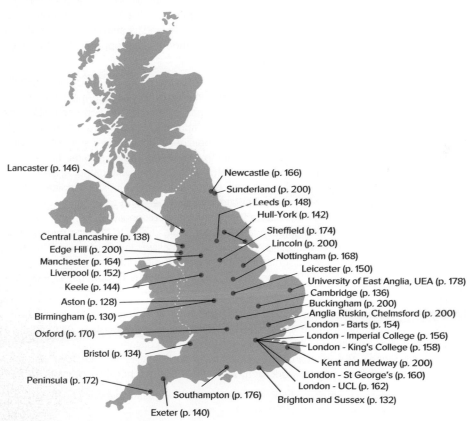

Lancaster (p. 146)

Newcastle (p. 166)

Sunderland (p. 200)

Leeds (p. 148)

Hull-York (p. 142)

Sheffield (p. 174)

Central Lancashire (p. 138)

Lincoln (p. 200)

Edge Hill (p. 200)

Nottingham (p. 168)

Manchester (p. 164)

Leicester (p. 150)

Liverpool (p. 152)

University of East Anglia, UEA (p. 178)

Keele (p. 144)

Cambridge (p. 136)

Aston (p. 128)

Buckingham (p. 200)

Birmingham (p. 130)

Anglia Ruskin, Chelmsford (p. 200)

London - Barts (p. 154)

Oxford (p. 170)

London - Imperial College (p. 156)

London - King's College (p. 158)

Bristol (p. 134)

Kent and Medway (p. 200)

London - St George's (p. 160)

Peninsula (p. 172)

London - UCL (p. 162)

Southampton (p. 176)

Brighton and Sussex (p. 132)

Exeter (p. 140)

Figure 8.1 Undergraduate medical schools in England.

▌Aston

The first cohort of Aston Medical School started in September 2018. Being a new medical school with a small cohort of students per year, it allows students to get to know everyone in their year group. This strong 'family' environment helps students to maximize learning experiences, feel supported, and develop true friendships.

University The university is located at the heart of Birmingham, the second largest city in the UK, which is perfect for people who enjoy a bit of London's bustle but also some fresh air. The medical school is situated within the university's main building, about 10 minutes away from the city centre. The school has opened a new clinical skills centre equipped, amongst other things, with ultrasound and ECG machines, and its affiliation with the Aston Medical Research Institute (AMRI) provides medical students with opportunities to obtain research experience if they are interested.

Course The MBChB programme is based on Leicester Medical School's curriculum (see p. 150), incorporating group-based learning and lectures, which are the mainstay of pre-clinical studies. The subjects are delivered in an organ, system-based approach. Students have compulsory group work sessions every day, and the contents are integrated with components of both basic science and clinical medicine, which prepare students for clinical years. Lectures are delivered in order, starting with an introduction to the block, then proceeding to physiology, embryology, and anatomy, and ending with pathology. Although lacking a dissection lab, the medical school's partnership with Leicester Medical School allows students to have at least one prosection session per term to enhance their anatomical understanding and to consolidate their learning. Additionally, students are able to gain early clinical experience in primary care settings, which helps to develop their professional communication and clinical skills. The course emphasizes interprofessional learning and communication. Medical students and students from other healthcare courses take part in group work and joint workshops, which provides a unique opportunity to establish interprofessional links.

Lifestyle On-campus accommodation is guaranteed for all first years; from the second year onwards, students usually move out to nearby off-campus accommodation. All major train stations and shopping centres are reachable within walking distance. The brand-new student union building was opened in 2019, with bars and study spaces available to all students. A common area and large group-work room within the medical school is accessible 24/7.

Factoid The university's main building is one of the UK's largest single brick buildings... so students easily get lost inside! See Table 8.2.

Table 8.2 Aston

Myth	Last choice for those missing their offer from Leicester
Reality	A new medical school striving to create the best doctors for tomorrow
Personality	Hardworking and aspiring
Best aspects	All staff are friendly and approachable, going the extra mile to assist students, and eager to get feedback from students to make the school better
Worst aspects	The lack of a dedicated teaching space (including simulation/dissection facilities) for medical students means it can get overcrowded at times
Requirements	**UCAT**; **A level** AAA–AAB, including chemistry and biology; third A level does not have to be a science subject; **GCSE** five Grade 6/Bs with maths, English language, chemistry, biology or double science

Course length	5 years	Structure	City/Campus
Type of course	Carbon fibre	Year size	120
Typical offer	AAA	Intercalated degree	BSc option for top decile students
Applicants	1,177	Student mix:	
Interviews	423	% Mature	10%
Offers	359	% International	17%

Uncompetitive	(rating: 2 of 5)	Competitive
Low living costs	(rating: 3 of 5)	High living costs
Working really hard	(rating: 4 of 5)	Not working/chilling out

Contact details	Aston Medical School, 295 Aston Express Way, Birmingham, B4 7ET Tel: +44 (0) 121 204 3000, Web: www2.aston.ac.uk/aston-medical-school

An insider's view …

Aston Medical School's ethos is widening participation into medicine and ensuring tomorrow's doctors reflect the societies which they will be serving in the future. We are committed to encouraging diversity and inclusivity with respect to ethnicity, gender, sexuality, disability, medical conditions, and socioeconomic background. It is essential that our doctors reflect the general population which they serve, which includes those with physical, mental, and other forms of disabilities which will not interfere with the medical student's fitness to practice. Towards this goal, we have put in place a comprehensive student support system which is there to ensure every student is given help and support when needed.

Birmingham

Although the medical school at Birmingham University is over 100 years old, the course and facilities are cutting edge. As the home of 11 Nobel laureates, there is a strong tradition of research which pervades the university. Studying at Birmingham makes for a fantastic educational and cultural experience.

University   Birmingham has a vast medical school situated on the Edgbaston campus, around a 20-minute bus ride from the city centre. The main Queen Elizabeth Teaching Hospital is next to the medical school and is one of 15 hospitals throughout the West Midlands that are used for clinical placements. The wide diversity of patients guarantees Birmingham students meet a broad cross-section of the population. There is a good public transport network and many hospitals have free 'shuttles' between other hospitals within their trust; travelling to placements is rarely an issue. Recent developments include a state-of-the-art-library and a 12-acre 'green heartland' at the centre of campus. Birmingham students can also benefit from their local rail service, as this is the only university in the UK to have its own station!

Course   The integrated course incorporates clinical exposure from the first term. The first two years (preclinical) are focused on core science. A typical preclinical week would comprise four days at the medical school in lectures (with hundreds of other medics!) and small-group tutorials (around 16 per group). Anatomy teaching benefits from a refurbished prosectorium, which contains 10 ventilated tables and individual flat screens for displaying X-rays and MRI scans. In the preclinical years, you receive GP teaching once a fortnight, where you can observe consultations, receive basic clinical teaching, and cover some clinical skills. The clinical years are mainly hospital-based, with a fortnightly GP attachment and occasional lecture at the medical school. Specialist rotations begin in the fourth year, at which point the group sizes get much smaller. With renowned research facilities within the medical school, such as the CRUK Birmingham Centre, many students choose to intercalate—an option that is available at any stage after your second year. There are a wide range of subjects on offer apart from the usual biomedical science subjects, including 'international health' and 'history of medicine'. Should you have a burning desire to study a course not offered here, Birmingham Medical School will also allow its students to go to other universities for this year.

Lifestyle   There are various catered and self-catering options for first-year campus accommodation, including rooms near the medical school on the Edgbaston campus. This campus is set within 250 acres of stunning parkland, benefitting from its own shops, bars, banks, and even art gallery!

In the unlikely event that the highly active MedSoc fails to keep you entertained, you're within easy reach of the city's highlights: the Bullring shopping centre (Europe's biggest), four bustling indoor and outdoor markets, and literally hundreds of restaurants offering a range of international cuisine. Huge stars regularly perform in the nearby NEC and NIA or, if you prefer something quieter, the Symphony Hall is one of Europe's finest concert halls. Is it any wonder that around half of Birmingham students choose to stay here after their studies?

Factoid   Sir Norman Haworth was awarded his Nobel prize for synthesizing Vitamin C whilst working at Birmingham Medical School. See Table 8.3.

Table 8.3 Birmingham

Myth	Old, overcrowded, and lost in a second-rate city		
Reality	Successful medics who thrive in one of the greatest places to be		
Personality	Modest, sociable, and outgoing city people		
Best aspects	Lifestyle; the UK's second-largest city offers as much as London, but with fewer crowds and at less expense; you will NOT be bored		
Worst aspects	There is a long way to travel for placements across the West Midlands (but travel reimbursements are available)		
Requirements	No admissions test; **A level** three A2s including chemistry and biology with predicted AAB; **GCSE** at least eight A*s with As in maths and English		
Course length	5 years	Structure	Campus
Type of course	Red brick	Year size	360
Typical offer	AAA	Intercalated degree	BMedSci
Applicants	4,000	Student mix:	
Interviews	1,000	% Mature	10%
Offers	800	% International	8%
Uncompetitive			Competitive
Low living costs			High living costs
Working really hard			Not working/chilling out
Contact details	University of Birmingham Medical School, College of Medical and Dental Sciences, University of Birmingham, Edgbaston, Birmingham, B15 2TT Tel: +44 (0) 121 414 3481, Web: www.medicine.bham.ac.uk		

An insider's view ...

Selection for interview is based purely on exam results. Candidates must have AAA grades at A level. We have used GCSE results as the 'tie breaker' to decide who gets offered one of the limited interview places. At the interview, we consider the candidate's work experience and non-academic activities, in the context of exploring the information provided in the personal statement. Exam results are not considered at this stage, so all candidates invited for interview have an equal chance.

▌Brighton and Sussex

As a small medical school, Brighton and Sussex Medical School (BSMS) has a real family feel. However, entry places have been recently increased, and alongside this it now has a state-of-the-art anatomy laboratory. Students belong to both the University of Brighton and the University of Sussex, yet all study as one cohort on the university campuses. With full access to the facilities of both universities and being located in the cosmopolitan city of Brighton there is something for everyone!

University BSMS opened its doors in 2003, boasting modern resources. Each campus has purpose-built lecture theatres, seminar rooms, and computer suites. The University of Brighton campus houses a fully equipped clinical skills area for use by all students; it is also one of only few medical schools to have access to a high-fidelity simulator patient. The purpose-built medical research centre situated at the University of Sussex ensures that BSMS is at the heart of new developments in all areas of medicine. In years three and four, study is based primarily in the Royal Sussex County Hospital in the centre of Brighton. This means you will never have far to travel and the familiar environment makes clinical study less daunting! In the fifth year, placements are further afield but accommodation is provided on most—and by this point, it's nice to see more of Sussex!

Course The integrated medical course at BSMS incorporates many teaching methods, including PBL and IT-based; there is an emphasis on small-group work. In the first two years a systems-based approach is used to provide students with core scientific know-ledge alongside clinical teaching, which begins in week one. Anatomy teaching is aided by both computer-based imaging classes and regular dissection, which is a selling point of BSMS. In the new dissection suite, each group of eight students is allocated a cadaver and dissects the particular system that is being studied at that time. Students are also given the opportunity to direct their learning with student-selected modules offered throughout the course. An intercalated degree is optional between the third and fourth years and can be undertaken at either the University of Brighton, Sussex, or elsewhere as an external student. There are modular assessments during the course, with major finals and elective in fifth year. A major component of the fourth year is an individual in-depth research project. You are assigned to a BSMS research team with whom you undertake a project of a medically relevant topic of your choice.

Lifestyle First-year medical students are guaranteed accommodation at either the Brighton or Sussex campuses which are next to each other in Falmer, a parkland area four miles from the city centre. The Sussex campus is shared with students from many other courses, offering a fantastic opportunity to socialize with non-medics! Both campuses have bars, restaurants, libraries, and sports/fitness facilities. Should you want to escape from it all, there is handy pedestrian access to an area of outstanding natural beauty: South Downs National Park. After the first year, students generally live in Brighton city centre where transport links are very good. Brighton is a rich city which will satisfy every personality. The dynamism of the festivals, events, and clubs on offer is tempered by the beautiful Sussex countryside, surrounding historic villages and relaxing hiking trails. Being by the sea is another bonus—you can't beat a lunch on the beach in-between clinics.

Factoid BSMS is taught on statistically the sunniest university campus in England! See Table 8.4.

Table 8.4 Brighton and Sussex

Myth	'New' touchy-feely medics, more into sunbathing than studying
Reality	A 21st-century course in a lively but relaxed city, with a lot of hands-on clinical experience
Personality	Laid-back, but able to get the job done
Best aspects	The family atmosphere and the location—Brighton is unlike any other medical school
Worst aspects	Lots of seminars teaching communication skills (although often an overlooked skill)
Requirements	**UCAT**; **A level** three A2s and one AS including A in A2 chemistry and biology; **GCSE** at least a B/Grade 6 in English and maths

Course length	5 years	Structure	Campus
Type of course	Plate glass	Year size	193
Typical offer	AAA or AAB and GCSE English and maths at Grade 5/C (contextual)	Intercalated degree	BSc/MSc

Applicants	1,927	Student mix:	
Interviews	762	% Mature	–
Offers	422	% International	–

Uncompetitive	Competitive
Low living costs	High living costs
Working really hard	Not working/chilling out

Contact details	Brighton and Sussex Medical School, BSMS Teaching Building, University of Sussex, Brighton, East Sussex, BN1 9PX
Tel: +44 (0) 1273 643529, Web: www.bsms.ac.uk

An insider's view ...

BSMS is committed to modern patient-focused education, with a high proportion of early clinical contact. The medical course has a strong science base benefitting from research-informed teaching, which equips our graduates with the ability to practice evidence-based medicine. The programme is delivered in an integrated systems-based manner using a variety of traditional and contemporary approaches, which we believe enhances the learning experience. The relative small size of BSMS means students and staff quickly get to know each other and the high proportion of small-group teaching means all students get the support they need. Student-selected elements are important aspects of the course and our students benefit in particular from a self-organized elective period and engagement with an individual research project in year four. We are therefore looking for enthusiastic and capable students with self-motivation directed to becoming one of tomorrow's doctors.

Bristol

Home to Banksy, Skins, and the Clifton Suspension Bridge, Bristol is a fantastic setting in which to study medicine. Once a major port, Bristol has enjoyed a rich and vibrant history with most of its unique architecture surviving to this day. Bristol also offers a six-year gateway to medicine course for students who did not take science A levels.

University The university offers university halls to first-year students at a variety of locations, some closer to campus than others. Those who live further from campus can use the dedicated university bus service between their halls and campus.

Over recent years, more study spaces have become available across campus, all with a modern look and feel. This includes the refurbished Biomedical Library, including its large social seating areas for those well-needed breaks from revision. Several of the libraries and learning spaces are also kitted out with cafes where you can grab lunch, snacks, and that necessary caffeine hit!

There are also many places where students can access support. Lecturers and tutors are readily available for academic queries. For any pastoral support, the medical school has dedicated pastoral staff available. The University of Bristol have their own GP service for university students and staff.

Course The MB21 curriculum, introduced in 2017, features a helical approach to case-based learning (CBL), delivered via group discussions, lectures, practicals, and clinical placements. Every year, each body system is revisited and supplemented with additional knowledge. This programme focuses more on independent study while providing plenty of early patient contact, and with anatomy taught via prosections.

In the first year, around 30% of your time is spent in lectures, 60% on independent learning, and 10% on placements. From the third year onwards, most of your learning occurs on hospital placements throughout Bristol and the South West (including Yeovil or Swindon), with accommodation provided for students who are placed outside of Bristol.

Students at Bristol also have the opportunity to contribute to research, designing posters, giving oral presentations, and attending local conferences. Assessments are in the form of written multiple-choice exams and practical exams (Objective Structured Clinical Examinations or OSCEs). Students also have the opportunity to intercalate after their third year, gaining an additional degree, in one academic year, in a variety of disciplines including anatomy, bioethics, and global health.

Bristol Medical School aims to produce doctors who excel in patient-centred care across community and hospital-based specialties and to prepare them for the rapidly changing world of twenty-first century healthcare.

Lifestyle After their first year, most students live in rented accommodation in the Redland or Clifton areas of Bristol. Nearby campus facilities are excellent. Both medical and university societies organize student events, and Bristol features a vibrant nightlife with the majority of bars and clubs located in the Triangle area or Park Street. Cabot Circus in the city centre features boutique shops, restaurants, and a cinema complex. In addition, Bristol Hippodrome and Colston Hall regularly features live musical and theatrical performances.

Factoid Dorothy Hodgkin, former Chancellor of the University of Bristol (1971–1988), was the first British woman to win the Nobel Prize in Chemistry. See Table 8.5.

Table 8.5 Bristol

Myth	West Country bumpkins dressed in Jack Wills on their Macbook Pros
Reality	A lively mix of hard-working medical students (some of whom wear Jack Wills and have a Macbook Pro)
Personality	Confident, relaxed, and eager to learn
Best aspects	Enthusiastic teaching and plenty to do in the great city of Bristol
Worst aspects	Hills … but just think of the free work-out
Requirements	**A level** three A2s including A in A2 chemistry and either biology, physics, or maths; **GCSE** Grade 7/A in maths, Grade 4/C in English. Minimum two weeks' work experience in care environment.

Course length	5 years	Structure	Campus
Type of course	Red brick	Year size	215
Typical offer	AAB	Intercalated degree	BSc
Applicants	3,696	Student mix:	
Interviews	1,027	% Mature	6%
Offers	711	% International	8%
Uncompetitive			Competitive
Low living costs			High living costs
Working really hard			Not working/chilling out

Contact details	Bristol Medical School, 5 Tyndall Avenue, University of Bristol, BS8 1UD. Tel: +44 (0)117 394 1649, Web: https://www.bristol.ac.uk/medical-school/

An insider's view ...

The research ethos of the University of Bristol underpins the teaching of the medicine course. With an appropriate core of medical knowledge and understanding, developing cognitive and transferable skills relevant to medical practice, students are prepared for their FY1 year and equipped for lifelong learning throughout their careers. Students can intercalate, studying for an additional year towards a second degree in a variety of subjects. Student-selected components form a large part of the course, allowing students to pursue specific areas of interest through project-based work. For the final three years of the course, students are immersed in clinical settings, benefitting from our unique Academy system, allowing them to experience a diverse variety of hospital environments and patient contacts—from the busy city centre to more rural-based hospitals.

▍Cambridge

The medical course at Cambridge is as traditional as punting on the River Cam or singing in King's College Chapel (see p. 158).

University As a collegiate university, Cambridge has no defined university campus. Instead, 31 colleges of varying size and character are dispersed across the whole town, each providing its own students with accommodation, canteens, and libraries. Preclinical lectures are at the New Museums site and Downing site in the middle of town, next to Pembroke College. There is nowhere in Cambridge that is more than a short bike ride away, and walking and cycling are the predominant modes of transport. In your clinical years you may take a short (20-minute) bus ride to the clinical school at Addenbrooke's Hospital, if you decide not to cycle.

Course In the first two years students are given a thorough grounding in the scientific principles of medicine. Rather than taking a systems-based approach, core medical sciences are explored separately through lectures and practical classes. Anatomy, physiology, and biochemistry are studied in the first year, followed by pharmacology, pathology, neuroscience, and head and neck anatomy the following year. Although this is an intense curriculum, the solid foundation it provides is ultimately invaluable. Whilst patient contact isn't a priority in the first two years, the Preparing for Patients Course gives students the opportunity to meet patients in GP practices and hospitals. The third year is dedicated to a specialist subject in which students earn their BA degree. Most choose to study a scientific discipline and take advantage of being at one of the most renowned research centres in the world by carrying out their own research project. There is also the chance to pursue a non-medical subject, from anthropology to zoology!

The true bastion of the Cambridge educational experience (and the silver bullet to the challenges posed by the rigorous course) is the supervision system. Students receive weekly supervisions in small groups from a specialist in each subject. Supervisors offer the opportunity to clarify and further discuss lecture material and also to deliver feedback on essays.

Provided all is well, all preclinical students stay in Cambridge for the clinical component of the course. The main teaching base is in the large Addenbrooke's Hospital, with some of the time spent in regional district general hospitals. The bulk of the learning is ward-based, through consultant-designated teaching and supervisions. Clinical sciences are taught through lectures called 'clinicopathological conferences', where experts from medicine, surgery, pathology, and radiology join forces to dive deep into clinically important topics. In parallel, great emphasis is placed on development of communication skills through critical appraisal in small-group sessions.

Lifestyle Students are usually offered college accommodation for the entirety of the preclinical (and sometimes clinical) course. In the first year you will usually have your own room on a corridor with other students who may or may not be studying medicine. Each college possesses its own perks and quirks (see p. 243), but all provide the facilities and the funding to enable their students to get involved in every conceivable extracurricular activity. The college bars and local pubs outnumber a growing but still modest selection of nightclubs, but this is more than made up for with extravagant formal halls or nights spent dancing at the college bops!

Factoid The famous end-of-year May ball held at St John's College was rated the seventh best party in the world, according to *Time* magazine. See Table 8.6.

Table 8.6 Cambridge

Myth	Brainy boffins in ivory towers isolated from patients		
Reality	Hard-working students with a desire to improve their clinical competence through scientific understanding		
Personality	Intense, competitive, organized		
Best aspects	Receiving personal tuition from some of the top scientists in the world is an extraordinary and once-in-a-lifetime privilege		
Worst aspects	The exams—they are just as bad as everyone says, only worse		
Requirements	**BMAT**; **A level** three A2s with chemistry plus either biology, physics, or maths (though three of these are preferred); **GCSE** at least Cs in science and maths		
Course length	6 years	Structure	Collegiate
Type of course	Stone	Year size	276
Typical offer	A*A*A	Intercalated degree	BA (compulsory)
Applicants	1,584	Student mix:	
Interviews	~1,200	% Mature	6%
Offers	340	% International	8%
Uncompetitive			Competitive
Low living costs			High living costs
Working really hard			Not working/chilling out
Contact details	University of Cambridge School of Clinical Medicine, Addenbrooke's Hospital, Box 111, Hills Road, Cambridge, CB2 0SP Tel: +44 (0) 1223 336700, Web: www.medschl.cam.ac.uk		

An insider's view ...

As expected from a leading international centre for scientific research, Cambridge's medical course is unashamedly scientifically orientated. This might not suit all tastes, but provides a fantastic opportunity for scientifically inclined students to excel. Our philosophy is that medicine progresses through the application of new scientific/technological developments in clinical practice. Medical training at Cambridge therefore differs sharply from elsewhere, retaining a clear division between an initial in-depth grounding in preclinical sciences and clinical training. The course is tough and highly competitive: we are looking for the most able students, with a particular interest in and flair for the sciences as well as vocational motivation.

▍Central Lancashire

The University of Central Lancashire (UCLan) Medical School was accredited by the GMC in 2020. The medical school was primarily set up for students from the North West who would not typically have the opportunity to study medicine. To that end, the university offers a certain number of fully funded scholarships to students from widening participation areas. Although the intake varies year to year, only 15 of 150 places are for UK students who are from North West of England or students on UCLan's BSc medical sciences foundation course.

University UCLan has several campuses, the primary one for the medical school in the first two years is the Preston main campus, between Manchester and Liverpool. Students can be placed in different campuses including Burnley, Blackburn, and Whitehaven in Cumbria.

Course The course reflects many others around the UK. The first two years focus on non-clinical aspects of medicine and encompass medical sciences as a whole including pharmacology, anatomy, physiology, biochemistry, and even more specialized subjects such as radiology. Students attend communication skills workshops and clinical skills training sessions, equipping them for the community and GP placements in the first year which each last two weeks and are undertaken in January and May/June. From the second year, students attend placements on a weekly basis. One of the really nice things about studying anatomy at UCLan is that instead of cadavers, 3D human models and virtual anatomy dissection tables are used.

In phase 2, which is the clinical phase, students spend their time focused on learning clinical practice. Years 3 and 4 are spent predominantly on the hospital wards, rotating through different specialties, alongside one teaching day, which also includes a significant component of 'flipped' teaching (where a group of students learns about a specific topic and then teaches the remainder of their cohort about the topic under the guidance of a suitable consultant). Students are randomly assigned to one of the partner hospitals, including but not limited to East Lancashire Hospitals NHS Trust, West Cumberland Hospital, and Royal Blackburn Hospital. In year 5, students take their elective, deepening their understanding on a favoured specialty or exploring medicine in a different country where they may go on to practice.

Being such a new medical school, UCLan has placed an enormous emphasis on the thoughts and ideas of its students. This means that if you have any feedback to give on any aspect of your experience, the school is eager to hear it and to make any adjustments that might be required.

Lifestyle Although the medical school is quite new, the university as a whole dates back to 1828, and the old buildings and structures are prominent within the city. The medical school is only a 10-minute walk from the city centre and therefore accessible to everyone who chooses to not live on campus. There is a variety of accommodation to choose from, both private and university-owned, with IQ KOPA and Ribble Brook House being the closest to the lecture theatres. The university has its own pub, which is a safe and convenient place to relax for the students. Because most of the medical students are international students, there is a very vibrant and diverse environment. To celebrate this diversity, the medical school and the medical society organize the international night event every year, which is a fantastic cultural exchange of food, dance, and a myriad of traditions.

Factoid Victoria Derbyshire, journalist and BBC television presenter, studied at the predecessor to UCLan, Preston Polytechnic. See Table 8.7.

Table 8.7 Central Lancashire

Myth	The medical school for people with more money than smarts		
Reality	A vibrant, passionate new medical school eager to contribute to the NHS workforce within North West England		
Personality	Excited and eager to help and learn		
Best aspects	Excellent teaching, superb anatomy suite, and kind and flexible academic tutors; international colleagues		
Worst aspects	Everything is spread out and getting around can be a challenge when it comes to clinical placements; restricted entry to UK medical applicants		
Requirements	**A level** AAB; 2:1 or above for graduate applicants with a year's work experience. UK applicants must be from the north west of England or currently studying UCLan BSc Medical Sciences Foundation Entry programme.		
Course length	5 years	**Structure**	Campus
Type of course	Plate glass	**Year size**	150 (~15 UK)
Typical offer	AAB	**Intercalated degree**	MRes
Applicants	–	**Student mix:**	
Interviews	–	**% Mature**	~20%
Offers	–	**% International**	90%
Uncompetitive	🏆 🏆 🏆 🏆 🏆		Competitive
Low living costs	💰 💰 💰 💰 💰		High living costs
Working really hard			Not working/chilling out
Contact details	The School of Medicine, University of Central Lancashire, Preston, Lancashire, PR1 2HE Tel: +44 (0)1772 891998, Web: www.uclan.ac.uk/schools/medicine/		

An insider's view ...

The University of Central Lancashire MBBS degree offers an innovative approach to medical education, training students to become professional, compassionate doctors. Students will benefit from a state-of-the-art curriculum, designed with local patients. We offer a warm, supportive, and multicultural learning environment, where every student is treated as an individual. You'll enjoy early patient contact and clinical placements in the NHS from Year 1.

Exeter

Exeter Medical School is one of two medical schools in the picturesque South West, whose campuses cover the Cornish coast (popular with surfers and ice cream lovers!) to Barnstaple and the North Devon Coast down to Exeter (popular for clubbing and sports fans) and Torbay, the English Riviera.

University Exeter Medical School was one of two medical schools (the other being Plymouth, see p. 172) that were created with the splitting of Peninsula Medical School in 2012, officially producing their first cohort of doctors in 2017. The medical school structure is unusual in being split over two sites in two counties, with students spending time in either Exeter's St Luke's campus and the Royal Devon and Exeter Hospital, or the Truro campus and the Royal Cornwall Hospital.

Course Exeter's course is regularly updated reflecting feedback from both students and tutors. While it still has the traditional preclinical and clinical divide (Y1–Y2 and Y3–Y5 respectively), all students have clinical placements and skills teaching from the beginning of the course, balancing academic work with hospital placements and clinical learning. Preclinical years use a PBL approach, with three-week rotations based around body systems. Each three-week block teaches appropriate anatomy, physiology, pharmacology; the spiral curriculum means that students are constantly reviewing and improving their knowledge. Students are tested regularly on their medical know-how with regular applied medical knowledge (AMK) tests and OSCEs to get them used to examining patients and recognizing signs. In recent years there has been a shift to providing more placement time for the clinical years, encouraging self-directed learning via online resources. Here, students can access the lessons particular to their placement weeks, rotating through Medicine, Surgery, Specialties, Acute, Chronic, and Palliative Care. Third- and fourth-year students spend the majority of their week in the hospital. AMKs continue regularly through these years and Exeter's finals (OSCEs) are at the end of year 4. Year 5 gives students choice in their placement, with preferences for each of their rotations in Immediate Care, Surgery, Medicine, and Specialty. Longer blocks give the students more of an opportunity to step into the role as a senior medical student, and the year ends with a six-week block in which the student shadows an F1 on their rotation. Student-selected components (SSCs) make up a full quarter of the course each year; students select from a large catalogue of projects, which have different themes depending on the student's stage. In later years, these become more longitudinal and culminate with conference days at the end of the year. Exeter students go on elective in the middle of their fifth year for six weeks, with a poster conference towards the end of the year.

Lifestyle Most medical students in Exeter start out at Rowancroft, the university's accommodation near St Luke's campus, and then find accommodation locally. Truro students find accommodation in advance in groups, often taking up student houses from those leaving Cornwall. St Luke's has an active student body with numerous medic societies, and a newly refurbished Cross Keys cafe for food and drink. If you want a bit of a change, then the non-medical Streatham campus is where you can join a range of societies—there's plenty to get involved with!

Factoid Harry Potter author J.K. Rowling used one of her professors at the University of Exeter as the basis for Albus Dumbledore. See Table 8.8.

Table 8.8 Exeter

Myth	The not-so-great spin-off series from Peninsula		
Reality	An innovative, adapting medical course taught on the beautiful southern coast		
Personality	Relaxed, but motivated (to direct their own learning)		
Best aspects	Clinically orientated curriculum gets you comfortable with skills early on		
Worst aspects	Transport during the winter with storms can be difficult		
Requirements	**UCAT; A level** three, with biology and chemistry		
Course length	6 years	Structure	Campus
Type of course	Stone	Year size	290
Typical offer	ABB	Intercalated degree	BSc/MSc/MClinEd
Applicants	1,400	Student mix:	
Interviews	800	% Mature	–
Offers	400	% International	5%
Uncompetitive	🏆 🏆 🏆 🏆 🏆		Competitive
Low living costs	💰 💰 💰 💰 💰		High living costs
Working really hard			Not working/chilling out
Contact details	College of Medicine and Health, St Luke's Campus, Heavitree Road, Exeter, EX1 2LU Tel: +44 (0)1392 724837, Web: https://medicine.exeter.ac.uk/medical-school/		

An insider's view ...

As a Russell Group University and the *Sunday Times* University of the Year, the University of Exeter Medical School builds on the success of the Peninsula College of Medicine and Dentistry. The course integrates the science and clinical aspects of medicine, ensuring an excellent education and student experience. Our students learn in a research-rich environment and our problem-based education model produces doctors who are recognized to be amongst the best-prepared to practice medicine.

Hull and York

Hull and York Medical School (HYMS) formed as a partnership between the universities of Hull and York and local NHS trusts in 2003. The medical school uses its relatively young age to its advantage, employing cutting-edge teaching facilities (including a £28 million health campus in Hull opened by the Queen in 2017) and a purpose-built curriculum to prepare future doctors for the demands of modern medicine.

University The medical school is based at both the Hull and York campuses—after accepting offers, students are divided equally between these base sites at random for the first two years. Teaching takes place at both university campuses; situated at 1½ miles from the city centre in York, 3 miles in Hull. The two campuses are one hour's drive apart; however travel between them is rarely required. From year 3, clinical placements are conducted in Hull, York, Grimsby, Scarborough, Scunthorpe, Middlesbrough, or Northallerton, with students rotating through most sites, which ensures exposure to different patient demographics and health providers.

Both university campuses have undergone significant redevelopments; the leafy Hull campus now features numerous state-of-the-art buildings including Allam Medical Centre which houses a simulated hospital ward, midwifery suite, operating theatre, and critical care unit. The updated anatomy facilities now enable Thiel embalming and plastination to prepare high-quality prosections. At York, £500 million has been invested in campus expansion and renovations of medical facilities.

Course The course is split into three phases; however, they are linked by the spiral curriculum (i.e. topics are revisited with increasing depth). Phase I (years 1 and 2) consists mostly of early clinical experience, lectures, skills and anatomy teaching, and SSIPs (student-selected modules). Structured small-group PBL is used to consolidate learning and set outcomes for independent study, while SSIPs provide the opportunity to study subjects in further depth by conducting academic and laboratory-based research projects. Phase II (years 3 and 4) is primarily clinical, with eight-week rotations through different specialties including one day per week in a GP surgery. Phase III (year 5) includes a six-week elective and formal work shadowing to prepare students for FY1. There is a great emphasis on optimizing the course, therefore student feedback is continually requested, and acted upon.

Students can also intercalate to attain an additional Bachelors or Masters degree after the second or third year, and are given the amazing opportunity to choose between one of the popular courses hosted by HYMS or even to intercalate at any other UK university.

Lifestyle The majority of York-based students live in the campus colleges for the first year, moving to privately owned accommodation in later years. Steeped in history, the enchanting city features stunning buildings, galleries, and cafés, which are complemented with numerous theatres, bars, and clubs by night. Hull-based students can choose between on- and off-campus accommodation, many of which are new developments, later moving to private accommodation. Hull was recently named as 'City of Culture' and also offers a vibrant and varied array of clubs, bars, cafés, creative hubs, and live-music venues that host international artists. The students' union is also award-winning. Despite these offerings, the cost of living in Hull remains among the lowest in the UK. During clinical years, accommodation at non-base sites is provided for free. University social life is fantastic at both Hull and York, which starts from the first day with an introduction to your new 'Medic parents' and numerous popular events organized by MedSoc. There are also many highly active medical and surgical societies and volunteering schemes to explore.

Factoid Students run a 'Teddy Bear Hospital', offering a health check for the teddy bears of primary school children, which helps put them at ease if they need to see a doctor. See Table 8.9.

Table 8.9 Hull and York

Myth	A northern GP factory valuing patient communication over science
Reality	An exciting course, continually appraised to offer the latest teaching methods and facilities
Personality	Dynamic, welcoming, and enthusiastic
Best aspects	Having two campuses and enjoying social activities at both, with keen (but friendly) inter-campus competition
Worst aspects	Having two campuses; lecture video-links can be problematic and the spread of hospital sites requires significant travel
Requirements	**UCAT**; **A level** three As including chemistry and biology; **GCSE** eight Grade 4/Cs including English and maths to Grade 6/B

Course length	5 years	Structure	Split campus
Type of course	Carbon fibre	Year size	231
Typical offer	AAA	Intercalated degree	BSc, MSc
Applicants	1,800	Student mix:	
Interviews	960	% Mature	20%
Offers	700	% International	5%

Uncompetitive	🏆 🏆 🏆 🏆 🏆	Competitive
Low living costs	💰 💰 💰 💰 💰	High living costs
Working really hard		Not working/chilling out

Contact details	Hull and York Medical School, The University of York, Heslington, York, YO10 5DD
	Tel: +44 (0) 870 1245500, Web: www.hyms.ac.uk

An insider's view ...

The HYMS course encourages you to be an independent learner who wants to see medicine through the patients' eyes from the start. The course features early, extensive patient contact and all learning is rooted in clinical situations. At interview we are seeking students with excellent communication skills and reasoning ability, who show they are flexible, non-judgemental thinkers with a genuine interest in medicine. The course particularly suits slightly older applicants—with many mature students and those coming from school who have had a gap year.

Keele

The Keele undergraduate medical school curriculum was developed in 2007, largely based on the Manchester curriculum. Keele also offers an additional health foundation year (A104) for applicants without the necessary science subjects required for entry into the standard five-year course.

University The purpose-built undergraduate medical school is based on the large and green Keele campus near Newcastle-under-Lyme. It includes several laboratories, plentiful IT facilities, and a student common room to socialize and study (or sleep!) in. The campus provides some great restaurants, bars, and sports facilities. Two of the three clinical years are mostly spent at University Hospital of the North Midlands, which is within walking distance of most rented accommodation, with a few placements at County Hospital in the clinical years. The other year is spent at the Royal Shrewsbury Hospital.

Course The systems-based curriculum is highly rated by its students. The curriculum is spiral, meaning that topics are revisited several times over the course with increasing complexity. Students are assigned to a weekly PBL group of 12 for their clinical cases. Alongside PBL there are lectures, seminars, practical classes, and regular tutor contact. Students are assigned to a different group for anatomy and lab, allowing a real mixing of the cohort as well as information learnt. Anatomy is taught by a combination of prosections, computer aids, and dissection. Although the first two years are traditionally preclinical years, hospital-based placements and clinical skills teaching, as well as a strong emphasis on the psychosocial aspects of medicine, begins from year one.

Third-year students are based at the hospital but return to the Keele campus for teaching one day a week. This is packed with applied sciences, anatomy, clinical pathology, and ethics seminars to complement clinical learning. To accompany timetabled learning there are also opportunities to 'sign up' to and get unique chances to see an area of personal interest or to address areas of weakness.

Students in the top third of the year can opt to do an intercalated Bachelors degree after the second year, or a Masters degree after the fourth year (most medical schools only offer a Bachelors as an intercalated degree).

Lifestyle The large green campus surrounded by beautiful Staffordshire countryside is a great place to study. Students in the first two years tend to live in university accommodation spread across campus and near the medical school (Barnes Block). Clinical students move to rented accommodation close to the hospital for their year in Stoke-on-Trent or Shrewsbury.

For the cinema, escape rooms, or local high-street stores and restaurants, Newcastle-under-Lyme town centre is a 15-minute bus ride from campus. The Intu Potteries shopping mall in Hanley is a short bus journey away too. Stoke-on-Trent rail station is halfway between campus and Hanley, meaning Manchester and Birmingham are easy to get to for even more activities! The medics' social calendar includes sports, trauma course day, research opportunities, themed nights out, and the infamous balls. In the third year, there is an extra special ball to commemorate being halfway through your medical degree, ingeniously titled 'the halfway ball'.

Factoid Keele Medical School was first suggested in the late 1960s; however, it was felt that the university was too small to support it. Not many medical schools can boast such an extensive planning period! See Table 8.10.

Table 8.10 Keele

Myth	An unknown, untested medical school in the middle of nowhere
Reality	A tried and tested course adapted to a beautiful rural setting
Personality	Eager, versatile students coming from every background imaginable
Best aspects	The family-like atmosphere fostered by the small size and campus setting; the friendly staff, doctors, and fellow students
Worst aspects	Learning sometimes feels undirected and causes undue stress about gaps in knowledge at exam times
Requirements	**UCAT**; **A level** three As at A2 including biology or chemistry, plus another different science subject (chemistry, biology, physics, maths/further maths/statistics) and an academic subject; **GCSE** at least five Grade 7/A with Grade 6/B in English, maths, and sciences

Course length	5 years	Structure	Campus
Type of course	Carbon fibre	Year size	172
Typical offer	A*AA–AAA	Intercalated degree	BSc/MSc MMedsci
Applicants	1,535	Student mix:	
Interviews	647	% Mature	33%
Offers	3,78	% International	4%

Uncompetitive		Competitive
Low living costs		High living costs
Working really hard		Not working/chilling out

Contact details	Keele University Medical School, Keele University, Keele, Staffordshire, ST5 5BG Tel: +44 (0) 1782 733642, Web: www.keele.ac.uk

An insider's view ...

As one of the smallest undergraduate medical schools in the UK, Keele offers a highly supportive learning environment in which students and staff work together to develop the knowledge, skills, and attitudes required by tomorrow's doctors. Our mission is to graduate excellent clinicians and our focus throughout the course is on making learning directly relevant to clinical practice. We welcome applications from students from all backgrounds who have a thorough understanding of the academic, organizational, and personal demands of a medical career. This understanding should be gained through school/university study, participation in health-based or caring work, and activities involving team working.

Lancaster

Situated in the North West of England and at the heart of 'Red Rose' country, the historic city of Lancaster began life as a Roman fort in 80 AD; it still has a lot to offer. Lancaster is surrounded by a diverse mix of city, coast, and countryside, with the Lake District and Morecambe Bay just a stone's throw away. The university is a vibrant place to study, with a top-ten UK ranking for both research and teaching, high student satisfaction ratings in the National Student Survey, and six times award-winning student accommodation.

University Lancaster is one of only a few remaining collegiate universities in the country. Each college has its own unique atmosphere and encourages a strong sense of identity amongst its students. The main campus, which sits on 360 acres of parkland, is one of the safest campuses in the UK and is only a 10–15 minute bus journey away from the town centre. The £41 million 'Health Innovation Campus' (HIC) has been built adjacent to the university's main campus, where the new medical school is based.

Course Lancaster is one of the newer medical schools in the UK, with the first cohort of students graduating in 2011. Lancaster has a PBL curriculum, with only one or two lectures or seminars a day, and students are expected to engage in plenty of independent study. They are assisted by a wide range of facilities to help them do this, including the Clinical Anatomy Learning Centre (CALC) on campus, which has virtual dissection facilities, and the clinical skills labs at each local hospital. Much emphasis is placed on communication skills, including regular sessions with 'simulated patients', played by actors.

   Clinical teaching begins in the first year, with weekly practical skills. Clinical placements begin at the start of year two, with students spending two days a week in medicine or surgery placements in the Morecambe Bay hospitals, Blackpool Victoria Hospital, and Royal Blackburn Hospital. Getting to placement is not a worry as the medical school endeavours to organize transport wherever possible. In the third year, students rotate through five specialties, supplemented by PBL and clinical teaching. Placement in the fourth year combines medicine, surgery, and the specialties, with students spending around three days in hospital and one day in a community setting (e.g. GP surgery). Final exams are at the end of the fourth year, and are followed by a five-week long elective. On their return, students enter the clinically intensive fifth year to prepare them for becoming junior doctors. Students also complete several special study modules, carrying out research in an area of their choice; 10–20% of students continue their research interests by intercalating between the fourth and fifth year.

Lifestyle The majority of first-year students live in halls of residence on the main university campus, before moving into private rentals in one of the student areas surrounding the city from the second year. Since Lancaster is so compact, just about wherever you choose to live lies within walking distance of the town centre, and placements are easy to get to. Lancaster University has a massive number of societies and sports teams to get involved with to keep you busy, and with the nine college bars on campus and the infamous university nightclub 'the Sugarhouse' in town, evenings will definitely not be quiet. The medical society (Lancaster MedSoc) also organizes regular social events, including the freshers' and winter balls, annual trips to other medical schools, the medic pantomime, and inter-year sporting tournaments.

Factoid James May, Andy Serkis (Gollum), and Jason Queally (Olympic gold medal-winning cyclist) all graduated from Lancaster University. See Table 8.11.

Table 8.11 Lancaster

Myth	Untried and untested, in an unknown university
Reality	An exciting opportunity to study medicine in a thriving university
Personality	Friendly, sociable, driven
Best aspects	As one of the smaller UK medical schools, students benefit from smaller teaching groups and form a close-knit community
Worst aspects	Placements in a few local (district) hospitals may limit the opportunity to observe more complex clinical cases in larger tertiary settings
Requirements	**A level** three, two of which must be biology, chemistry, or psychology; **GCSE** at least 15 points from nine GCSEs (A*–A/Grade 7–9 = 2 points, B/Grade 6 = 1 point), with at least B/Grade 6 in English, maths, and science, and minimum C/Grade 4 in other subjects.

Course length	5 years	Structure	Collegiate
Type of course	Carbon fibre	Year size	129
Typical offer	AAA	Intercalated degree	BSc or MSc
Applicants	986	Student mix:	
Interviews	525	% Mature	17%
Offers	286	% International	3%

Uncompetitive	🏆 🏆 🏆 🏆 🏆	Competitive
Low living costs	💰 💰 💰 💰 💰	High living costs
Working really hard		Not working/chilling out
Contact details	Lancaster Medical School, Furness Building, Lancaster University, LA1 4YG. Tel +44 (0) 1524 5 94547, Web: www.lancs.ac.uk	

An insider's view ...

At Lancaster Medical School, students learn through problem-based learning and extensive clinical experience, with an emphasis on effective communication skills and medicine in the community. The first clinical placement occurs in year 1 and students are on the wards and in GP practices from the beginning of year 2. The admissions process consists of three stages: (1) academic aptitude—only applicants who meet the academic entry requirements progress beyond stage 1; (2) non-academic criteria—the personal statement is assessed to determine those who most ably demonstrate the required non-academic criteria; and (3) multiple mini interview (MMI)—interviewees are ranked according to their MMI score and offers are made to the highest-scoring applicants.

Leeds

Leeds has a highly adaptable medical course, with SSCs running throughout. These allow students, from an early stage, to concentrate on the areas of medicine that interest them. Leeds has a lively and vibrant feel with a highly respected nightlife.

University The medical school is located on the main university campus, about one mile north of the city centre, directly connected to the Leeds General Infirmary (LGI). The recently refurbished Worsley Building houses the medical and dental schools. It provides a welcoming place to study, eat, and chill out, with large artworks that inspire hashtags galore. Hospitals for the clinical years are close by, with students going to LGI on campus and St James's University Hospital (Jimmy's) two miles away. Other hospitals include Bradford, Pontefract, and Dewsbury, all of which are a short train ride away. There is opportunity to volunteer for placements further afield to really experience the beauty of Yorkshire. Being based on the main campus gives ready access to the excellent university facilities, including numerous shops, cafes, and bars. The sports centres are famous for accommodating the Chinese Olympic team in 2012, and the Brownlee brothers during their studies at Leeds. Leeds University has a very active student union that helps improve students' lives locally and nationally.

Course The first two years are mainly campus-based, with the curriculum comprising of lectures, practical anatomy teaching, PBL, and small-group learning. Teaching is mainly by scientists, with occasional lectures by doctors. Anatomy is taught by experts, using professionally dissected specimens or 'prosections'. Patient contact begins in the first year with visits to patients' homes and then increases throughout the course. The final two years are fully clinical, incorporating small-group ward-based teaching with lectures between placements. Every year includes SSCs, allowing students to choose the courses that most interest them. While these are mainly medical, there are diverse opportunities for non-medical interests to be explored (e.g. creative writing, innovative design, complementary therapies). There is a strong drive towards research, with health research modules in every year of the course. Optional intercalated degrees are open to all students, usually between the third and fourth year. A foundation course with an additional year at the start is also available.

Lifestyle Students often spend their first year in halls on or near the campus, before moving to privately rented houses in the student area around the north-west of the campus (Hyde Park, Woodhouse, or Headingley). Leeds has a good system of public transport and many people cycle using newly installed bike lanes. The social life is superb with an endless variety of university societies and sports teams. Leeds University Union has something for everyone! Outside the university, Leeds is a great hub for music, arts, and the theatre; there are excellent opportunities for climbing, walking, cycling, and camping in the beautiful Yorkshire Dales nearby.

Factoid St James's Hospital is one of the largest teaching hospitals in Europe and famously opened its doors to film-makers for the documentary television series 'Jimmy's' in the 1990s. See Table 8.12.

Table 8.12 Leeds

Myth	The armpit of the north, known only for wool and beer
Reality	A dynamic medical school with a strong research record, based in a large and lively city with excellent social and cultural offerings
Personality	Lively and outgoing
Best aspects	Award-winning anatomy lecturers, huge focus on student support, and stunning libraries
Worst aspects	The brutalist architecture of the Worsley Building is in essence a giant cinderblock
Requirements	**BMAT**; **A level** three As at A2 including chemistry or biology; **GCSE** six Grade 5/Bs including English, maths, and sciences

Course length	5 years	Structure	Campus
Type of course	Red brick	Year size	225
Typical offer	AAA	Intercalated degree	BA or BSc
Applicants	2,487	Student mix:	
Interviews	1,056	% Mature	7%
Offers	417	% International	8%
Uncompetitive	🏆 🏆 🏆 🏆 🏆		Competitive
Low living costs	💰 💰 💰 💰 💰		High living costs
Working really hard			Not working/chilling out
Contact details	Worsley Building, University of Leeds, Leeds, LS2 9JT Tel: +44 (0) 113 343 7194, Web: www.medicinehealth.leeds.ac.uk		

An insider's view ...

Leeds offers one of the best undergraduate medicine courses (the MBChB) in the UK, that will prepare you for a successful transition to working as a doctor and give you a great start to your career. In addition to the many strengths of our course, such as our integrated wet anatomy teaching, clinical placements, and SSC programme, Leeds students will see patients at every stage of their career on the course, with a range of experience in hospitals, community, and GP surgeries. We are mapping skills for success as a new doctor (career development, patient safety, leadership) through the course, taking our students from the start of their university course to graduation as a doctor.

Leicester

Situated at the heart of England, Leicester is known for its ethnically diverse population, superb curry houses, and an orange-coloured cheese (Red Leicester). The university has a proud tradition of high-quality research and teaching at both undergraduate and post-graduate levels and is a vibrant place to study.

University The medical school building is based on the main university campus, which is a short walk south of Leicester city centre. The campus has just finished an extensive re-furbishment including a brand-new medical school building and a new library. Currently a multi-million-pound refurbishment project is underway in the students' union building (complete with cafes, shops, and O_2 nightclub). There's also a large park south of the campus (and a large cemetery to the north to help motivate you in your medical studies!). In the clinical years, about half the time is spent in Leicester's three large hospitals (Royal Infirmary, General, and Glenfield) while the other half is spent at affiliated hospitals which range from 30 miles away (Kettering) to 65 miles away (Boston). Free accommodation is provided at all affiliated hospitals and, with smaller teaching groups, the standard of teaching is very high. Needless to say, having a car (or friends with cars) is a big asset in the later years.

Course Leicester follows a lecture- and systems-based course complemented by seminars, laboratory practicals, and cadaveric dissection. There is a strong emphasis, from an early stage, on integrating clinical teaching into the curriculum, including communication skills, history taking (using actors as simulated patients), and clinical examination; it's no surprise that Leicester graduates are known for their bedside manner! Along with the core teaching there are seven student selected modules to teach you more about areas that interest you the most. The clinical course begins from the third year, with longer apprentice-style placements in Medicine, Surgery, and General Practice, based in hospitals and GP practices. Year 4 builds on this by focusing on specialty blocks such as Obstetrics and Gynaecology, Child Health, Cancer Care, and Psychiatry. Finally, year 5 is comprised of an extended foundation assistantship, designed to fully prepare you for work as a foundation doctor. After finals in the final year there is a seven week elective studying any specialty in any medical setting (usually overseas).

About 10% of students spend a year in research towards an intercalated BSc after the second year, or an intercalated MSc after the third or fourth year.

Lifestyle The majority of first-year students live in one of the university halls of residence. These are situated in Oadby, a leafy suburb with regular bus links to the city and campus 3½ miles away. In later years most medical students rent houses in one of the student areas surrounding the university and within a gentle walk of campus; the most popular of these is Clarendon Park. The social life is excellent, with numerous university societies and teams; the medical society is also very active, with regular socials including the famous 'pyjama pubcrawl' at the start of each year. Since students account for over 12% of Leicester's term-time population, the city centre has developed accordingly, giving it a nightlife that is hard to beat. Recent redevelopments include the Highcross shopping centre and a new cultural quarter. Being in the centre of the country, the city is very accessible, with great train and road links (via the M1, M69). For the outdoorsy types, Rutland Water and the Peak District are within 50 miles.

Factoid Sir Alec Jeffreys discovered DNA fingerprinting at Leicester in 1984. See Table 8.13.

Table 8.13 Leicester

Myth	Students learn more about communicating with patients in foreign languages than they do about medical science		
Reality	A culturally rich and redeveloped city-centre university campus with a medical school proud of both its science and communication teaching		
Personality	A sociable bunch, as good at communicating with each other as they are with patients		
Best aspects	Relaxed atmosphere, regular small-group teaching, and a highly structured course		
Worst aspects	Some of the 'award-winning' campus architecture is hard to appreciate		
Requirements	**UCAT**; **A level** three A2s including chemistry or biology, plus one other science from biology, chemistry, physics, or psychology; **GCSE** Grade 6/Bs in English, maths, and either double science or chemistry and biology.		
Course length	5 years	**Structure**	Campus
Type of course	Plate glass	**Year size**	290
Typical offer	AAA	**Intercalated degree**	BSc, MSc, or PhD
Applicants	2,309	**Student mix:**	
Interviews	1,095	**% Mature**	18%
Offers	701	**% International**	5%
Uncompetitive	🏆 🏆 🏆 🏆 🏆		Competitive
Low living costs	💰 💰 💰 💰 💰		High living costs
Working really hard			Not working/chilling out
Contact details	Leicester Medical School, George Davies Centre, Lancaster Road, Leicester, LE1 7HA. Tel: +44 (0) 116 252 2969, Web: www.le.ac.uk/medicine		

An insider's view ...

Leicester Medical School prides itself on its friendly and caring approach to students. Leicester's results in the National Student Survey confirm that it is an excellent place to study. The integrated course structure of Phase I builds knowledge and skills in a logical manner, providing an excellent basis for full-time clinical attachments. The entire course emphasizes a patient-centred approach and our graduates are well equipped to cope with the demands of the Foundation Programme. The course is demanding but students find plenty of time to enjoy their social lives through the medical students' society and many other groups.

Liverpool

Liverpool's School of Medical Education is a welcoming, supportive, and progressive place to study. The teaching methods are innovative and it is one of the most affordable places to live as a student. As the Beatles sang, 'Don't pass me by'.

University The medical school is on the city side of the main campus by the Royal Liverpool University Hospital, about five minutes from the city centre. It has some excellent resources including the internationally renowned Human Anatomy Resource Centre (HARC), 24-hour libraries, and the new Centre for Excellence in Developing Professionalism (CEDP) that aims to develop and improve medical education. During the clinical years most of the attachments are within the city (including the well-known Alder Hey Children's Hospital) and those further away are mostly accessible by public transport. The university's support services are extremely helpful with immediate access to financial and pastoral assistance.

Course An integrated teaching model using a 'spiral curriculum' is at the heart of Liverpool's pioneering medical education programme. It has been designed to encourage independent thinking and clinically relevant learning using a mix of traditional lectures, CBL, HARC sessions, communication skills workshops, and a staged programme of research skills development that builds on previous knowledge year on year.

First-year teaching includes a system-based approach (e.g. cardiology, respiratory), where each block encompasses basic and clinical sciences to emphasize the structure and function of the human body under 'normal conditions'. This year also provides an introduction to the foundations of research. Years two to four are focused on learning to diagnose and manage illness, through a combination of hospital, community (e.g. GP), CBL, and lecture-based teaching. Final exams are taken at the end of year four, leaving the whole of year five for intensive clinical experience (i.e. learning the job of an FY1 (see p. 9)).

At the end of year four, students are given the opportunity to complete a four-week elective, which is often spent overseas; the timing of this is ideal since it is before the summer holidays, allowing for some well-deserved travelling! At the end of years three or four, students can also choose to take an intercalated degree to complement their learning. The medical school also offers a year in China to spend time at the sister university Xi'an Jiaotong-Liverpool University (XJTLU).

Lifestyle Liverpool students can benefit from the city's status as a capital of culture, as well as the relatively low living costs. Most students live in university halls of residence for their first year, allowing easy access to a wide range of social and sports events. During term time there is also a student bus providing access to the city centre. From year two, most students live near Smithdown Road with its cheap rental costs, local supermarkets, and cosy cafes with wi-fi. Nearby Sefton Park is Liverpool's equivalent of Central Park—it is stunning in summer, with community music festivals and lots of space to relax or work. Despite its coastal location, the city is surprisingly accessible to the rest of the UK, with London only 2½ hours away by train. For a weekend away, you can pop over to Dublin or the Lake District!

Factoid Set up in 1874, the lively Liverpool Medical Students' Society (LMSS) predates the founding of the University. See Table 8.14.

Table 8.14 Liverpool

Myth	PBL—Playstation-based learning		
Reality	PBL allows the relevant science to be learned in the context of clinical medicine and encourages communication and social skills		
Personality	Genuine, open-hearted, and supportive; co-operative, not competitive		
Best aspects	The LMSS gives a real sense of community and helps students feel supported across all aspects of the course		
Worst aspects	Long hours in the hospital in year five, including occasional on-calls		
Requirements	**UCAT**; **A level** three A2s including chemistry with either biology, physics, or maths and a third academic subject; **GCSE** Grade 6/Bs in English, maths, and science		
Course length	5 years	**Structure**	Campus
Type of course	Carbon fibre	**Year size**	315
Typical offer	AAA	**Intercalated degree**	BSc or MSc
Applicants	3,000	**Student mix:**	6%
Interviews	2,500	**% Mature**	8%
Offers	1,350	**% International**	

Uncompetitive	Competitive
Low living costs	High living costs
Working really hard	Not working/chilling out

Contact details Admissions Enquiries, School of Medical Education, Cedar House, Ashton Street, Liverpool, L69 3GE
Tel: +44 (0) 151 795 4370, Web: www.liv.ac.uk

An insider's view ...

Liverpool medical graduates are excellent team workers with highly-developed communication skills and the knowledge and understanding required of any doctor entering foundation training. The final year of training at Liverpool is recognized as being excellent preparation for the Foundation Year 1 and beyond, while the problem-based learning approach to the curriculum develops appropriate skills in lifelong learning. Liverpool graduates leave university with the professional attitudes recognized as important by the NHS in the twentieth-first century. We consider candidates from all backgrounds. Applicants are expected to be motivated, thoughtful, caring, and compassionate individuals with the academic potential necessary to complete the programme.

London—Barts

Barts London (BL) is a medical school with centuries of tradition, producing graduates such as William Harvey, Robert Winston, and *Monty Python* actor Graham Chapmen. BL students benefit from 'the city' experience, and the cultural diversity of the East End offers a unique opportunity to treat diseases rarely seen in the rest of the UK.

University The medical school is situated on one main campus (Whitechapel) with two other locations. Whitechapel is the site for all lectures and PBL meetings (where you'll spend most of your time). This site is also where the modern library facilities can be found, in the beautiful setting of a renovated church, as well as the prestigious Royal London Hospital which is home to the state-of-the-art clinical skills lab and simulation centre, allowing students to perfect their practical procedures. The campus in Mile End (15-minute walk from Whitechapel campus) is responsible for holding anatomy and physiology practicals. Clinical skills sessions are held at Barts Hospital, located in the centre of London (20-minute tube ride from Whitechapel campus), which is steeped in historical beauty and only a short walk from St Paul's Cathedral.

BL students have a choice of hospitals, both 'in-firms' and 'out-firms'. The in-firm hospitals include Barts Hospital (a tertiary cancer centre), the London Chest (specialist cardiac and chest unit), and The London (home to the air ambulance on BBC's *Trauma*). The out-firms extend into Greater London and Essex, but are all easily assessable via public transport and accommodation is available for the placement's duration.

Course An integrated course at Barts provides a broad range of learning techniques including PBL, lectures, prosection (with optional dissection module), clinical skills, and placements. PBL supplements lectures nicely by covering similar topics with a systems-based approach, where relevant anatomy and physiology is taught at the same time through practicals, providing students with structured and focused teaching. Patient contact is also present from the first week, with an emphasis on communication skills; giving students vital exposure to various clinical scenarios, essential for the third year onwards. The first year concentrates on healthcare within the community (GP), with hospital placements coming in year 2, easing you into this setting. The spiral curriculum revisits topics/systems each year which enhances knowledge previously covered in the course, helping to reinforce key concepts.

Lifestyle The majority of first-years live in university halls of residence situated in either Whitechapel or Barbican; this is guaranteed for everyone who does not have a home postcode within London. After this, students tend to find private accommodation with friends. Barts has an amazing sense of togetherness spanning throughout all five years. This begins with a 'Mummies and Daddies' event at which you'll be given your own adopted family who can help guide you through your first year, with all the tips and tricks of the trade. The BL students association is at the centre of this close-knit community, organizing countless events and having many societies to get involved with. Barts are notorious for their outstanding RAG volunteer work, consistently raising over £50,000 every year. Together with QM, they often outcompete their London counterparts during RAG charity week.

Factoid Barts and The London is a union of the oldest medical school in the UK (The London) and the oldest remaining hospital (Barts Hospital) founded in 1123. See Table 8.15.

Table 8.15 London—Barts

Myth	The 'soft' option of London medical schools		
Reality	We produce 'the best doctors in London' according to the General Medical Council during a previous visit		
Personality	Incredibly welcoming and always eager to get involved		
Best aspects	Diversity and sense of community; strengthened by the BL Students' Association and the fantastic pastoral system		
Worst aspects	London is expensive (grants/maintenance loans are available and East London is less costly than other areas of the capital)		
Requirements	**UCAT**; **A level** three A2s including two sciences; **GCSE** six Grade 777666/ AAABBB including English, maths, and science		
Course length	5 years	Structure	City/Campus
Type of course	Plate glass	Year size	324
Typical offer	A*AA	Intercalated degree	BMedSci or BSc (optional)
Applicants	1,655	Student mix:	
Interviews	1,134	% Mature	19%
Offers	767	% International	12%
Uncompetitive			Competitive
Low living costs			High living costs
Working really hard			Not working/chilling out
Contact details	Barts and The London School of Medicine and Dentistry, Student Office, Garrod Building, Turner Street, Whitechapel, London, E1 2AD Tel: +44 (0) 207 882 8157, Web: www.qmul.ac.uk/smd/		

An insider's view ...

Barts and The London is dedicated to producing doctors able to meet the challenges of twenty-first century medicine. We are looking for students who are able to work hard and who are self-directed and enthusiastic to learn, but who are also willing to immerse themselves in the abundant extracurricular activities within the school. There are opportunities to work with world-class scientists, as well as being exposed to some of the best clinical medicine in Britain. BL is the 'Olympic medical school', being sited three miles from the 2012 Olympic stadium and park. Do you have what it takes to be part of it?

London—Imperial College

Imperial College is one of the largest, most competitive, and most prestigious medical schools in the country. It was formed from several mergers including Imperial College and the medical schools of St Mary's and Charing Cross. Its reputation has grown dramatically since, both in the UK and across the world.

University Like many universities in London, the facilities are widely distributed. Preclinical teaching is split between the South Kensington (Imperial) campus and the Hammersmith (Charing Cross Hospital) campus. The central library in South Kensington has an extensive medical section, which is open 24 hours a day; libraries are also available at each of the teaching hospitals. Clinical years are divided between 16 hospitals in the North West Thames Deanery including the teaching hospitals of St Mary's, Hammersmith, Chelsea and Westminster, Charing Cross, and Northwick Park, numerous smaller hospitals, and a few placements outside of London. All of the hospitals are readily accessible by underground train or bus, so a car is rarely necessary.

Course The six-year systems-based course includes a compulsory BSc. The two preclinical years consist of lectures, seminars, and practicals alongside some problem-based learning (see p. 92) and interactive e-learning. Anatomy is taught by a mixture of dissection, prosection, group tutorials (i.e. 'living anatomy'), and online videos. Throughout the course all lectures are available online, which complements the learning objectives and aids revision. Clinical experience begins in year one along with teaching in communication skills. There is a month-long hospital placement in the second year. An influx of Oxbridge students joins the year as the clinical phase begins in year three; this is hospital-based with medical and surgical placements supported by weekly lectures.

The fourth year is devoted to the BSc and a 15-weeks-long research project. While most of these will be in standard medical subjects (e.g. immunology) a few are available for global health and management. The selection expands year by year, with some of the latest BSc fields being biomedical engineering, management, and medical humanities. Depending on grades and funding, a handful of students may be offered a three-year PhD to follow on from their BSc. The fifth year begins with an intense pathology course, rumoured to be the best in the country, followed by student-selected specialty modules and rotations through the major clinical specialties, which continue into the final year. Year six also includes an eight-week elective and work experience in preparation for graduation.

Lifestyle First-year students are guaranteed university halls of residence which are split between Kensington and Acton (the newest campus). Students then pursue private accommodation for the rest of their studies. Student membership (with a symbolic annual fee) also gives access to a state-of-the-art gym that includes an Olympic-sized pool, squash courts, rock-climbing wall, sauna, steam room, and jacuzzi. The social life is intense; in fact, Imperial has an entire union devoted to medical students, with its own buildings, bar, sports teams, and societies. Together with the main student union there are over 300 clubs and societies (and with just 20 signatures you can create your own!). Whether you are drawn to museums, galleries, bars, bands, or sports fixtures you will find that you have far more options than you have time for.

Factoid Sir Alexander Fleming (discovered penicillin), David Livingstone (African explorer), and Lord Ara Darzi (surgeon and former Minster for Health) all spent time at the institutions that make up Imperial College School of Medicine. See Table 8.16.

Table 8.16 London—Imperial College

Myth	The training ground of arrogant surgeons		
Reality	A multicultural mix of friendly students from many backgrounds who are proud of Imperial and the career opportunities it offers		
Personality	Motivated, hard-working, outgoing, sociable, able to cope with a big medical school in a huge city		
Best aspects	Ability to explore your artistic side with languages and humanities courses; over 300 societies and one of the largest Students' Unions		
Worst aspects	Expectations are high and the workload is unbalanced, heaviest in the 2nd and 5th years		
Requirements	**BMAT; A level** three A2s including two sciences (must include chemistry and biology)		
Course length	6 years	**Structure**	City
Type of course	Stone	**Year size**	345
Typical offer	A*AA (A* chemistry or biology)	**Intercalated degree**	BSc (compulsory)
Applicants	2,474	**Student mix:**	
Interviews	868	**% Mature**	0%
Offers	612	**% International**	7.2%
Uncompetitive	🏆 🏆 🏆 🏆 🏆		Competitive
Low living costs	💰 💰 💰 💰 💰		High living costs
Working really hard			Not working/chilling out
Contact details	Imperial College Medical School, Sir Alexander Fleming Building, South Kensington, London, SW7 2AZ Tel: +44 (0) 20 758 95111, Web: www.imperial.ac.uk		

An insider's view ...

In short, we want the very best, who will become superb doctors and leaders in their chosen field. Competition to gain entry to medical school remains fierce. We want our students to have a very good basis in and understanding of the scientific principles that underpin medicine. These are often the key principles that medical professionals return to when dealing with difficult problems. Thus, the emphasis on science within our curriculum and the opportunity that every student has to obtain a BSc is entirely appropriate. I am not, however, looking for 'anoraks'. I am looking for well-rounded individuals who have the ability to communicate well, become great clinicians, and make a real contribution to the future of the profession.

London—King's College

The jewel of King's College London School of Medicine is the teaching provided by the world famous Guy's, King's, and St Thomas' Hospitals (working together as King's Health Partners Academic Health Sciences Centre).

University The main hub of the medical school is based at Guy's Campus, south of the River Thames next to London Bridge. For preclinical students, the vast majority of teaching is at Guy's. There is one main library open for the majority of the day, as well as a 24-hour library for the night owls. At Guy's there is also the Gordon's Museum, one of the largest pathology museums in the world, which has a collection of 8,000 pathological specimens going back to 1608. Students can relax on campus in 'The Shed' or Guy's Bar. Medical students at King's also have access to libraries and other facilities at King's four other central London campuses, including the historic Maughan Library on Chancery Lane.

Course The integrated medical curriculum is divided into three stages. Stage 1 is a year long and consists of four modules that introduce basic science through a mixture of lectures, small-group tutorials, and online content. Anatomy is taught in the dissection room through full-body dissection, supported by the largest UK medical anatomy museum. Stage 2 spans years 2 and 3, and has a heavier clinical component integrated with lectures and small-group sessions delivered both centrally by the university and locally in placement hospitals. Stage 3 (years 4 and 5) is majority clinical, culminating in a 'transition to F1' placement to prepare you for your first job. In the clinical years students can be placed across hospitals in Kent and East Sussex as well as London. King's has a focus on communication skills and strong medical humanities modules. Students also have access to the Chantler Clinical Skills Centre, one of the largest centres of its kind in the UK, where they can practice their clinical skills on anatomical models.

SSCs are offered throughout the course and an optional BSc is available after years 3 or 4, with 14 undergraduate degree programmes at King's and the chance to intercalate elsewhere If your choice of course is not available. During the 12-week elective in the final year, students can exploit the numerous institutions that are partnered with King's, including Johns Hopkins and Emory University in the USA.

Lifestyle The vast majority of medical students live around campus. This includes halls at Wolfson House and Great Dover Street (a 10-minute walk from campus). After the first year, you could either reapply for halls and become a senior student or rent accommodation around London. During clinical training, halls-style accommodation is provided for hospitals outside of London. Guy's campus itself is close to many restaurants, bars, and the famous Borough Market.

King's has an abundance of societies one can join, ranging from writing for the *GKT Gazette* (established 1872!), mentoring school children through the SHINE programme, or getting involved with organizing shows or plays. Volunteering also plays a big role in the student life at King's, with opportunities locally and globally. If none of these take your fancy, then playing sport for the medical school might appeal; it can involve competing to win the Macadam Cup (the annual competition between the medical school and the university itself). King's Medical Students' Association and the student union put on plenty of socials and formal balls throughout the year.

Factoid The Colonnade Gardens on Guy's campus have the world's only life-size statue of the nineteenth-century poet (and surgeon apprentice) John Keats, who studied medicine there. See Table 8.17.

Table 8.17 London—King's College

Myth	'Too big'—a large and faceless London medical school		
Reality	A large London medical school with a strong community, where anyone can find their place		
Personality	Practical and hard-working		
Best aspects	Peer support networks, from senior students teaching OSCEs to mental health welfare from colleagues, makes you proud to be a GKT medic		
Worst aspects	A little bit further from the centre of London and still pricey		
Requirements	**UCAT**; **A level** three including chemistry and biology; **GCSE** Grade 6/B in English and maths		
Course length	5 years	Structure	City/Campus
Type of course	Red brick	Year size	320
Typical offer	A*AA	Intercalated degree	BSc
Applicants	2,664	Student mix:	
Interviews	1,032	% Mature	28%
Offers	871	% International	19%
Uncompetitive			Competitive
Low living costs			High living costs
Working really hard			Not working/chilling out
Contact details	Student Admissions Office, King's College London, Hodgkin Building, Guy's Campus, London Bridge, London, SE1 1UL Tel: +44 (0) 20 7848 6501, Web: www.kcl.ac.uk		

An insider's view …

Undergraduate medical students at King's College London School of Medicine study in an institution with research excellence while gaining a broad clinical experience in a very diverse community within London. King's Health Partners is a pioneering collaboration between the Medical School, King's College, and three of London's most successful NHS Foundation Trusts. The partnership aims for excellence in clinical medicine, research, and education through a new Education Academy. These links give medical students access to extensive clinical experience and active translational research. This is seen in the very broad programme of student-selected components (SSCs), where students can choose from over 800 SSCs ranging from languages and humanities to research and careers, the elective programme, and the opportunity for self-designed attachments.

London—St George's

St George's, University of London (SGUL), founded in 1733, is the second-oldest university in the UK to formally train doctors. Despite its history, it is less traditional than other London medical schools and ideally suited to students wanting 'something different' in a central location. It is the UK's only university which is solely dedicated to medicine and health sciences.

University St George's is a specialist medical college of the University of London. In fact, it is the only UK university to share a site with a hospital. You will find student physiotherapists, radiographers, paramedics, biomedical scientists, and healthcare scientists (to name a few) training here as well. This is an opportunity to learn alongside the colleagues you will be relying on as a doctor in years to come. Perhaps unsurprisingly the university is much smaller than most others. Its small size may explain St George's reputation as a friendly, caring community of student clinicians.

St George's boasts a rich history of contributions to medicine with alumni including Henry Gray (of *Gray's Anatomy* fame) and Edward Jenner (the father of vaccination). St George's has been ranked best for graduate prospects in the UK for three years running (2017–2019) by *The Complete University Guide*. It has also been ranked best in the world for the quality of citations for research influence by *The Times Higher* World University Rankings in 2017 and 2018.

Course The first two years (also known as the clinical science years) consist of six modules which are taught via lectures, small-group teaching, as well as practical sessions. A new clinical problem is introduced every week, with the week's teaching centred around it. There are three clinical practice years: transitional year (T/third year), penultimate year (P/fourth year), and final year (F/fifth year). T year is divided into six five-week blocks whereby you alternate between teaching and clinical placements on Medicine, Surgery, and General Practice. P year is entirely clinical and you will be expected to rotate through a number of clinical firms, spending five weeks on each. This is by far the longest year of the course. F year aims to prepare you to become an F1 doctor and includes a number of clinical rotations and assistantships, as well as an SSC and an elective period.

A previous Quality Assurance Agency (QAA) inspection awarded SGUL 23 out of a possible 24 points for teaching—the highest score of any medical school in London and the third highest in the UK after Oxford and Cambridge.

Lifestyle St George's Students' Union is smaller than many others but you will still find it difficult to be bored. As well as the usual array of societies and sports clubs, St George's has a particularly strong selection of community and charity projects.

In any event, London has plenty to keep students entertained: world-famous sights, huge shopping centres, bars and restaurants of every variety, and peaceful parks. Transport is easy since the whole city is connected by a single underground tube system, and it helps that the hospital and medical school are found on the same site.

Factoid St George's is home to the award-winning Channel 4 TV show *24 Hours in A&E*. You just need to be at the right place at the right time and who knows, you might make it onto the TV one day! See Table 8.18.

Table 8.18 London—St George's

Myth	Tedium in Tooting—nothing to do		
Reality	One of the world's top 10 coolest neighbourhoods (*The Lonely Planet 2017*), in the more affordable Zone 3		
Personality	Laid-back for London medical students		
Best aspects	A whole university dedicated to healthcare makes for an amazing learning environment		
Worst aspects	Everyone is a healthcare student, so there is a danger of becoming institutionalized		
Requirements	**UCAT**; **A level** three including chemistry and biology; **GCSE** five Grade 6/Bs including English, maths, and sciences		
Course length	5 years	Structure	City
Type of course	Plate glass	Year size	184
Typical offer	AAA–A*AA	Intercalated degree	BSc (optional)
Applicants	1,500	Student mix:	
Interviews	700	% Mature	25%
Offers	400	% International	7%
Uncompetitive	🏆 🏆 🏆 🏆 🏆		Competitive
Low living costs	💰 💰 💰 💰 💰		High living costs
Working really hard			Not working/chilling out
Contact details	St George's, University of London, Cranmer Terrace, London, SW17 0RE Tel: +44 (0) 20 8672 9944, Web: www.sgul.ac.uk		

An insider's view ...

St George's is the only UK university dedicated to healthcare. As such, it is small and friendly and has a strong emphasis on the practical aspects of becoming a doctor. From day one, medical students learn to work with students from allied health professions such as radiography and healthcare science students, mirroring the workplace environment. Clinical skills are taught as early as first year, and students hugely benefit from being on the same site as St George's Hospital, where most of our teaching takes place. Being a major trauma centre in London, St George's Hospital covers a large population of around 2.6 million over south-west London and Surrey. As a result, students are guaranteed to always see some interesting cases and have plenty of opportunity to get involved and learn.

London—University College (UCL)

UCL Medical School (UCLMS) offers research-led, world-class medical teaching in the heart of London. The medical school emerged from the amalgamation of the Middlesex, University College, and Royal Free Hospitals, combining a rich history of science and medicine into a single institution.

University UCL is the oldest and largest constituent college of the University of London, opening its doors as early as 1828. It was the first non-secular university in Britain and the first to admit women on equal terms with men, whilst the Royal Free Hospital was the first to admit women for training in medicine specifically.

The medical school spans three London campuses incorporating the three teaching hospitals of the Royal Free in Hampstead, the Whittington in Archway, and University College Hospital in Bloomsbury. In addition to learning hubs at each teaching hospital site, the medical school boasts a renovated medical library in the historic Cruciform Building and a purpose-built student centre with over 1,000 new study spaces.

Course The medical degree programme is divided into two phases with an additional intercalated BSc between Phases 1 and 2. Material in Phase 1 (years 1 and 2) is delivered through lectures, tutorials, and laboratory sessions, with extensive use of online materials. Phase 1 anatomy is taught through full cadaveric dissection (~eight students per cadaver), alongside prosection and computer simulations. Professional development is emphasized throughout the programme so students develop the background, skills, and attitudes necessary to practice medicine, and a comprehensive selection of science and non-science student selected components are also offered throughout. The intercalated BSc takes place in the third year, with UCL offering a wide range of courses, ranging from neuroscience to philosophy. All medical students are required to undertake an intercalated degree. Those with a particular interest in research may then choose to undertake an intercalated PhD by entering UCL's competitive MB PhD programme after the third or fourth year of their course

Phase 2 (years 4 and 5) integrates the knowledge of basic sciences into clinical practice through a range of clinical attachments in teaching hospitals, district general hospitals, and within general practice and the community. This experience is further refined in Phase 3 (year 6) of the programme. These two phases draw extensively on the facilities of leading partner healthcare institutions such as Great Ormond Street Children's Hospital, Moorfields Eye Hospital, and the National Hospital for Neurology and Neurosurgery. Most of these sites are within close proximity to the main UCL campus, although the furthest placements are over an hour's drive away. For placements further afield, travel expenses are covered or hospital accommodation is usually provided to students for free. Finals examinations take place in March of Year 6, following which students go on an eight-week elective, most taking this opportunity to study overseas in a contrasting healthcare environment.

Lifestyle All first-year students are offered accommodation in halls of residence. Much-needed breaks from studying can include anything London has to offer as the UCL campus is just minutes from the West End and Oxford Street. UCL has 140 clubs and societies run by students, as well as its own theatre: the Bloomsbury Theatre. Transport around central London is easy to negotiate—just grab an Oyster card and enjoy the underground and 24/7 bus service. If all else fails, it rarely hurts to walk. However, driving in London is not recommended.

Factoid UCL is frequently ranked in the top 10 QS World University Rankings for Medicine. See Table 8.19.

Table 8.19 London—University College (UCL)

Myth	Posh rugby players who hate King's College London
Reality	An eclectic mix of students with a healthy streak of inter-London competitiveness, receiving research-led teaching in the heart of London
Personality	International students through to Londoners born and bred; reputation and location attracts students wanting to work and play like no others
Best aspects	UCL teaching hospitals see some of the rarest diseases in the world, and diseases you might never see outside of London: malaria, TB, and Ebola
Worst aspects	The costs of living in central London
Requirements	**BMAT**; **A level** three including chemistry and biology; **GCSE** Grade 6/B in maths and English, Grade 5 in a modern foreign language

Course length	6 years	Structure	City
Type of course	Red brick	Year size	330
Typical offer	A*AA (reduced offers via Access UCL Scheme)	Intercalated degree	BSc (compulsory)
Applicants	2,883	Student mix:	
Interviews	863	% Mature	7%
Offers	709	% International	37%

Uncompetitive		Competitive
Low living costs		High living costs
Working really hard		Not working/chilling out

Contact details	Medical Admissions Office, UCL Medical School, UCL, Gower Street, London, WC1E 6BT
	Tel: +44 (0) 20 7679 0841, Web: www.ucl.ac.uk

An insider's view ...

We want students who are academically gifted, good communicators, and are willing to join proactively in the academic, clinical, and social life of the medical school and university. Our course has the best features of a modern integrated course whilst maintaining traditional components where appropriate. There is a strong emphasis on scientific excellence and the translation of science into clinical practice. We wish to train the clinical leaders of the future, producing doctors prepared for practice in the NHS, for the forefront of medical science, and for the wider global health community.

Manchester

Manchester may conjure up images of football, curry, and rain, but it has a medical school with one of the most innovative courses in the UK. The emphasis on problem-based learning (PBL) allows for a more mature approach to learning. The course allows for a flexible lifestyle, and those with a background in European languages can continue learning them and study abroad.

University The medical school building, called the Stopford Building, is in the heart of the university campus and includes a comprehensive medical library and purpose-built PBL rooms perfect for group study. Years 1 and 2 are spent entirely in Manchester, and from Year 3 onwards you are classed as a clinical student and based entirely in hospital. Clinical teaching is split between four base teaching hospitals: Central Manchester (Manchester Royal Infirmary), South Manchester (Wythenshawe), Salford Royal, and Lancashire (Royal Preston Hospital). Each base has several smaller hospitals attached, where students may rotate around as part of placements. Accommodation is often available at the more distant sites. All Manchester-based students spend time at The Christie, a world-renowned specialist cancer hospital right on their doorstep!

Course The Manchester curriculum adopts a problem-based learning (PBL) approach along with using research methods to answer more specific questions. PBL is structured around clinical cases and organized by systems (gastrointestinal, cardiovascular, etc.). For the first year, PBL sessions are in groups of 12, with a weekly case supported by relevant lab work, lectures, and anatomy tutorials, including full-body dissection with one cadaver and one teaching clinician per group. Patient contact begins from the first semester and increases during the 'intermediate' phase starting at Year 2.

About 100 students from St Andrews join for Years 3 to 5, as the PBL approach continues in smaller groups assigned to specific hospitals. In clinical years, the PBL teaching is referred to as 'themed case discussions' (TCD), where the scenarios are entirely clinical (unlike in the first two years). TCD is supplemented by clinical teaching, ward attachments, and online teaching to ensure appropriate clinical exposure. Being based in the hospital allows students to gain hands-on experience, both via the clinical skills facilitators and clinicians on the wards. Throughout the course, SSC blocks allow students to develop exposure to areas of personal interest, and this includes an 11-week project option in Year 3 and a six-week medical elective in Year 4 which can be in the UK or abroad.

Manchester has a huge research centre and students can take an intercalated Bachelor's or Master's degree in medical subjects after the second, third, or fourth year. There is also the European Option Programme (students with A level standard French, German, or Spanish study the language for four years and spend 16 weeks at a European partner hospital in Year 5) and a Diploma in Global Health.

Lifestyle University accommodation is guaranteed in the first year and most live in Fallowfield, about 10 minutes from campus by bus (a discounted year pass is available). Most students move to private accommodation in Fallowfield or neighbouring Withington from the second year onwards.

The university has invested vast amounts in improving the campus including computing resources, sporting facilities, theatres, a concert hall, museum, and gallery. The large student population means that there are a wide variety of charity, student, and sporting clubs, including numerous medics' societies that organize regular socials to suit the medics' often busy timetable. The city itself also has a lot to offer including the internationally renowned music and club scene (see the film *24-Hour Party People*) and two well-known football teams. Cheshire, the Peak district, and the Lake district are all just a stone's throw away.

Factoid With over 40,000 students, most of whom live near the Oxford Road, it is unsurprising that this is the busiest bus route in Europe. See Table 8.20.

Table 8.20 Manchester

Myth	DIY medical teaching allows students to effectively communicate their lack of real knowledge		
Reality	Truly well-rounded students who learn to think like a doctor from day one		
Personality	Self-directed study attracts outgoing, determined, and mature students able to take responsibility for their learning		
Best aspects	Case-based PBL brings medical learning to life and allows you to pursue your interests; small groups builds strong friendships and team-working skills		
Worst aspects	Unmotivated students can struggle with PBL		
Requirements	**UCAT**; **A level** three, with A in chemistry and at least one other science or maths; **GCSE** at least seven Grade 7/As and minimum Grade 6/Bs in English, maths, and at least two sciences		
Course length	5 years	Structure	Campus
Type of course	Carbon fibre	Year size	397
Typical offer	AAA	Intercalated degree	BSc/MSc/MRes
Applicants	3,000	Student mix:	
Interviews	1,500	% Mature	11%
Offers	850	% International	7%
Uncompetitive		Competitive	
Low living costs		High living costs	
Working really hard		Not working/chilling out	
Contact details	Manchester Medical School, Stopford Building, Oxford Road, Manchester, M13 9PT Tel: +44 (0) 161 306 0460, Web: www.medicine.manchester.ac.uk		

An insider's view ...

Applicants are expected to demonstrate high standards in both academic and clinical achievements. They will have a strong ethical framework; a strong sense of responsibility (for patients and communities); an empowering sense of fairness (needs of a diverse society, both locally and internationally); and the ability to become a leader and agent of change. They will also need to demonstrate caring-work experience, commitment, communication, and team-working skills. The enquiry-based learning course offered will use flexible learning methods, lectures, dissection, seminars, skills laboratories, and clinical learning in hospitals and community settings, which will be delivered from the start of the course.

▌Newcastle

Newcastle is one of the largest and oldest medical schools in the UK, with over 300 students in each year on the standard five-year MBBS programme, and an additional ~25 places available for postgraduate students on the accelerated four-year MBBS programme.

University Unlike most universities, Newcastle has its campus and medical school in the centre of the city. Newcastle offers excellent sporting facilities with a revamped £30 million sports centre situated right next to the medical school, in addition to some great refurbished outdoor facilities in easy-to-access locations around town. The medical school is also right next door to one of the newest and largest accommodation halls the university offers: Park View, with its very lively social scene. Clinical placements are split predominantly between four clinical bases: Tyne, Teesside, Wear, and Northumbria. Many of these placements require students to travel by driving, car-sharing, or the Metro. Some of the hospitals offer travel bursaries and accommodation, and all have libraries and computing facilities, with some even providing free printing for medical students.

Course Newcastle has an integrated spiral course taught using lectures, small-group seminars, laboratory practicals, and significant clinical exposure. The first and second years focus on medical sciences, clinical skills, and ethics in a systems-based and case-led approach. Anatomy is taught in small groups using prosections and computer-based models rather than dissection. There is early clinical and community exposure through regular general practice and hospital visits. In the second year, students have the unique opportunity to spend a semester abroad and study at the medical school's campus in Malaysia! Students can undertake two four-week placements of their choice in the third and fourth years, in their SSCs, before the eight-week elective. Whilst the third and fourth years focus on clinically based practice and clinical decision making, the fifth year aims to bring everything together and transition students into being FY1s. An optional intercalated degree is available for students after the second year (BSc/BA) or fourth year (MSc/MRes), including the option to intercalate at external institutions if their subject of choice isn't available at Newcastle University.

Lifestyle Newcastle medical students benefit from some of the cheapest accommodation and lowest cost of living in the country. Accommodation is mostly hall-based and spread out across the city at varying distances from the campus. Most students opt for privately rented accommodation after year one, living usually in Jesmond (£££), Sandyford (££), or Heaton (£). Jesmond is by far the most popular amongst students due its close proximity to many pubs, bars, and restaurants along Newcastle's famous Osborne Road. In years three, four, and five medical students usually tend to live nearer their clinical base unit. Students only tend to move out of Newcastle if they are based in Carlisle or Tees. The social life is nothing less than impressive: alongside the active students' union, numerous societies, and sports teams, the famous nightclubs and bars of the city centre are right on the doorstep. The city also offers easy access to a range of museums, galleries, shopping centres, and even the seaside, which is only a 15-minute commute away! Public transport is also one of Newcastle's many strengths, with the city boasting its own Metro rail system. This fast and cheap transport method is popular amongst students for getting to many parts of the North East, even serving Sunderland.

Factoid The university owes its existence to the medical school, established in 1834, and joining Durham University in 1851. In 1937 it became King's College, Durham, and then Newcastle University in 1963. See Table 8.21.

Table 8.21 Newcastle

Myth	More booze than brains		
Reality	A unified medical school with an excellent record in research and teaching, offering a diverse selection of study sites to suit all types		
Personality	Lively, fun grafters		
Best aspects	The opportunity to study in a wide variety of geographical and socioeconomic areas		
Worst aspects	Travelling to clinical placements; and finding the right work–life balance		
Requirements	**UCAT**; **A level** three, with some subject exclusions		
Course length	5 years	Structure	City/Campus
Type of course	Plate glass	Year size	342
Typical offer	AAA	Intercalated degree	BSc
Applicants	2,500	Student Mix:	
Interviews	1,100	% Mature	10%
Offers	684	% International	7%
Uncompetitive	🏆 🏆 🏆 🏆 🏆		Competitive
Low living costs	💰 💰 💰 💰 💰		High living costs
Working really hard			Not working/chilling out
Contact details	Claremont Road, Newcastle upon Tyne, NE1 Tel: +44 (0) 191 222 6000, Web: www.ncl.ac.uk		

An insider's view ...

The case-based integrated approach that our curriculum follows means that in the 'pre-clinical' years all teaching is delivered in the context of clinical cases and all content has clinical relevance. The pure science elements of the curriculum are de-emphasized, and so our admissions policy does not require applicants to have studied science at A level. Our clinical training is not based on the traditional '-ologies' but rather focuses on core competencies and knowledge that will enable successful transition to FY1, and is achieved in close partnership with our regional NHS trusts. Selection is aimed at finding bright, motivated individuals who want to develop into doctors willing to view their patients as members of society and not just as a collection of symptoms.

Nottingham

Nottingham combines the academic rigour of a traditional medical course with extensive clinical experience, uniquely integrated with CBL and full-body dissection. The course includes an obligatory intercalated degree (BMedSci) but unlike other medical schools, this is squeezed into five years, rather than requiring an extra year out.

University The large and green main university campus is a 10-minute bus ride away from the city centre, with the medical school, based in the Queen's Medical Centre (QMC), on the outskirts of main campus; the newer and eco-friendly Jubilee campus is a 15-minute walk away. There is a regular and free university bus service that runs between campuses. The majority of the first two years are spent in the QMC lecture theatres, seminar rooms, anatomy suite, and laboratories, with access to the dedicated medical library, 24-hour computer room, student cafes, and purpose-built clinical skills centre. The QMC, Nottingham City Hospital (15 minutes by bus), and Derby hospitals (30 minutes by car or bus) accommodate the majority of students for clinical placements, whilst others are allocated to district hospitals, which although further away, offer free student accommodation.

Course The course is split into two parts: the BMedSci phase and the clinical phase. During the BMedSci phase, students are taught through lecturers, seminars, workshops, CBL, clinical teaching, and practicals. Anatomy is taught through full-body dissection in small groups, supported by lectures and seminars. Clinical and patient contact is emphasized from the very beginning, with regular sessions spent in the hospital or GP surgery. In Year 3, students undertake a supervised research project for the BMedSci. Halfway through Year 3, students start the clinical phase of the course which includes placements in various trusts and specialties as well as student-selected modules. In Year 5, students sit their final exams and have the opportunity to go on a six-week elective! Upon returning there is a period dedicated to shadowing a junior doctor before graduation.

Lifestyle First-year students are guaranteed a place in university accommodation, most of which is on the main or Jubilee campus. Each hall has its own common room, library, social events, and sports teams, giving a strong sense of community. In later years most students move into private accommodation in neighbouring Lenton or Dunkirk; this is where you find most medics, so it doesn't get lonely! The Students' Union offers over 200 societies, teams, and social events—there's definitely something for everyone. However, if that's not enough, there are also medics' societies, social events, and a medic family/mentor system. Nottingham city centre is large enough to have a wide range of shops, restaurants, pubs, and clubs but small enough that it's very easy to get around. There is so much to do in Nottingham—from the buzzing nightlife, incredible theatres, and cinemas (including a cute, retro, pre-World War 2 cinema!) to the grand Nottingham Castle and Sherwood Forest from the tale of Robin Hood. There are excellent transport links, with the buses and trams most used by students. The Peak District is also just a short drive away.

Factoid MRI was discovered by Sir Peter Mansfield, a professor at the University of Nottingham, who's own abdomen was the first MRI image of organs within the body! He later became the university's first scientist to receive the Nobel Prize for Medicine. See Table 8.22.

Table 8.22 Nottingham

Myth	The unoriginal choice after Oxbridge and London
Reality	The right choice for applicants looking for a solid grounding in research and clinical science
Personality	Work hard, play harder!
Best aspects	The stunning campus with rolling hills and lakes; intercalated degree without adding an extra year to your studies
Worst aspects	The intensity of the clinical phase and short holidays; the challenge of completing a BMedSci project within the five-year course
Requirements	**UCAT**; **A level** three including chemistry and biology; **GCSE** six Grade 7/As and Grade 6/B in English

Course length	5 years	Structure	Campus
Type of course	Red brick	Year size	206
Typical offer	AAA	Intercalated degree	BMedSci (compulsory)
Applicants	2,179	Student mix:	
Interviews	1,000	% Mature	3%
Offers	628	% International	12%

Uncompetitive	Competitive
Low living costs	High living costs
Working really hard	Not working/chilling out

Contact details	Faculty of Medicine and Health Sciences, University of Nottingham Medical School, Queen's Medical Centre, Nottingham, NG7 2UH Tel: +44 (0) 115 823 0000, Web: www.nottingham.ac.uk

An insider's view ...

Nottingham has a high number of applicants and so attracts outstandingly able students onto both its A level and graduate-entry course. The interviews are designed to select the best communicators and most vocationally motivated students. Our teaching philosophy is to put the patient at the centre of the student's learning, with clinical experience from week one. The integrated BMedSci degree provides an opportunity for the more scientifically minded student to excel. Although our course is tough and very competitive, Nottingham is a friendly place of learning, nurturing the lifelong skills required to be a good doctor.

Oxford

If you're going to study medicine, where better than the place where doctors first discovered the living cell, understood the circulatory system, or treated patients with penicillin?

University Medicine at Oxford goes back over 700 years, so they must be doing something right. As a collegiate university its medical students are taught both by individual colleges and the medical school. In the first three years you will feel as if you have two homes: your room in college and the Medical Sciences Teaching Centre. The latter is a modern complex with lecture theatres, laboratories, and computer suites. This alone dispels the myth that Oxford is as resistant to change as *Staphylococcus* is to antibiotics. One of the most valuable and unique aspects of the course is the weekly meetings with your college tutor, during which your essays are used as the basis of discussion. You'll have no trouble writing these as Oxford boasts the second largest library in the United Kingdom.

Course The preclinical course unashamedly focuses on the scientific basis of medicine and there is little patient contact. The course has not yet capitulated to the PBL movement embraced by other medical schools and teaching still comes from lectures, practical classes, and college tutorials. Preclinical disciplines such as physiology, anatomy, and pathology are each individually examined by short-answer and essay papers. Anatomy is taught using prosected specimens but there are full-body dissection opportunities as well. The third year revolves around a research project which you choose, and leads to a BA(Hons) degree in Medical Sciences.

After the third year, as long as you have passed everything up to that point, you can progress onto your clinical studies in Oxford, although there is the opportunity for a few students to move to London to finish their clinical training, if they wish to do so. In Oxford, teaching is based at the John Radcliffe Hospital and the surrounding district general hospitals and GP practices. The medical elective is three months long, longer than most medical schools, although by this time you'll feel as if you've earned a placement in the sun!

Lifestyle Oxford has every society known to mankind and a few others (korfball or quidditch anyone?!). The collegiate system means that you can pursue an activity casually at college level, or more seriously as part of the university team. Many students try rowing and there are dedicated novice events to help them give it a go. Osler House, the clinical students' club, offers support to students and lots of socializing opportunities. Medical students tend to live in their colleges (spread around Oxford) throughout the preclinical course, but many choose to rent houses closer to the hospital in later years. Driving is almost impossible as parking is scarce, but nothing in Oxford is more than a short cycle ride away.

Factoid Medicine at Oxford is packed with traditions. In the first year you'll be treated to 'dissection drinks' (i.e. drinks disguised as bodily fluids), while clinical medics put on an annual pantomime in which the star is invariably a pink elephant named Rita. Honestly. See Table 8.23.

Table 8.23 Oxford

Myth	Geeks safe from skin cancer as they rarely leave the Oxford spires to see daylight
Reality	Three science-intense years followed by three patient-centred years—the best of both worlds
Personality	Gifted musicians, varsity sports stars, student journalists, world debaters, or just students interested in science … anything goes!
Best aspects	The tutorial system, where you regularly get 1:2 or 1:3 teaching
Worst aspects	First- and second-year exams are awful, but almost all students pass first time
Requirements	**BMAT**; **A level** three, with chemistry and one other science or maths; **GCSE** Cs in sciences/maths if not offered at A level

Course length	6 years	Structure	Collegiate
Type of course	Stone	Year size	150
Typical offer	A*AA	Intercalated degree	BA (compulsory)
Applicants	1,792	Student mix:	
Interviews	425	% Mature	<1%
Offers	170	% International	3%

Uncompetitive 🏆 🏆 🏆 🏆 🏆	Competitive
Low living costs 💰 💰 💰 💰 💰	High living costs
Working really hard	Not working/chilling out

Contact details	Medical Sciences Office, John Radcliffe Hospital, Headington, Oxford, OX3 9DU Tel: +44 (0) 1865 285783, Web: www.medsci.ox.ac.uk

An insider's view …

The course is intended for students with a particular enthusiasm for the science that supports medicine and its continuing advancement. It provides more in-depth knowledge than you will immediately need for the clinical stage of your training and is designed to provide you with an understanding and enthusiasm for science and scientific method that will serve you well both now and later in your career.

Peninsula

Plymouth University Peninsula Medical School opened in 2002 as a joint enterprise between the University of Exeter and the University of Plymouth. In 2012 they separated into different medical schools becoming the University of Plymouth Faculty of Health and Human Sciences.

University The medical school is split across three sites in the South West of England: Plymouth, Taunton, and Torbay. Medical students spend their first two years in Plymouth before rotating for clinical placements in years three, four, and five. Plymouth has a central, city-based university with a large student population and vibrant scene; the modern campus is located close to the historic Barbican and natural seafront area of the Plymouth Hoe. The refurbished medical school has an abundance of high-quality clinical skills resources like plastic arms for practicing cannulation and even a state-of-the-art 'Anatomage Table'. There is also a university building located on the hospital grounds which is equipped with life-like simulation suites, surgical scrubbing areas, and lots of very friendly and supportive clinical educators to enhance your learning.

Course The course leaders place a heavy emphasis on patient-focused teaching, professionalism, and communication skills. Overall, staff are extremely supportive while constantly challenging you to improve and improving themselves by responding to feedback and new evidence and advances in medical education. Every year, student-selected units (SSUs) provide something a little different based on specialist interests—from attending intensive spinal surgery placements to life drawing and even sailing around Cornwall in an old tall ship, you have lots to choose from!

The first two years are preclinical, where students learn through Enquiry Based Learning ('EBL' known elsewhere as PBL) group work, which is case-based learning. This is supplemented by lectures and clinical skills sessions. Group sizes are very small and interactive, so students are well supported in their self-directed learning. There is no preclinical dissection or prosection; however, there is heavy use of radiological imaging and living anatomy which is used to improve communication with patients.

The third and fourth years are organized into 'pathway' weeks within encompassing blocks. Each week is spent studying a different specialty (e.g. respiratory), while receiving relevant block teaching from specialists. Short placements do result in a loss of continuity as students move departments so often, but it also means there is an unrivalled spectrum of specialists to learn from. For every rotation you are guaranteed a clinical reasoning session with a specialist consultant or registrar. The fifth year is spent rotating (every six weeks) through preferred specialties, working closely with and learning how to become a foundation doctor. This includes a medical elective which you can take anywhere in the world! An intercalated BSs/MSc is available between the fourth and fifth years for the top 15% of each year, based on medical school exam grades.

Lifestyle Accommodation is easily available and first years are all guaranteed rooms in university halls. Students at Peninsula are surrounded by the beautiful Dartmoor countryside and gorgeous South West Coastline. It's not unusual to wake up in the morning, smell the sea air, hear the seagulls, and think 'I'm on holiday'. MedSoc makes the most of the beautiful countryside by organizing surf trips and camping on Dartmoor, and you can even try expedition medicine courses!

Factoid A 30-minute drive from any locality will get you to a beach suitable for surfing, sunbathing, or Dartmoor, the largest national park in England! See Table 8.24.

Table 8.24 Peninsula

Myth	BM BS—Bachelor of Mooching, Bachelor of Surfing
Reality	A fresh, new, innovative medical school, not afraid to train doctors a little differently … and allow time for some surfing
Personality	Reflective and compassionate
Best aspects	Being taught by doctors, not scientists—everything you learn is clinically relevant
Worst aspects	The location is a double-edged sword; quite far away from … everywhere else
Requirements	**UCAT**; **A level** three including biology and chemistry, physics, maths, or psychology; **GCSE** seven Grade 4/Cs including English, maths, and science

Course length	5 years	Structure	Campus
Type of course	Carbon fibre	Year size	156
Typical offer	A*AA—-AAA (AAB for widening access participants)	Intercalated degree	BSc
Applicants	1,679	Student mix:	
Interviews	1,024	% Mature	10%
Offers	476	% International	4%

Uncompetitive		Competitive
Low living costs		High living costs
Working really hard		Not working/ chilling out

Contact details	Peninsula Medical School, The John Bull Building, Tamar Science Park, Research Way, Plymouth, PL6 8BU
	Tel: +44 (0) 1752 437 444, Web: www.pcmd.ac.uk

An insider's view …

Peninsula offers an exciting and challenging undergraduate medical programme, which is forward-thinking and focused on patients and improving health. It offers an integrated, clinically-led curriculum that promotes meaningful interactions with patients from an early stage. The curriculum emphasizes activity-based, structured, small-group learning methods and learning in the clinical environment and from patient encounters, coupled with extensive support for independent learning. Students develop an integrated knowledge and understanding of the sciences, of clinical, communication, and leadership skills, and of personal and professional values that underlie safe and effective medical practice.

Sheffield

Sheffield has been nicknamed the 'largest village in England'. Despite being a lesser-known city, Sheffield is well connected, with Leeds and Manchester less than an hour away by train, and London a mere two hours away. With over 60,000 university students, new students are unlikely to feel isolated in this city. The thriving student community also means that the past image of an industrial town is rapidly developing into that of a vibrant, up and coming city.

University The medical school is part of The Royal Hallamshire Hospital, one of two major teaching hospitals in the city. Sheffield Teaching Hospitals NHS Trust have a strong research base, with world-leading research in neurology and orthopaedics. Several smaller hospitals are also used for teaching and a car is often necessary to reach these clinical placements. The medical school has an on-site Health Sciences Library and café. Other university libraries are a 10-minute walk away and remain accessible 24/7 for those inevitable late-night cramming sessions.

Course The preclinical course is based on physiological symptoms and integrates problem-based learning with key elements of traditional 'chalk and talk' teaching methods. This hopefully means everyone finds a mode of teaching which appeals to them. Clinical experience is introduced from the first semester and all second-year students undertake a six-week research attachment. Anatomy is a well-taught part of the course, utilizing human cadavers. There are no January exams for the first two years, and so everything is tested in June; leaving Christmas relatively stress-free but also leaving you unable to benchmark yourself against the year group before the summer exams. Formal teaching by the medical school is complemented by peer-led sessions in which senior students help teach those in earlier years. Clinical training begins in the summer of the second year, focusing on history taking and examination-related skills. Sheffield is unique in permitting students two seven-week electives. Sheffield have reflected the growing popularity of intercalated degrees by offering many research-based BMedSci or Master's projects. If none of these take your fancy, there is the option of doing a BSc degree in another university. With one of the highest student to foundation doctor retention rates, once you've tried this city you'll never want to leave!

Lifestyle There is no shortage of things to do in the 'steel' city! The number of student opportunities is only limited by your imagination. Whether you're interested in sports, theatrics, or volunteering, you'll find something of interest. As well as university-run societies, medics also have their own sports teams and societies, created to work around the medical teaching timetable. Activities include a legendary bar crawl, annual ball, and medics' ski trip. With the Peak District only 20 minutes away, students have the best of city and country life on their doorstep. Particular highlights include shopping at Meadowhall Centre, catching a performance at the world-famous Crucible Theatre, a trip to the busy West Street (with more bars than streetlights), or a Saturday night out in the legendary Pop Tarts (surely the best student union in the country!).

Factoid Although Oxford (see p. 170) claims to have used penicillin first, they were actually beaten by a Sheffield pathologist nine years earlier—keep up guys! See Table 8.25.

Table 8.25 Sheffield

Myth	Shabby town, decent training … but you probably wouldn't …		
Reality	Reliable, quality clinical education and a social life to match—you probably should …		
Personality	Simply banterful		
Best aspects	Full cadaveric dissection and the opportunity to go on elective twice		
Worst aspects	Longer term times than other medical school means less time to spend sunbathing in the summer		
Requirements	**UCAT**; **A level** three including chemistry or biology and at least one other science; **GCSE** five Grade 7/As with Grade 6/B in English language, maths, and at least one science		
Course length	5 years	Structure	Campus
Type of course	Red brick	Year size	306
Typical offer	AAA	Intercalated degree	BMedSci
Applicants	2,350	Student mix:	
Interviews	1,300	% Mature	7%
Offers	800	% International	6%
Uncompetitive	🏆 🏆 🏆 🏆 🏆		Competitive
Low living costs	💰 💰 💰 💰 💰		High living costs
Working really hard			Not working/chilling out
Contact details	The Medical School, University of Sheffield, Beech Hill Road, Sheffield, S10 2RX Tel: +44 (0) 114 271 3349, Web: www.sheffield.ac.uk		

An insider's view …

The Sheffield curriculum's integration of medical sciences and clinical medicine is important in successful learning, and we promote the acquisition of basic clinical skills from the very beginning of the course through contact with patients. We have a very well-developed programme that utilizes patients as educators, and this is founded on the belief that patients are valid and reliable assessors of students' professional behaviours and clinical skills. We combine traditional teaching methods of lectures and bedside teaching with a longitudinal thread of problem-based learning.

▌ Southampton

If you want sun and sea without studying in the Caribbean, perhaps you should look closer to home. Although medicine in Southampton spans decades rather than centuries, the medical school has achieved a reputation for its atmosphere and interactive course.

University The medical school is based in Southampton General Hospital where facilities include two large lecture theatres, smaller seminar rooms, a large library, clinical skills rooms, numerous computer suites, and a cafeteria. Students are based in the separate 'Academic Block', but this proximity to wards means exposure to hospital life from day one. Despite years four and five being taught mainly in the Academic Block, teaching is initially split between the South Academic Block and Highfield campus (which are within walking distance of each other). Once on campus, students can use all the university facilities, from the Hartley Library to the Jubilee Sports Centre.

Course Southampton is renowned for pioneering the interactive, hands-on approach to medical education. This structure has been adapted by other medical schools (such as Brighton and Sussex Medical School and Cardiff University) with great success. Medical students meet patients weekly from the first few weeks of the programme through units called Medicine In Practice (MIP). Students gain experience in both hospital and general practice, which reinforces teaching from lectures as well as allows them to learn practical skills (e.g. examinations, history taking). The course begins with two preclinical years in which basic sciences (e.g. anatomy, biochemistry) are structured according to major physiological systems (e.g. cardiovascular). Students can also select modules to learn about medical humanities, foreign languages, and research. Teaching is a mixture of lectures, seminars, tutorials, and prosection practicals. The main clinical component of the course begins in year three. Students spend year four studying an area of interest in depth, with many choosing to pursue an intercalated degree, most commonly between years three and four. In common with many medical schools, Southampton students are sent far and wide, such as Portsmouth and Winchester, with the option to go to Jersey in the final year. This range of hospitals means the student to doctor ratio is kept low and you won't find yourself as one of ten students attached to a single firm.

Lifestyle The medical student cliché 'work hard, play hard' is certainly apparent in Southampton. The university famously boasts 300 societies, within which there are sports (from kite surfing to extreme ironing!), volunteer work, and theatrical and musical groups. Some medical students find their timetables are not always compatible with these activities (despite every Wednesday afternoon being free in the first three years), hence the creation of unique medical clubs. These include everything from medics' netball, hockey, and rugby to the choir, and a host of other volunteering groups. Medic groups are a great opportunity to meet students from other years, compete against other medical schools, and take time out from life on the wards. If you're looking for places to escape to, how about half an hour's drive to 375 square kilometres of New Forest National Park or a short ferry ride across to the Isle of Wight?

Factoid The university has grown from just 700 students in 1862 to over 20,000 students spread across seven campuses today. See Table 8.26.

Table 8.26 Southampton

Myth	A student beach holiday, funded by the taxpayer		
Reality	A structured, time-intensive course, with no rules against studying on the beach		
Personality	Fun, friendly, and outward-looking		
Best aspects	Patient contact from day one—daunting but the best way to learn		
Worst aspects	An incredibly exam-orientated course		
Requirements	**UCAT**; **A level** three including chemistry and biology; **GCS**E six Grade 7/As including maths and science, and Grade 6/B in English.		
Course length	5 years	Structure	Campus
Type of course	Plate glass	Year size	205
Typical offer	AAA	Intercalated degree	BSc
Applicants	3,000	Student mix:	
Interviews	-	% Mature	Unknown
Offers	350	% International	7.5%
Uncompetitive			Competitive
Low living costs			High living costs
Working really hard			Not working/chilling out
Contact details	Southampton General Hospital, Tremona Road, Southampton, SO16 6YD Tel: +44 (0) 2380 796 586, Web: www.som.soton.ac.uk		

An insider's view ...

The School of Medicine is committed to the highest quality of provision in pursuit of excellence in biomedical sciences and clinical research. We have a reputation for academic excellence in all aspects of teaching and research. Should you wish to study basic science or clinical research, the School of Medicine in Southampton will give you a great environment in which to develop your skills and provide the foundation upon which to build an exciting research career.

University of East Anglia (UEA)

Whilst Norwich Medical school at UEA is relatively new, it has already established itself as a highly reputable medical school, and a great place to study.

University The UEA campus is located about two miles west of Norwich city centre. Set in over 300 acres of parkland, it is the perfect blend of city and student life. There is a fantastic clinical skills lab, study space, and lecture theatre located at the Bob Champion Building, close to the main teaching hospital (Norfolk and Norwich), which is a 10-minute walk from the campus-based medical school. PBL and seminars take place on campus. Each lecture/seminar and PBL rooms are fully equipped with all you need for a great learning environment. Most teaching staff are located in this same building and readily available for any queries. The ground floor consists of the all-important 'student social space' with microwaves, vending machines, and hot- and cold-water facilities.

Course The course is delivered in system-based modules, with each being followed by module-specific secondary-care placement. During the campus-based teaching, your 'typical' learning week will be based around a presentation or condition relevant to the module and covered through lectures, seminars, anatomy workshops (dissection), and GP placement. Perhaps the most distinguishing feature of UEA is its strong emphasis on clinical attachments. From week one in the first year students have hands-on contact with patients in both primary and secondary care. This gives you, as a student, a great insight into conditions, on-the-job experience, and help to develop communication skills. Secondary-care placements are primarily at Norfolk and Norwich Teaching Hospital, as well as two district hospitals for which transport is provided. In later years, the opportunity arises for residential placements from Northampton to Southend-on-Sea, where transport and accommodation are also provided.

UEA makes the most of PBL, a student-centred learning style based on group activity (of 8–10 students), with clinical scenarios as the focal point. Collaboratively, you construct the week's learning outcomes, dividing them between yourselves, and producing a write-up and presentation. In parallel to clinical-based teaching, there are opportunities to conduct research, undertake audits, and study topics which particularly interest you, which help you develop lifelong learning skills. Either after the third or fourth year, UEA offers the opportunity for you to intercalate and pursue Masters degrees, including in clinical education, research, molecular medicine, cognitive neuroscience, and health economics. Intercalating provides the chance to focus on an interest, publish work, and gain points towards your foundation year.

Lifestyle On-campus accommodation is only guaranteed for the first year of study. UEA has a variety of excellent halls, some with en-suite rooms. The iconic Ziggurats have incredible views over the lake to watch the sunrise/set. The city of Norwich itself is a mixture of culture and entertainment, against the beautiful backdrop of countryside and coast. The Sainsbury's Centre for Visual Arts holds famous works by Henry Moore and Francis Bacon. The prestigious Large Common Room (LCR) and Waterfront venues are run by the UEA student union and attract massive touring bands and artists, having previously featured Coldplay, Ed Sheeran, and the Red Hot Chilli Peppers. UEA boasts a multi-million-pound 'Sportspark' offering a 50-metre swimming pool, gym, 400-metre athletics track, indoor climbing wall, and gymnastics centre, all available at discounted student rates.

Factoid The Sainsbury's Centre, an art gallery and museum on UEA's campus, is the Marvel Avengers headquarters. See Table 8.27.

Table 8.27 University of East Anglia (UEA)

Myth	All smiles and no brains		
Reality	New, exciting course producing doctors who cure and care		
Personality	Outgoing, down-to-earth team players		
Best aspects	Sports, societies, and events outside of medicine help maintain an important work–life balance		
Worst aspects	The large number of assessments that must be completed after every module		
Requirements	**UCAT**; **A level** three including biology or chemistry; **GCSE** six Grade 7/As including maths and science		
Course length	5 years	Structure	Campus
Type of course	Carbon fibre	Year size	208
Typical offer	AAB	Intercalated degree	BSc or MRes
Applicants	1,400	Student mix:	
Interviews	1,000	% Mature	10%
Offers	600	% International	5%
Uncompetitive	🏆 🏆 🏆 🏆 🏆		Competitive
Low living costs	💰 💰 💰 💰 💰		High living costs
Working really hard			Not working/chilling out
Contact details	The Undergraduate Admissions Office, Norwich Medical School, Faculty of Medicine and Health Sciences, University of East Anglia, Norwich, NR4 7TJ. Tel: +44 (0)1603 591515, Web: www.uea.ac.uk/medicine		

An insider's view ...

Studying medicine at UEA will be exciting and rewarding. Medicine is ever-changing and constantly fascinating. The people you will meet—students, academics, clinicians, as well as the many patients you will see—make medicine a special course and a wonderful, if demanding, career. The five years of your course will fly by! Make the most of the opportunities to learn; work with your colleagues; plan your elective and consider an intercalated degree. Do also make time to enjoy yourself outside medicine by participating in sports or clubs, and time with friends.

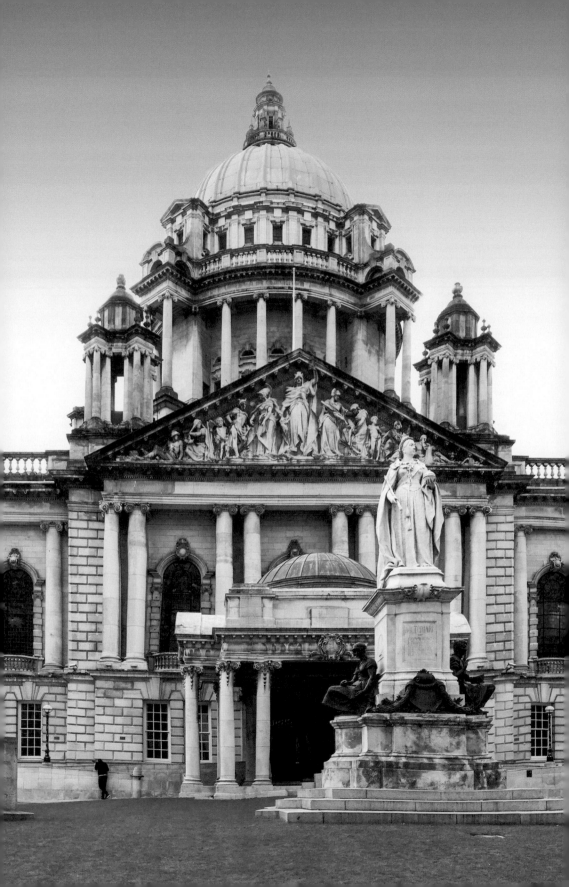

Northern Ireland

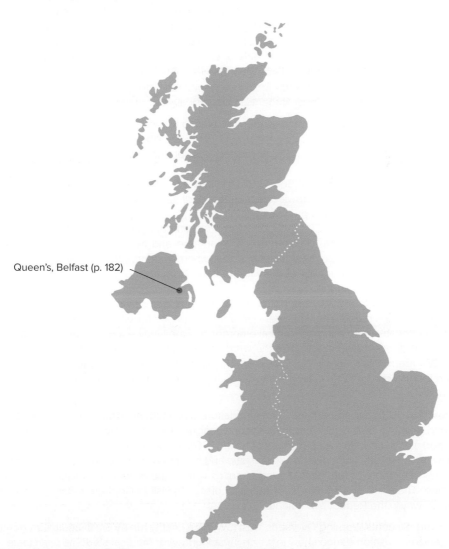

Queen's, Belfast (p. 182)

Figure 8.2 Undergraduate medical schools in Northern Ireland.

Queen's, Belfast

Belfast is a very up and coming city with a big personality, and Queen's University Belfast (QUB) is one of its cornerstones. It is a progressive university with strong leadership and vision for the future, so much so that it was awarded 'Entrepreneurial University of the Year' in 2009. Over the past five years there has been a growing number of students from outside of Northern Ireland and a diverse range of different nationalities entering QUB.

University The first two years are based at the Medical Biology Centre (MBC) on the university campus, which is a 15-minute walk from the city centre. The campus itself has numerous facilities including a new library, and is in the process of building a new, state-of-the-art students' union. There is also a not-for-profit shop, various cafes, and bars. including the speakeasy bar, all within a short walk of each other. Clinical teaching takes place at 14 different hospitals; six of these are within 10 miles of the university (the others are 19 to 83 miles from campus) and all offer free accommodation. The majority of hospitals can be reached by bus; however, most students in the clinical years do have a car.

Course The medical curriculum has been updated to reflect how healthcare priorities and delivery is changing both locally and internationally. Healthcare systems are developing stronger emphases on primary and secondary care partnerships, and on prevention and population health.

During years one and two students build the basics for their practice through a systems-based approach, with core knowledge taught through lectures and practicals—QUB has a great anatomy centre which provides anatomy teaching through full cadaveric dissection. Early clinical contact and CBL group work ensures students are consistently linking their scientific knowledge with clinical practice. Years one and two provide a foundation for practice which leads into years three and four when students are immersed in practice. In the clinical years, students begin with rotations in medicine and surgical specialties. The fourth year follows the cycle of life through paediatrics, obstetrics, mental wellbeing, and care of the elderly. A quarter of clinical practice is in the primary care setting, spread throughout the course. The final year is all about preparing for practice: ensuring students feel comfortable managing the clinical emergencies they may encounter as a new doctor. The GMC licensing exam will form the written finals at the end of year four and the final OSCEs are in February of the final year. This is followed by the assistantship, working with foundation doctors—aiming to make the transition from student to foundation doctor seamless.

Lifestyle QUB now guarantees accommodation to all students since the construction of brand-new city-centre halls. From the second year, most students move to cheap, privately rented accommodation which ranges between £200 and £300 a month, the cheapest cost of living in the UK. The social life is fantastic and has really developed within the last few years, with plenty of reasonably priced bars as well as more upmarket places in the city centre. There are also hundreds of beautiful places to visit in Northern Ireland or a short drive away in the Republic of Ireland.

Factoid Students Working Overseas Trust (SWOT), a charity run by QUB medical students, organizes a fashion dance show in which most fourth-year medical students participate. It usually raises over £50,000 a year which is taken to hospitals in the developing world by students on their electives. See Table 8.28.

Table 8.28 Queen's, Belfast

Myth	Narrow-minded locals who aren't adventurous enough to study further from home
Reality	QUB offers every possible opportunity for adventure and broadening your horizons, regardless of how far you are from home
Personality	Friendly students who are always up for having 'craic', but always apply themselves when the crucial time comes
Best aspects	Exposure to patients from early on in the first year; the huge selection of clubs and societies; the long holidays; the cheap cost of living
Worst aspects	Large tutor groups (eight to ten students); and it can feel separate from other medical schools in the UK
Requirements	**UCAT**; **A level** three A2s including chemistry and at least one other science or maths, and AS biology; **GCSE** must include Grade 4/Cs in maths and physics or double award science

Course length	5 years	Structure	Campus
Type of course	Red brick	Year size	262
Typical offer	A*AA–AAAa	Intercalated degree	BSc or MSc
Applicants	1,300	Student mix:	
Interviews	700	% Mature	27%
Offers	500	% International	10%
Uncompetitive		Competitive	
Low living costs		High living costs	
Working really hard		Not working/chilling out	
Contact details	School of Medicine, Queen's University Belfast, 73 University Road, Belfast, BT7 1NN Tel: +44 (0) 289 024 5133, Web: www.qub.ac.uk/mdbs		

An insider's view ...

Queen's Belfast is unique in that it is the only medical school in Northern Ireland. Although it has educated doctors who work on all five continents, many of its alumni work within the health service in Northern Ireland. As a result there is a strong family atmosphere with good relationships between hospital doctors, general practitioners, and the medical school. These deep loyalties facilitate and ensure that our students are welcomed and well taught and, as a consequence, many of our students complete their foundation training in Northern Ireland. Students who are outgoing, flexible, keen to participate in and embrace the experiences offered, and who can balance work and social life adapt well to our course.

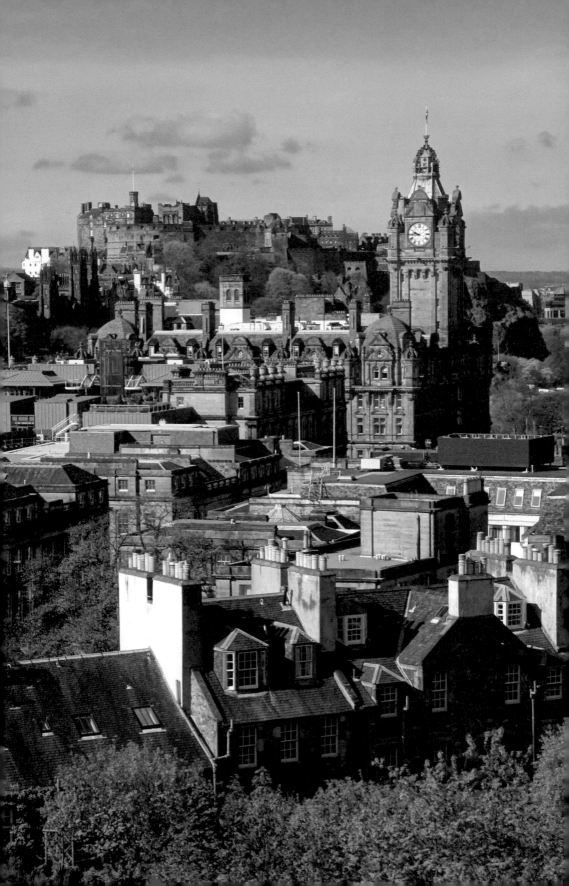

Scotland

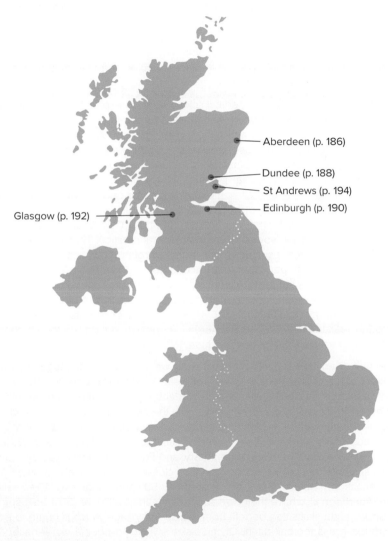

Aberdeen (p. 186)

Dundee (p. 188)

St Andrews (p. 194)

Edinburgh (p. 190)

Glasgow (p. 192)

Figure 8.3 Undergraduate medical schools in Scotland.

▌Aberdeen

Founded in 1495, the University of Aberdeen has a long and rich history of medical dis-covery and innovation. Students in Aberdeen have the opportunity to study medicine in a thriving medical school which is consistently ranked highly in both Scotland and the UK.

University The first three years take place in the purpose-built Suttie Centre, which houses a lecture theatre, IT suite, anatomy teaching area, and clinical skills centre. The Foresterhill Health Campus is home to Aberdeen Royal Infirmary, Aberdeen Maternity Hospital, and the Royal Aberdeen Children's Hospital, which gives students early access to experienced teachers who are experts within their specialty. In years 4 and 5, the clinical years, all stu-dents undertake a remote and rural placement which will see you spend some time in Raigmore Hospital in Inverness. However, you may also have the chance to experience unique opportunities even further afield in places such as Fort William, the Western Isles, or even Orkney and Shetland!

Course After a term of lectures in medical sciences, disease processes, and clinical skills, systems-based teaching begins with clinical cases to enhance learning. This means you are taught about the appropriate anatomy, physiology, and biochemistry of each of the body systems as well as the disease processes. Students are then able to begin to rec-ognize symptoms and appreciate what investigations and treatments to use. Early patient contact begins from the start of year 1 with 'patient partners'. This allows you to explore patients' symptoms and perform clinical examinations for each of the systems studied in a safe and monitored environment before starting your clinical attachments, which begin in the second term of year 1. The Foundations of Primary Care course also begins in the first year and introduces the specialist area of general practice. This aims to generate an appreciation of the physical, psychological, and social roles of humans as individuals within the setting of society, with particular reference to health. In addition, SSCs are integrated into the course and allow students to work in small groups on a chosen topic. Students are allowed to take time out of their medical studies and choose from a wide range of subjects including art, languages, and teaching. Aberdeen also offers students the chance, after the third or fourth year, to pursue a particular area in depth whilst studying for a further qualifi-cation at undergraduate (BSc) or postgraduate (MSc) level.

Lifestyle Aberdeen itself is a vibrant coastal city with a thriving local economy which can satisfy every cultural taste. Here you will find plenty of shopping opportunities, museums, art galleries, and concert halls. With a large student population (there are two universities within the city), there is also a lively nightlife, with the city having received several awards for safety in the city centre. Halls of residence are available for all first-year students at Hillhead Student Village on the main university campus. A free shuttle bus is available be-tween the Hillhead Student Village, the library, and Foresterhill. However, by the second year, most students rent private accommodation closer to the medical campus.

Aberdeen Student Union Association boasts over 50 sports clubs and 140 societies. The medics at Aberdeen also have their own social community, with over 50 medic-specific so-cieties. Sports enthusiasts can benefit from the Sports Village which is home to a full-size indoor artificial-grass football pitch, Olympic-size swimming pool, a water-based hockey pitch, and both indoor and outdoor athletic training facilities.

Factoid The world's first full-body MRI scanner was invented and built by a team at the University of Aberdeen. See Table 8.29.

Table 8.29 Aberdeen

Myth	Off the map and even further off the radar
Reality	Easily accessible via car, train, or plane … and worth getting to
Personality	Dedicated, interested, and supportive
Best aspects	The excellent standard of tutorial-based (including ward) teaching
Worst aspects	The food-stealing seagulls
Requirements	**UCAT**; **Highers** AAAAB at S5 including chemistry and at least two of biology, physics, and maths; **A level** three including chemistry and at least one of biology, physics, or maths; **NAT5/GCSE** Grade 5/C in English and maths

Course length	5 years	Structure	Campus
Type of course	Stone	Year size	208
Typical offer	**Highers:** BBB **A level:** AAA	Intercalated degree	BSc/MSc
Applicants	1,900	Student mix:	
Interviews	1,000	% Mature	30%
Offers	540	% International	8%
Uncompetitive	🏆 🏆 🏆 🏆 🏆		Competitive
Low living costs	💰 💰 💰 💰 💰		High living costs
Working really hard	🧑‍💻 🧑‍💻 🧑‍💻 🧑‍💻 🧑‍💻		Not working/chilling out
Contact details	Medical Admissions, University of Aberdeen, Polwarth Building, Foresterhill, Aberdeen, AB25 2ZD Tel: +44 (0) 1224 437923, Web: www.abdn.ac.uk/medicine		

An insider's view …

The School of Medicine and Dentistry is a vibrant part of the university with distinction in research and an impressive reputation for its teaching. The medical curriculum has been recently updated and provides a high-quality learning experience, with integration of science and clinical teaching. We have a new £21-million teaching building that provides our students with state-of-the-art facilities for learning clinical skills and anatomy. As the most northern medical school in the UK, we have a special interest in remote and rural healthcare, and our students have the option of following a 'remote and rural' track in the fourth and fifth years, with clinical attachments scattered across the Highlands and Islands. The Aberdeen programme also features a six-week student-selected option in medical humanities in year three, giving students the chance to broaden their horizons outside of medicine. Our graduates are well prepared for life as junior doctors and we take considerable pride in their progress and achievements.

Dundee

The Lonely Planet ranked Dundee in its top 10 list of places in Europe to visit, and the medical school consistently performs well in UK league tables.

University The medical school is located in Ninewells Hospital, about a 30-minute walk from the main university campus Within the medical school itself there is a library and IT suite, several teaching rooms, and two lecture theatres, along with the main social area. There is a café within the medical school as well as a clinical skills centre, where you will spend much of the first three years learning about patient examinations, consultation skills, and procedural techniques. For the first couple of months your teaching will be on the main campus, where most of the time you'll be in the Medical Science Institute (MSI), with its main lecture theatre and dissection rooms. At times you may also be placed in Perth Royal Infirmary (PRI), which is about 30 miles away but easily reached by the X7 bus (or you may be one of the lucky ones with a car). However, these trips are pretty sporadic in the first few years. In the fourth and fifth years you can be placed in hospitals throughout Scotland.

Course The course is divided into two main parts: Years 1–3 form the Systems in Practice (SIP) years, and Years 4 and 5 form Preparation in Practice (PIP). During SIP you learn about the basic science behind each body system, as well as learning in more detail about different medical conditions, how they present and how they are managed. You will also start learning clinical skills through simulation in the clinical skills centre. Teaching is structured with a mixture of lectures, tutorials, clinical skills teaching, dissection, and ward-based teaching. In Years 4 and 5 you spend your time out on clinical placements, putting the theory you've learned during the first three years into practice. These can be in various hospitals throughout Scotland and will include at least two GP placements as well. The main final exams are taken at the end of the fourth year, which gives you more of a relaxed fifth year to really get to grips with clinical skills before you start working. At some point in Year 5 you will also undertake an eight-week medical elective, with common destinations including Australia, New Zealand, and South Africa.

Throughout the five years you will undertake several SSCs, where you will get to have some choice over optional modules to take, which may be a specialty that you're particularly interested in or an area you want to learn more about. There is also the option to undertake an intercalated honours degree between the third and fourth years, with several different courses available to choose from.

Lifestyle First years generally live in one of the student halls. Heathfield and Belmont are right on campus, Seabraes is about a five-minute walk from campus, and West Park is halfway between Ninewells and the main campus. Most choose to stay on campus as it is next to the union, gym, and main library, as well as being five minutes from the town centre. From the second year onwards, students generally rent private accommodation in the West End and city centre, which is significantly cheaper than most other places in the UK. Dundee is nice and compact, so nothing is ever too far away, and there's a big student population, so the place really feels like your own.

Factoid Dundee University Medical School is the origin of the internationally used, and widely feared, Objective Structured Clinical Examination (OSCE). See Table 8.30.

Table 8.30 Dundee

Myth	Dundee students do more self-reflecting than their bathroom mirror		
Reality	A course that teaches you to manage patients instead of pathology and disease		
Personality	Relaxed and friendly		
Best aspects	Clinical experience right from the start; first-hand experience with patients on the wards earlier on than most other medical schools		
Worst aspects	The challenging fourth year, including a research project and finals		
Requirements	**UCAT**; **Highers** five at S5 including chemistry and another science; **A level** three A2s including chemistry and another science; **GCSE** Grade 6/ Bs in biology, maths, and English if not taking A2		
Course length	5 years	Structure	Campus
Type of course	Red brick	Year size	169
Typical offer	**Highers:** AAAAB **A level:** AAA	Intercalated degree	BMSc
Applicants	1,642	Student mix:	
Interviews	668	% Mature	13%
Offers	388	% International	8%
Uncompetitive	🏆 🏆 🏆 🏆 🏆		Competitive
Low living costs	💰 💰 💰 💰 💰		High living costs
Working really hard	🪑 🪑 📖 🛋 💉		Not working/chilling out
Contact details	Medical School Office, University of Dundee Medical School, Level 9, Ninewells Hospital, Dundee, DDI 9SY Tel: +44 (0) 1382 632640, Web: www.dundee.ac.uk		

An insider's view ...

Dundee has a leading international reputation in medical education. It is home to the world-famous Clinical Skills and Cuschieri Surgical Skills Centres, both of which provide integrated skills programmes from expert clinical tutors in the undergraduate curriculum. The medical school is part of the College of Medicine, Dentistry, and Nursing, giving students the chance to learn with and about other professions working in the healthcare sector. Dundee was one of the first medical schools to work with the NHS to involve medical students in learning about patient safety. We want students from a wide variety of backgrounds who want to excel in medicine and who want to work with the school to ensure that they are aware of their own professional limits.

Edinburgh

Edinburgh's prestigious medical school is set in the heart of the beautiful capital of Scotland, in the shadow of Arthur's Seat—an extinct volcano. Despite the city's vintage, it has a modern and innovative course with an excellent international reputation for medical education and research.

University The medical school buildings are close together but span three centuries; the oldest is mostly used for preclinical teaching while the newly built Chancellor's Building, attached to the New Royal Infirmary, is the preferred location for clinical teaching. Libraries abound, with one at each hospital and a newly redeveloped central library, with a 24-hour computer lab, overlooking the popular Edinburgh Meadows. The Anatomy Resource Centre and cadaver specimens are also available for private study. The three main hospitals for clinical experience are the New Royal Infirmary, the Royal Hospital for Sick Children (both near the city centre), and Western General (two miles from the centre). A few students go to more far-flung hospitals (up to 50 miles away) which have good public transport and free accommodation.

Course The first two years follow a systems-based approach taught by lectures, problem-based learning (PBL), and tutorials that amount to two to five hours of teaching per day. Anatomy is taught using professionally prepared prosections. Alongside the medical sciences there is teaching on communication skills and psychosocial and ethical principles. Contact with patients begins in the first year, focusing on families and the elderly, whilst students attend a general practice once a week in the second year, undertaking clinical examinations (OSCEs) at the end of the year. The second-year timetable is less demanding than the first year, with more self-directed learning. All students now intercalate in their third year: options include Anatomy, Physiology, Surgical Sciences, and a variety of other courses. Selection to competitive courses is based on average academic performance in the first two years. Students can also opt to complete their intercalated degree at a university outside of Edinburgh.

Clinical teaching also follows a system-based approach in the fourth year and then a specialty-based approach (e.g. paediatrics, psychiatry) in the fifth and sixth years. The teaching is a mixture of clinic and ward-based shadowing and lectures. Throughout the course there are SSCs including a 14-week research project in the fifth year and an eight-week elective in the sixth year (often spent overseas).

Lifestyle Most first-year students live in university accommodation, including the catered Pollock Halls of residence, whilst a large number of self-catered flats are spread across the city. From the second year, most students move into privately rented flats which can be expensive. Public transport networks are widespread and easy to use for both university commitments and for getting home at night. Outside of university there is Edinburgh's renowned cultural high life, including castles, theatres, galleries, festivals, and, of course, the 'Fringe'. The surrounding area is also stunning, with beaches, hills, mountains, and even skiing.

Factoid Infamous body-snatchers Burke and Hare sold exhumed bodies to Edinburgh Medical School in the early nineteenth century. Ironically, Burke's body was donated to the medical school after his hanging: his skeleton is still on show today. See Table 8.31.

Table 8.31 Edinburgh

Myth	Little England—there are so many English students you'll be lucky to even meet a Scot		
Reality	A great mix of pleasant and multi-talented students from throughout the UK and across the globe		
Personality	Professional, competitive, but always helpful		
Best aspects	Internationally renowned professors and world-class research; student selected components/research opportunities; self-directed learning		
Worst aspects	Incredibly variable level of feedback on exam performance		
Requirements	**UCAT**; **Highers** five at S5 including chemistry and two of biology, mathematics, or physics; **A level** three A2s including chemistry and one of biology, maths, or physics		
Course length	6 years	Structure	Campus
Type of course	Stone	Year size	212
Typical offer	**Highers:** AAAAB **A level:** AAA	Intercalated degree	BSc or BMedSci
Applicants	2,551	Student mix:	
Interviews	Graduates only	% Mature	5%
Offers	537	% International	10%
Uncompetitive	🏆 🏆 🏆 🏆 🏆		Competitive
Low living costs	💰 💰 💰 💰 💰		High living costs
Working really hard			Not working/chilling out
Contact details	College of Medicine and Veterinary Medicine, The University of Edinburgh, The Chancellor's Building, 49 Little France Crescent, Edinburgh, EH16 4SB Tel: +44 (0) 131 242 6407, Web: www.ed.ac.uk		

An insider's view ...

Edinburgh—as all UK medical schools—is required to select those with the greatest aptitude for medical studies from those with high academic ability. It measures academic ability not only through examination grade achievements but also the UCAT aptitude test, and gives equal weighting in selection for appropriate personal qualities, career exploration, and all other forms of non-academic achievement.

Glasgow

Glasgow Medical School is a particularly Scottish institution, almost as famous as deep-fried Mars Bars and 'Auld Lang Syne'.

University In earlier years of the course, most vocational and PBL teaching takes place in the purpose-built Wolfson Medical School Building, which is found in the heart of Glasgow's vibrant West End. To compliment the objectives of the new integrated curriculum, it boasts its own PBL rooms, communication skills areas, clinical skills suite, seminar rooms, and a library with 24-hour access for medical students—perfect for last-minute crammers.

Opened in 2014, the Queen Elizabeth Teaching and Learning Centre houses the ultimate training environment for later years. It offers state-of-the-art teaching facilities and a Clinical Innovation Zone, with the ability to use modern DNA sequencing techniques! The café will cater for your desperately needed hourly coffee.

Starting from day one, clinical teaching occurs across 25 teaching hospitals and around 200 GP practices throughout the west of Scotland. Most students do not own a car early on, and thus depend on Glasgow's extensive public transport network.

Course In recent years, Glasgow boldly opted to end its traditional preclinical/clinical medical course and embark on a new, innovative curriculum.

Early on in the course, the majority of the knowledge is imparted through PBL sessions which take place twice every week. These are complemented by lab classes and lectures. Clinical skills sessions also commence during this time, with visits to hospital wards and GP practices for students to start practicing their skills; some even have a go at diagnosis and simple procedures and investigations.

In years one and two, weekly vocational studies sessions are also held in which GPs lead tutorials so students learn the communication skills, attitudes, and values expected of them as doctors. For the second half of the course, students are based in local hospitals and progress through 10 five-week clinical attachments.

The course follows a 'spiral curriculum' where content is revisited at different stages with increasing depth and clinical focus.

A total of three five-week SSCs are undertaken to personalize one's learning experience. Students inclined towards an intercalated degree can apply for one after their third year, although entry is competitive. Glasgow students also enjoy two short (four-week) electives, at the end of year three and again after year four, with many choosing to complete their elective overseas, making it an enjoyable yet beneficial experience.

Lifestyle Students mainly live in the city's West End. In their first year, most students live in halls of residence, which are shared with students from other faculties. This raises the possibility of meeting people whose life does not centre on a circuit of hospitals. Glasgow has two student unions, each with its own style and regular followers. The university sports centre is on campus and £15 a month buys students unlimited access to state-of-the-art facilities, 53 sports clubs, and over 100 exercise classes per week. If only the curriculum left more time to enjoy them!

Factoid The University of Glasgow was founded in 1451 is often considered to be the 4th oldest university in the English-speaking world. See Table 8.32.

Table 8.32 Glasgow

Myth	Famous for the booze, less famous for medicine		
Reality	A highly reputable institution providing a modern curriculum of PBL, labs, and lectures to produce competent doctors of the future		
Personality	Sociable hard-workers who aren't afraid to let their hair down		
Best aspects	Small-group work, allowing you to meet lots of new people		
Worst aspects	You can rarely leave home without an umbrella		
Requirements	**UCAT**; **Highers** five or six at S5 including chemistry and biology and either maths or physics; **A level** three A2s including chemistry and one of biology, maths, or physics; **GCSE** Grade 6/B in English and biology (if not taken at AS/A2)		
Course length	5 years	**Structure**	Campus
Type of course	Carbon fibre	**Year size**	282
Typical offer	**Highers:** AAAAA/ AAAABB **A level:** AAA	**Intercalated degree**	BSc
Applicants	2,063	**Student mix:**	
Interviews	859	**% Mature**	19%
Offers	543	**% International**	14.5%
Uncompetitive	🏆 🏆 🏆 🏆 🏆		**Competitive**
Low living costs	💰 💰 💰 💰 💰		**High living costs**
Working really hard			**Not working/chilling out**
Contact details	Wolfson Medical School Building, University of Glasgow, University Avenue, Glasgow, G12 8QQTel: +44 (0) 141 330 6216, Web: www.gla.ac.uk		

An insider's view ...

In Glasgow, we view our medical students as our future colleagues and, while we expect high standards of behaviour, we consider their well-being of paramount importance. Our students learn in a purpose-built, award-winning medical school building while still gaining early clinical experience. In years three to five, they obtain a wealth of clinical experience in 24 hospitals and ~200 general practices in the west of Scotland.

St Andrews

The golfing greens at St Andrews aren't the only courses that are world-class.

University As the third oldest university in the English-speaking world, tradition runs deep in St Andrews, with a record of hundreds of years of providing excellent medical education. Students benefit from the new medical school building opened in 2010, which lies in the heart of the science campus in North Haugh. The university is closely integrated with the small town, so you are never more than a short walk away from teaching facilities, your accommodation, or the ancient town centre. The medical school building houses all the teaching facilities you will need for your three years at St Andrews. A huge range of medical models and dissection specimens are available, and the enthusiastic staff and lecturers are always happy to discuss any questions you might have.

Course The curriculum is based around eight to ten lectures weekly, along with tutorials, laboratory sessions, clinical skills sessions, and dissection sessions to provide a foundation in the medical sciences. In the first year, tutorials are based around clinical reasoning scenarios; in the second year, around ethical dilemmas in medical practice; and in the third year, time is spent consolidating neurological structure and function. Throughout the three years at St Andrews, there are also patient communication tutorials involving both real and simulated patient interactions, often with feedback on filmed interactions. Clinical experience moves from community hospitals and GP attachments in the second year to larger hospitals, specialty attachment, and clinical reasoning in the third year, allowing plenty of experience and confidence building in patient interaction as well as history taking and examination skills. Up to 40% of a week can be taken up with clinical skills, and all lectures and teaching have a strong theme of clinical medicine.

The last term is mainly concerned with conducting a critical review or laboratory dissertation in an area of your interest. Your medical degree will not finish at St Andrews. Instead, after three years you will graduate with a BSc in Medicine, when you will be able to continue your studies at any of the other Scottish medical schools or at Manchester (see p. 164) or Barts (see p. 154) in England. This is nothing to worry about—just tick a box on applying and the universities do the rest. You will then complete your training at your chosen medical school, earning an MB ChB.

Lifestyle St Andrews is the world's smallest big town. One in three of the population has something to do with the university, so you soon feel part of a tight-knit community when walking through St Andrews. Perched on the beautiful north-east Fife coast and set next to the spectacular St Andrews golf courses (which students can learn on and play at greatly discounted rates), the wide beaches and ancient ruins provide the backdrop for spectacular library breaks, and the town is amply endowed with a large number and variety of pubs. Whilst the town does not compete with large cities for social venues, there are well over 100 student societies—from AstroSoc to Tunnocks teacake appreciation, events from techno nights and student music festivals to knitting and 'pints and politics'. St Andrews also has regular buses running to Glasgow and Edinburgh, and train links are only five minutes out of town.

Factoid The town was originally called Kilrymont (Cennrigmonaid) until St Regulus supposedly brought the remains of St Andrew to the town which would be renamed in his memory. See Table 8.33.

Table 8.33 St Andrews

Myth	Privately educated southerners too busy finding their Kate/William to enter a hospital		
Reality	Keen and friendly students in a busy social town with a particularly strong international student mix—where no one mentions the royals		
Personality	Friendly, sociable, and keen for a post-exam sea swim		
Best aspects	Dissection; close-knit student atmosphere; and the unique student lifestyle		
Worst aspects	Having to leave after three years		
Requirements	**UCAT**; **Highers** five at S5 with an A in chemistry and one of biology, physics, or maths; **A level** three A2s with an A in chemistry and one of biology, physics, or maths; **GCSE** five Grade 7/As with maths, biology, and English at Grade 5/B if not offered at AS/A2		
Course length	6 years	Structure	City
Type of course	Stone	Year size	131
Typical offer	**Highers:** AAAAB **A level:** AAA	Intercalated degree	BSc (compulsory)
Applicants	1,031	Student mix:	
Interviews	453	% Mature	3%
Offers	361	% International	15%
Uncompetitive	🏆 🏆 🏆 🏆 🏆		Competitive
Low living costs	💰 💰 💰 💰 💰		High living costs
Working really hard			Not working/chilling out
Contact details	The Bute Medical School, University of St Andrews, St Andrews, KY16 9TS Tel: +44 (0) 1334 463599, Web: medicine.st-andrews.ac.uk		

An insider's view ...

The programme at the St Andrews Medical School offers the chance to obtain two degrees for the price of one in offering everyone a BSc in Medicine as well as a MBChB at the end of the course. This is the only medical school in Scotland to do this, offering a distinct choice for students wishing to study in Scotland. By definition it offers a course strong in the basic medical sciences and one that is based on research-teaching linkages in all its aspects. Evidence base informs what is taught and students learn research skills as part of their coursework. All students undertake a research project in their final year and the teaching in the school is informed by medical education research undertaken by the staff. The school has been praised by the GMC for the strength of its anatomy teaching, which is done by full-body dissection. The school consistently comes at the top of the student satisfaction tables, which reflects the highly supportive and interactive programme on offer. The school strives to achieve the feeling of being part of one big family, which is helped by being a school of modest size based in a small country town on the east coast of Scotland.

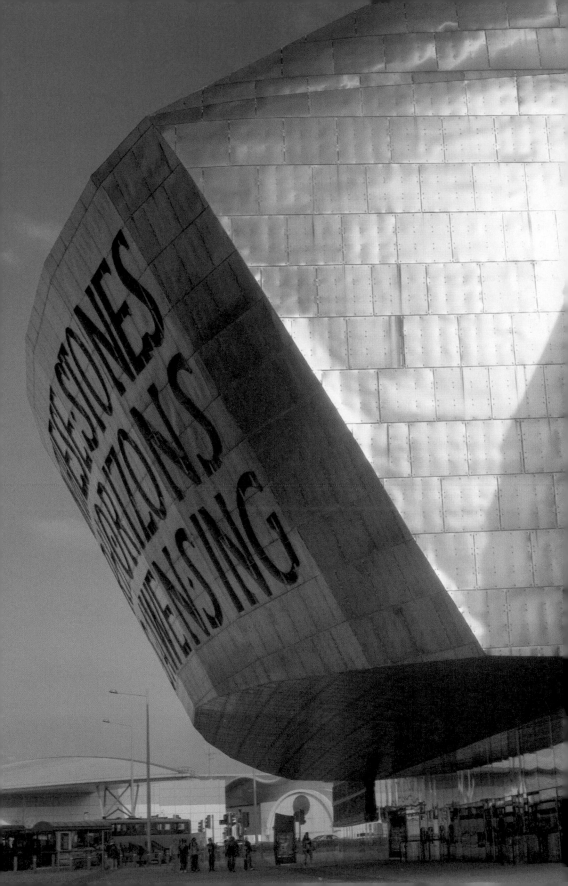

Wales

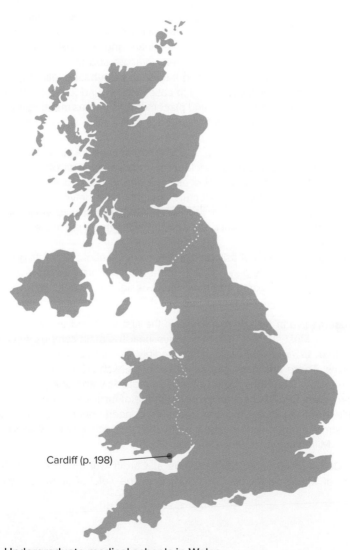

Cardiff (p. 198)

Figure 8.4 Undergraduate medical schools in Wales.

■ Cardiff

Cardiff is home to the only undergraduate medical school in Wales. It is based in a thriving cosmopolitan city just a short drive from both the Brecon Beacons and beautiful Welsh coastline.

University Cardiff is widely considered to be the most prestigious university in Wales; and with over 30,000 students, it is one of the largest academic institutions in the UK. It is also one of the largest medical schools, accepting over 300 students every year.

Course The course begins with a 'platform for clinical sciences' module which encompasses general subjects such as biochemistry and physiology taught using a range of methods including labs, workshops, group seminars and lectures. These subjects are then integrated with placements from first year interspersed throughout the year. From the second part of Year 1, students are taught through case-based learning. This involves a group of 10 students and a facilitator. Each case lasts around 2 weeks, during this time students may have associated lectures and placements as well as meeting with their group to cover key aspects of the case. Each case ends with a case wrap-up allowing the key learning points and discussion.

Intercalated degrees are available to academically successful students and take place after the third or fourth year. Options include a range of subjects offered at Cardiff and nearby universities such as Bangor. The elective period takes place at the end of the final year. The clinical course includes lectures taught at the University Hospital of Wales. Students are allocated placements in south-east Wales in the third year and across the country in the fourth and fifth years. It goes without saying that a car makes life much easier in the clinical years.

A definite highlight is the emphasis on clinical communication: students get lots of practice meeting patients and role playing early in the course. Cardiff encourage medical students to get involved in research and have many designated weeks allocated to student selected components, which students to pursue their own academic interests.

Lifestyle Students live in halls of residence in the first year and usually rent privately in subsequent years. Most students live in Cathays, near the main campus. Accommodation can cost less than £75 per week, which is incredibly favourable when compared to other university towns. There are many clubs and societies, with particularly successful teams in netball and rugby. The rugby team remains unbeaten by any other medical school for the last seven years. Cardiff offers an excellent range of facilities, as befitting a capital city. These include the usual shops, theatres, galleries, concert venues, and nightlife. There is an awesome atmosphere on international rugby days, especially when Wales play at home in their famous Millennium Stadium—definitely worth a visit!

Factoid In 2007, Professor Sir Martin Evans at Cardiff was awarded the Nobel Prize in Physiology of Medicine for his contributions to the field of stem-cell research. See Table 8.34.

Table 8.34 Cardiff

Myth	An old-school establishment favouring Welsh students
Reality	A dynamic and constantly evolving course with a broad mix of students like any other, but a friendly Welsh charm like no other
Personality	Very approachable, with a strong sense of community
Best aspects	Great lifestyle; friendly staff and students; low living costs
Worst aspects	Students can be sent anywhere in Wales for placements from the fourth year
Requirements	**UCAT**; **A level** three A2s including chemistry and biology; **GCSE** Grade 6/Bs in top nine subjects including English, maths, and sciences

Course length	5 years	Structure	Campus
Type of course	Red brick	Year size	300
Typical offer	AAA	Intercalated degree	BSc
Applicants	2,400	Student mix:	
Interviews	860	% Mature	10%
Offers	450	% International	9%

Uncompetitive		Competitive
Low living costs		High living costs
Working really hard		Not working/chilling out
Contact details	Cardiff University School of Medicine, Cardiff University, Cardiff, CF14 4XN Tel: +44 (0) 29 2074 2020, Web: http://medicine.cf.ac.uk	

An insider's view ...

These are exciting times for Cardiff University School of Medicine. The Cochrane Building provides state-of-the-art clinical skills, simulation, and library facilities for our students. And investment in new support staff and academic appointments leave us better placed than ever before to meet the demands placed on us by students, funders, and the NHS.

New UK medical schools

In an effort to expand the number of doctors working in the NHS, the government increased the number of medical school places available in the UK. This has resulted in expansions of existing medical schools, but also the emergence of new medical schools in a bid to address the workforce shortfall.

The GMC undertakes a thorough review and quality assurance process, to ensure that all medical schools (new and old) meet and maintain rigorous educational standards. Between 2017 and 2020, Buckingham (see p. 201), Central Lancashire (see p. 138), Exeter (see p. 140), Lancaster (see p. 146), and Plymouth (see p. 172) universities were approved as bodies able to award UK medical degrees. The following institutions are now in the process of establishing medical schools in the same way: Anglia Ruskin, Aston (see p. 201), Edge Hill, Kent and Medway (see p. 202), ScotGEM (a joint venture of St Andrew's (see p. 194) and Dundee (see p. 188), and the University of Sunderland.

Risk or opportunity? This should be good news for medical school applicants, as more places should mean more chances of success. Some of the new institutions are based in sought-after areas (Birmingham, London), giving you the opportunity to study medicine in attractive (and traditionally highly-competitive) locations. New medical schools are unlikely to carry institutional inertia, and may offer more adaptable up-to-date learning experiences. You might also expect newer facilities and the latest resources to aid in your training, and enthusiastic staff going the extra mile to make their new medical school a success. You will play an exciting and important role in this adventure.

While each new medical school curriculum is usually modelled on that of another institution, it is impossible to immediately replicate everything perfectly in a different location. Students at new medical schools are more likely to experience last-minute changes or logistical difficulties as the new school staff get used to training student doctors for the first time. These new medical schools often arise from less well-known universities, which might mean less infrastructure, facilities, and financial support for students. Teething problems will undoubtedly be ironed out, particularly as new courses will likely be under extra scrutiny, but this may come as little consolation if you feel that your own learning experiences are adversely affected.

Applying to a new medical school You may find it harder to learn about these courses and there may be less information available online. There might not yet be any graduates and perhaps only one or two intakes working their way through the medical school course. You might wish to reach out to these students and the admissions office, as with all other medical schools, acknowledging that the pool of individuals you can contact will be smaller.

With this in mind, you may decide to include a new medical school as one of your four UCAS choices, but think carefully, especially if applying to more than one. Attend the open days, and be sure to cast a critical eye. Which hospitals are the medical students attached to? Are these hospital doctors accommodating of students? Are you competing for clinical access with a neighbouring medical school? If new buildings and technology are being promised, will they be available for your specific intake? When does the school expect to receive GMC approval for its course, and which medical school is acting as a contingency school to ensure you will graduate with a UK medical degree?

The amount of information available for these courses will continue to increase with time, but we have included below what is currently available as of 2020.

Anglia Ruskin/Chelmsford School of Medicine

The Anglia Ruskin School of Medicine features a purpose-built £20-million state-of-the-art skills lab, GP simulation suite, anatomy suite, and lecture theatre. Teaching at Anglia Ruskin is by a systems-based approach, based on the Chelmsford campus in Essex.

In the first year, the basic underlying scientific principles of medicine are taught, including all of the underlying cardiology, gastroenterology, and respiratory system detail. Medical students are able to dissect Thiel-embalmed cadavers, aiding their understanding of anatomy with virtual dissection and 3D-printed models derived from CT scans as well as using ultrasound to apply their learning to living tissue. There is a practical laboratory component as well as some clinical exposure, and time to consolidate your knowledge independently is built into the course structure. In years 2 and 3, there are more specific teaching blocks, though significantly more time is dedicated to application of knowledge in a clinical context. Hospital placements will cover the Essex region of Basildon, Broomfield, Colchester, and Harlow, alongside various GP and community settings in the region.

Intercalation is possible between the third and fourth years. Years 4 and 5 adopt a case-based approach to learning medicine with more clinical exposure, culminating in a 'preparation for practice' block that serves to prepare graduates for their foundation post.

Anglia Ruskin require applicants to take the UCAT. A typical offer would be conditional upon attaining grades AAA at A level. Applicants who meet the criteria of their Widening Access to Medicine Scheme would receive an offer of grades ABB at A level. Graduate entrants would be expected to attain an honours degree with a minimum 2:1 classification.

The year size is ~100 students, and in the 2019/20 admissions cycle 1,185 applications were received, of which 600 were interviewed and 297 made offers. Forty per cent of the students were over 21 years old and none were international.

Buckingham Medical School

The University of Buckingham Medical School is the first independent, not-for-profit medical school in the UK, led by the Dean of Medicine, Professor Karol Sikora.

As an educational charity it does not receive any government funding, relying soley upon university fees, and hence the tuition fee of ~£37,500 per year for both home and international students alike. A tuition fee loan (e.g. £6,165 in September 2017) can be received, in addition to annual repayable maintenance loans to help towards living costs (based on household income). However, this still leaves the costs out of reach of most applicants. For those who can afford it, Buckingham provides another opportunity to study medicine in the UK if you miss out on your other offers (see also p. 325).

Buckingham Medical School opened its doors in 2015 for the first cohort of 67 students, and will now receive students at its central campus, as well as a satellite campus in Crewe. Uniquely among medical schools, Buckingham offers a four-and-a-half-year degree as opposed to the usual five-year degree. The curriculum includes a clinical skills course from the outset and ensures a string clinical component in each area of medicine from year one, with good staff to student ratios in the first two years. Teaching is modular, starting from the basic cellular biology underpinning medicine and progressing to larger organ systems. Buckingham includes a strong public health narrative in its course as well as having an emphasis on team working and pharmacology. The final part of the course Is entirely clinical and includes rotations through all of the major areas of internal medicine. These are based within Milton Keynes Hospital, as well as Bedford Hospital, St Andrew's Healthcare, and various general practices around the Buckingham area.

Students can apply directly without going via UCAS, and need at least AAB at A level (including chemistry or biology), although no admissions test is required (UCAT or BMAT). Up to five selection days are held per year, where multiple mini interviews are conducted to select successful candidates. In 2015, 250 applicants were eligible for interview and 67 offers accepted.

Edge Hill Medical School

Edge Hill Medical School is partnered with Liverpool, which is acting as its contingency school until it receives full GMC accreditation. The medical school is based in Orsmkirk (Lancashire), in between Liverpool and Manchester.

The curriculum follows a similar approach to the other new medical schools, based within its established interdisciplinary Faculty of Health, Social Care, and Medicine. The first year mainly focuses on the life sciences, with an exploration of main body systems in health. The second year places a greater emphasis on the patient and introduces students to clinical medicine in a hands-on manner. The third year emphasizes the importance of team work within medicine, exposing students to the multidisciplinary approaches to medicine through caring for specific patient groups. In the fourth year, there is a greater clinical focus for students, while the fifth year is designed entirely to prepare students for practice with a focus on acute medicine, assistantships, and a specialist placement. The university has received very high student satisfaction scores across disciplines, and has been rated as one of the safest campuses in the north west.

A level entry requirements are AAA–A*AB including chemistry and biology (if A*AB, A* must be in chemistry or biology). Five grade 6/Bs at GCSE are required including English, maths, and science. UCAT and multiple mini interviews are used as part of the selection process. A foundation-entry medicine course is also available for those meeting widening participation criteria who can enter with AAB at A level. Approximately 30 offers will be made each year.

Kent and Medway Medical School

The Kent and Medway Medical School (KMMS) opened its doors to its first cohort in 2020, basing its programme on the one used by the established Brighton and Sussex Medical School. BMBS degrees will be jointly awarded by the University of Kent and Canterbury Christ Church University, the two campuses where medical school teaching is delivered. Both campuses boast high-quality accommodation and bespoke teaching and learning facilities for medical students.

The five-year integrated programme utilizes individual patient studies to cement the science taught and introduces students to the use of an ePortfolio from an early stage—a useful addition given the prevalence of the ePortfolio in higher medical training. The first two years of the course take a systems-based approach using lectures, tutorials, clinical symposia, cadaveric dissection, e-learning, and clinical simulation. Intercalation is offered between the third and fourth years, but is not mandated. Years 3, 4, and 5 are clinically focused and predominantly based in an acute care hospital in Kent and Medway. Placements are given across the full breadth of medicine and surgery, mental health, primary care, and community services to ensure comprehensive experience for all students.

The KMMS's standard offer requires sitting the UCAT and AAB at A level (including chemistry or biology), or a 2:1 for graduate applicants. KMMS received 1,537 applications and gave 300 interviews in its first year, with a year group of ~100. Candidates eligible for widening participation may be considered for lower conditional offers of BBB.

Lincoln Medical School

Lincoln Medical School opened its doors to students in 2019. Students are registered with Nottingham University from where they will receive their award, and follow their curriculum, enhanced with a 'Lincolnshire flavour'! As a result of this, students receive lectures from academic staff at both institutes. This offers students the best of new modern Lincoln Medical School, while receiving a highly renowned Nottingham University degree.

The five-year course at Lincoln mirrors that at Nottingham, being split into preclinical and clinical phases—the initial phase focusing on the underlying science and the latter on clinical application of the same. Lincoln University boasts a brand-new anatomy teaching centre, as well as clinical skills practice spaces and established links across Lincolnshire Partnership NHS Foundation Trust sites, including Lincoln County Hospital, Grantham and District Hospital, and Pilgrim Hospital (Boston).

Lincoln require applicants to sit the UCAT and state that their usual A level offer is AAA (or AAB contextual offer) including biology (or human biology) and chemistry. Six GCSEs at grade 7/A, including science, are required. You can apply to both Nottingham University and Nottingham University (Lincoln) courses via UCAS, but will only need to be interviewed once if invited, and may receive offers from one or both. Approximately 90 places will be available.

Sunderland School of Medicine

Sunderland School of Medicine opened its doors in 2019 and is working in partnership with Keele University while the initial set of students make their way through the programme before GMC accreditation is complete.

Sunderland's five-year MBChB programme involves a PBL spiral curriculum in which basic topics are built upon, year on year, to help cement the underlying medical science. Sunderland University is unique in that it integrates medical teaching with that for pharmacists, nurses, paramedics, biomedics, and physiological scientists, allowing for tremendous interdisciplinary opportunities.

The programme focuses on providing teaching in small classes, although it also employs lectures and seminars, with a strong component of self-directed learning. Anatomy is taught using state-of-the-art anatomical models along with virtual cadaveric dissection coupled to ultrasound teaching in living tissue, and cadaveric dissection based at the Sunderland Royal Infirmary site. Sunderland boasts world-leading modern facilities, with a patient diagnostic suite, a living lab (immersive simulation room, with two seven-bedded simulation wards), and three multi-user laboratories.

The first and second years are based primarily at City campus and provide a smattering of clinical exposure along with the bulk of the preclinical science. Intercalation with an MSc is available after the second and fourth years and can be completed either at Sunderland or at another university. Years 3 to 5 are based in Sunderland and South Tyneside and are predominantly comprised of the clinical placements of the degree. Year 5 is the preparation for professional practice year and is comprised of extensive student apprenticeships. The elective gives you the opportunity to experience medicine anywhere in the world, including at Sunderland's campus in Hong Kong.

All new students are guaranteed free accommodation for the first year and half-price accommodation in Year 2.

The University offers a summer medical school for Year 12s, and year 13s undertaking a gap year. Student cohorts from under-represented groups who complete this summer school will be guaranteed an interview. See www.sunderland.ac.uk/open-days/medicine-summer-school for further details.

Applicants must sit the UCAT, and AAA are required at A level, including chemistry or biology, and five grade 7/As at GCSE, with at least a grade 6/B in English, maths, and science. Resits are taken under certain circumstances. The selection process includes a multiple mini interview and maths test, for ~50–100 places per cohort.

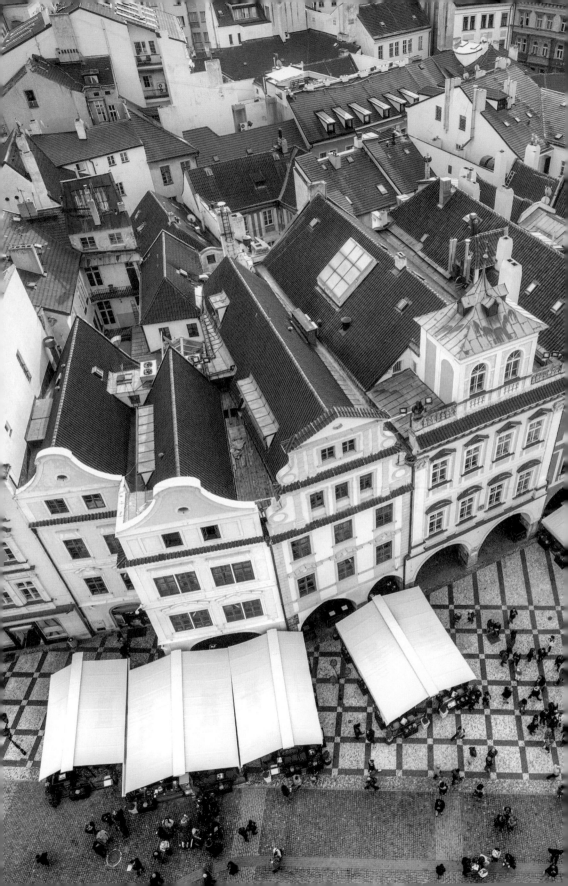

Overseas

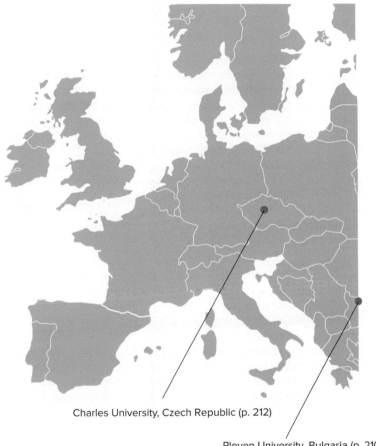

Charles University, Czech Republic (p. 212)

Pleven University, Bulgaria (p. 210)

Figure 8.5 Undergraduate medical schools overseas.

▋ Studying abroad

Applying to universities abroad has become a relatively common consideration for UK students, with increasing availability of English-taught courses across many countries. Hence the inclusion of two European medical schools as examples in this book.

Why study abroad? Many students who decide to study at international medical schools find themselves exploring these options if they haven't taken the correct choice of A levels, or have missed out on admissions criteria of their chosen UK medical schools. International medical schools are an option in these circumstances, for individuals still wishing to enter medical school without 'losing' any additional time. While the admissions criteria may be less stringent, the courses are no less work (and often more traditional (stone—see p. 102)), and you will still need to reach the same safe standard for clinical practice by the time you finish your course.

Entry requirements The entry requirements and fees vary widely across the medical schools and from country to country; the quality of online information is a good way to test the likely accessibility of each medical school for foreign students. You should follow this up with a telephone call to the admissions office. If you are considering studying abroad for up to six years, as in the UK, you should visit the medical school before making the final decision. This can often be a planned visit in conjunction with the admissions office, at which time the admissions test can also be taken. Each medical school often has its own admissions test, which does not necessarily require you to have completed any particular exams to sit it. Indeed, sitting the admissions test and receiving an unconditional offer, even prior to receiving an invitation to interview at a UK medical school, could provide you with additional confidence for these assessments and a concrete back-up plan if you don't get your UK preferences.

Practical requirements There are practical considerations when deciding if studying abroad is right for you. This includes your ability to learn a new language, because while the course may be taught in English, in order to interact with locals you will need to learn the language to a conversational standard. Visiting the medical school and speaking with existing students also allows you to gauge the standard of English used by teaching staff (often, but not always, excellent).

There is also the additional burden of travelling and living abroad. For established universities with a long history of receiving UK students, there are often student societies to support new incoming students and help them settle in. Nevertheless, leaving home and starting university can already be a stressful experience, and the added strain of doing this abroad where friends and family are a plane journey away can be too much for some. Medical students attending these universities are self-selecting; they may be mature, highly independent students, who have spent time abroad, perhaps on a gap year, or who have completed a previous degree.

Returning to practice in the UK You need to find out the success rate of qualifying students returning to practice medicine in the UK. Some UK medical schools accredit courses which are taught abroad, such as St George's University London (Cyprus) and Barts/QMUL (Malta), and are in the process of receiving GMC approval to award these as UK medical degrees in their own right (see www.gmc-uk.org). Many graduates of international medical schools will still be eligible to register with the GMC in the same way as UK graduates, with no additional barriers to jobs. With the introduction of the UK Medical Licensing Assessment (UKMLA; www.gmc-uk.org/education/medical-licensing-assessment) international students, from the 2023–24 intake onwards, will sit the new exam alongside those from UK medical schools. This should maintain equality of job opportunities at Foundation Year 1 for home and international medical graduates. That said, you may not be formally guaranteed a job like UK graduates.

Beyond Europe If you are not geographically restricted, you may want to consider options further afield, including the USA and the Caribbean (such as St George's University in Grenada, West Indies). St George's University London also have international programmes based in London and Nicosia, which can include clinical placements in Israel or North America. The application processes are unique to each school, can be competitive, and are usually eye-wateringly expensive (cumulative fees can easily surpass £250,000). That said, generous loans and scholarships are usually more readily available, and you will have easier entry into practicing within the US healthcare system after qualification, where the earning potential can be many-fold greater than for UK-equivalent doctors. The US Department of State's EducationUSA network offers students from the UK comprehensive and current information about opportunities to study at accredited universities in the USA (www.fulbright.org.uk/going-to-the-usa/undergraduate/educationusa-advice), while the Sutton Trust US programme directly supports high-achieving state-school students from low- and middle-income families across the UK to apply to, and secure funding at, top US universities (http://us.suttontrust.com).

Pleven University, Bulgaria

Bulgaria is a destination most people don't think of when looking to study medicine abroad but is definitely one that should be considered a strong contender. The degree is also recognized in the UK and Europe, allowing graduates to obtain full registration with the GMC.

University Medical University (MU)—Pleven is based in north-west Bulgaria, a two-hour drive from Sofia airport. The centre holds the da Vinci Surgical System (a robotic system that operates while controlled by a surgeon using a console), and comprises of two auditoriums with built-in audiovisual displays, as well as a library for students. There are two main public university hospitals where students spend their clinical years, as well as in the city's acclaimed state-of-the-art private hospital, Sveta Marina. The university's main faculty buildings and hospitals are easily accessible and all within walking distance of each other.

Course The academic year for the English course commences in February. Each year comprises of two semesters: February–July and September–January. The first two years of the degree are centred on preclinical basic science. Clinicals start from the third year, and the final (sixth) year is the internship, based entirely in hospital.

There are lectures and practical classes that students must attend to pass the semester and proceed to the examinations. Each student receives a student book (studentka knizhka) at the beginning of the degree that must get signed off by both the practical teacher and professor of each subject at the end of each semester. Exam grades are then recorded annually in this book. During the first three years of the course, students take compulsory Bulgarian language classes. These are extremely beneficial and of paramount importance due to the fact that patient contact is solely in Bulgarian, as most of the population of Pleven does not speak English.

Similar to Charles University in Prague (see p. 212), MU—Pleven offers the Erasmus programme to students, allowing them to travel to another country to study medicine or perform research for a semester or year.

On graduating, students will have to translate and legalize their documents in order to register with the GMC. After receiving their licences to practice, graduates can start applying for jobs, with no additional barriers compared to any UK-graduated applicant.

Lifestyle Many students choose to move into private accommodation as it is generally luxurious, spacious, and inexpensive. Students can expect to get a two-bedroom apartment within walking distance to the university, hospitals, and town centre for on average £300 a month. Student hostels are also available for a bargain price of £35 a week. Bulgaria is one of Eastern Europe's most attractive destinations, with stunning mountains and go-to ski resort. The Black Sea is another wonderful place to relax in the summer, and it is also worth seeing the breathtaking Rila Monastery (a UNESCO World Heritage Site), the seven Rila lakes, and the Belogradchik rocks. Pleven itself is a small, safe, tranquil city. Given its proximity to the border of Romania, it is easy to travel to the latter's beautiful capital, Bucharest, by car or coach. Transport is incredibly cheap, which is perfect for students who are likely to be travelling on a budget.

Factoid The main bacterium used for yoghurt production is *Lactobacillus bulgaricus,* which was first identified by Bulgarian doctor Stamen Grigorov in 1905, and is part of the normal flora of the gastrointestinal tract of mammals living in Bulgaria! See Table 8.35.

Table 8.35 Pleven University, Bulgaria

Myth	Charles University's poorer cousin		
Reality	A wonderful setting to live and study medicine for students from around the world		
Personality	Flexible and independent		
Best aspects	Ability to gain full registration and licence to practice with the GMC		
Worst aspects	Airline tickets can be expensive; and patient contact is exclusively in Bulgarian		
Requirements	Passing an admissions exam set by the university		
Course length	6 years	Structure	City
Type of course	Stone	Year size	120
Typical offer	Entrance exam	Intercalated degree	No
Applicants	500	Student mix:	
Interviews	–	% Mature	20%
Offers	300	% International	100%
Uncompetitive	🏆 🏆 🏆 🏆 🏆		Competitive
Low living costs	💰 💰 💰 💰 💰		High living costs
Working really hard			Not working/chilling out
Contact details	Medical University—Pleven 1, Sv. Kliment Ohridski Str. 5800 Pleven, Bulgaria Tel: +359 64 884 153, Web: http://www.mu-pleven.bg/index.php/en		

An insider's view ...

Medical University—Pleven offers a full-time six-year course of training in the specialty of medicine, entirely in English. The admission requirements for citizens of countries which are members of the EU/EAA are based on their achievements in the subjects of chemistry and biology at high-school level and entrance tests, organized by MU—Pleven. The university calendar is arranged so that the academic year starts in February. The students also attend classes in the Bulgarian language for the first three years in order to be able to communicate with patients in the University Hospital throughout their clinical studying and state clinical practice (internship). Our mission is to train professionals not only prepared to meet the challenges of medical science but also to realize the motto of the university—'Non sibi sed omnibus' ('Not for oneself but for all')—by instilling the value of service and ideals of humanity in our students.

Charles University, Czech Republic

With the introduction of the UKMLA in 2023, graduates of Charles University should be able to register with the GMC just as a UK graduate would be able to. Students from Charles University will take the new exam alongside graduates from UK medical schools.

University The First Faculty of Medicine is based in the heart of Prague, half an hour's drive from the main airport. Charles University has faculty buildings and teaching hospitals spread across the city, all of which are within walking distance or easily accessible via the incredibly reliable (and cheap) public transport network.

Course The first three years of the course are dedicated to the basic sciences of medicine. Subjects (including everything from pathophysiology to Latin terminology) are taught separately, rather than being systems-based, through formal lectures and practical classes. Students at Charles are encouraged to pursue independent learning; nevertheless, tutors in each subject are always available to clarify any problems that you may encounter. The Charles medical course offers cadaveric dissection to assist in anatomy teaching, as well as practical microscopy courses and autopsy demonstrations. The recently renovated faculty library provides a fantastic work space beside the ever-helpful Student Affairs Department (which is a constant source of support for administrative matters). The preclinical course also includes a medical Czech language course, which although not essential for daily life in Prague, is extremely helpful for communicating with patients during the clinical years.

The latter half of the degree is based upon clinical rotations through various medical specialties at the city's main hospitals. A typical day involves small lectures in your class group, followed by ward rounds, case studies, and training of practical skills. In the final year, you take a series of State final exams in internal medicine, surgery, paediatrics, and obstetrics and gynaecology in order to qualify as a doctor.

The Erasmus programme offers an exciting opportunity during any of the first five years to study medicine abroad and to experience the lifestyle, culture, and university life of another country in Europe. It can be undertaken preclinically (research-based) or clinically (hospital/clinic-based placement).

Most subjects end with an oral examination, which is particularly useful for professional qualifications later on in your medical career. In order to 'complete' the subject and attend the final oral examination, there are a series of small 'credit' tests throughout the semester and other requirements (such as attendance to practical classes) which help to keep you on track with studying for big exams.

Lifestyle University accommodation is available for the whole medical course, but most students choose to live in private accommodation around the city. Prague is a vibrant and exciting city with lots to do, and has a large international community of both students and professionals. The beautiful hills of the countryside surrounding Prague contrast with the historic quarters, which boast some of the most attractive architecture in the world. As the capital city, there is something to suit all tastes: pubs, restaurants, nightclubs, cafes, opera, ballet, and theatres, all at a fraction of the price in the UK. Whether sightseeing along Charles Bridge, shopping in the markets of the Old Town Square, or enjoying a walk along Petrin Hill, there's never a dull moment. Being in Central Europe also gives easy access to visit neighbouring Vienna or Berlin for weekends or to enjoy some skiing on the local slopes.

Factoid Jan Purkyne, of the Purkinje fibres of the heart and Purkinje cells in the cerebellum, graduated from Charles in 1819 and became the Head of Physiology. See Table 8.36.

Table 8.36 Charles University, Czech Republic

Myth	A last resort for those who fail to get the grades for a UK medical school		
Reality	An internationally renowned medical faculty, producing doctors who go on to practice in whichever country they choose.		
Personality	Adventurous and open-minded		
Best aspects	The degree allows registration with the GMC and professional recognition across most of the world; the opportunity to live and work in one of the finest cities in Europe, with easy and cheap opportunities to travel		
Worst aspects	You are not guaranteed an FY1 job in the NHS (although this has not been an issue in recent years); the €13,000 a year course fees, on top of travel, can make Prague expensive		
Requirements	Passing an admissions exam set by the university		
Course length	6 years	**Structure**	City
Type of course	Stone	**Year size**	120
Typical offer	Entrance exam	**Intercalated degree**	No
Applicants	1,195	**Student mix:**	
Interviews	243	**% Mature**	Unknown
Offers	150	**% International**	100%
Uncompetitive	🏆 🏆 🏆 🏆 🏆		Competitive
Low living costs	💰 💰 💰 💰 💰		High living costs
Working really hard			Not working/chilling out
Contact details	Charles University—First Faculty of Medicine, Kateřinska 32, 121 08, Praha 2, Czech Republic Tel: +420 224 961 111, Web: www.lf1.cuni.cz/en		

An insider's view ...

First Faculty of Medicine, with almost 1,200 staff members and 3,400 students, represents the largest medical faculty in the Czech Republic. It is an integral part of Charles University from its foundation by the King of Bohemia and Emperor of the Holy Roman Empire Charles the Fourth in 1348. As such, it is also the oldest medical faculty in Central Europe. Studying medicine in Prague is not only a chance to study in a beautiful and historical city that is, according to many people, the most beautiful metropolis in Europe; it is a chance to get an MD degree that is accepted in both the USA and EU.

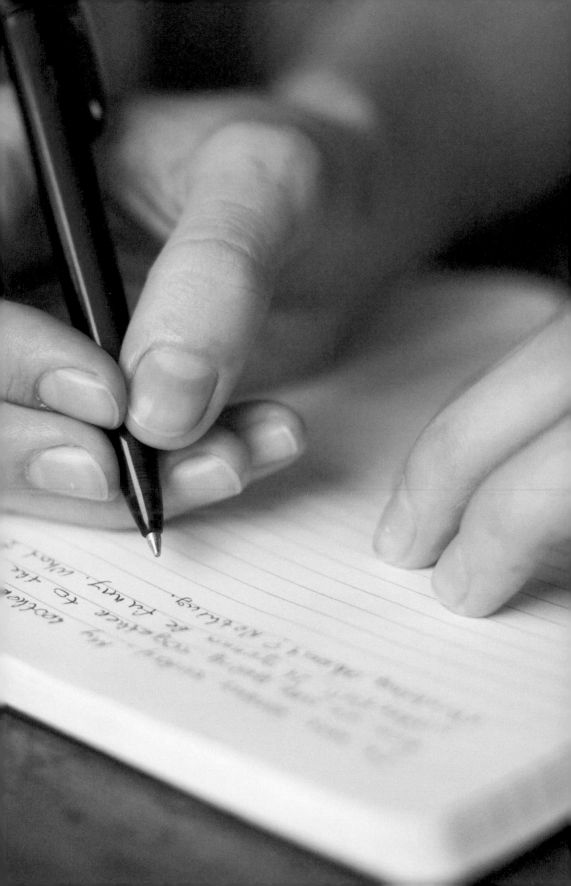

9

Perfecting the UCAS form

The UCAS application form

All applications to British medical schools are handled by the Universities and Colleges Admissions Service (UCAS), including those to graduate-entry courses (see p. 252). UCAS only permits online applications, so it is important to become familiar with the website (www.ucas.com) as early as possible.

Your passport to an interview

Your UCAS form *is* your application. It is one of the major hurdles you have to overcome to get an offer from a medical school, along with achieving excellent A levels (see p. 22), admission test (see p. 74), and the interview or assessment centre (see p. 304). Until you are invited to interview, all that the medical schools know about you is what is written on your UCAS form and your admission test results. There is limited space to make *your* application stand out, so you have to make the most of every available character.

> ### Key points
>
> The UCAS form is the culmination of all your hard work: school reference (see p. 218), predicted A levels, GCSE and AS grades, work experience, and extracurricular activities. Every word needs to support the case that you will make an excellent doctor.

Some general tips

- **Deadlines** Applications for medicine (and dentistry, veterinary science, and Oxbridge) have an earlier deadline. This is usually 15 October, but check the UCAS website to be certain.
- **Courses** Although there are five spaces on the UCAS form, you can only apply to four medical schools. The other space can be used as a backup option (i.e. a non-medical course). Biomedical science is a common choice as a backup because it prepares you outstandingly well for application to graduate-entry medicine.
- **Deferred entry** If you wish to defer your entry for a gap year (see p. 34), you can indicate this on your application, but check with medical schools before doing so. Some have policies on deferred applicants and others require agreement beforehand.

> ### Key points
>
> The UCAS deadline for medicine is earlier than for other courses, usually 15 October. Start early and try to finish about a week before this date to avoid the risk of last-minute technical problems.

Mechanics of the form

The online UCAS form is quite simple to use, but there are a few things to note.

- **Registration** This takes less than 10 minutes. Keep a careful note of your username, password, and personal ID.
- **Email confirmation** You will need to confirm that you have provided a valid email address. Use a professional-looking address as this is seen by medical school admissions staff.

- **Payment** The application fee is around £25 if you are applying to two or more courses. This is paid online by debit/credit card.

UCAS Track

An online system called UCAS Track is provided to manage and follow your application. This means you can expect to see offers/rejections shortly after decisions are made. You can also use UCAS Track to update personal details and add course choices. Be aware that it is only usually final decisions (e.g. offers/rejections) that appear on UCAS Track. Medical schools will communicate with you directly (e.g. by post) about interview arrangements, but keep a close eye on UCAS Track just in case.

Non-medicine courses

Although most applicants choose a related discipline (e.g. biomedical science) as their fifth option on the UCAS form, this is by no means necessary.

A student's experience ...

I applied to a law course in addition to four medical schools, and was worried the law school would think I was uncommitted given my medicine-orientated personal statement. The law course agreed to accept a letter explaining my unusual choice of courses. I explained that I really wanted to work in a profession where I could use my skills to solve problems that make a difference to people. Both medicine and law provided these opportunities. I relied on some legal work experience, which probably helped, and ended up with offers from the law course and two medical schools. The challenge now is to choose!

- **Choose carefully** Even if you don't want to study a non-medicine subject, think about this additional choice. There is nothing to gain from choosing an option you could never imagine accepting, let alone feeling as if you ought to accept it if your medical applications don't work out.
- **Don't rush** Although medical school applications are required by the early UCAS deadline, this is not necessary for many other courses. If you leave the fifth choice blank, you can add another course through UCAS Track right up to the standard deadline.
- **Nothing to lose** There is nothing to lose from choosing a non-medicine subject. It will not prejudice your medical school application; universities cannot see where else you applied until after making offers.
- **Justifying your personal statement** One obstacle is that your personal statement must be written for medicine. Admissions tutors for other courses might struggle to assess your suitability (and commitment) for their subject. Don't be afraid of writing separately to these courses explaining your reasons for applying in this way.

Key points

If you think you want to go directly into higher education, then use the remaining UCAS fifth choice. You can always take the graduate route (see p. 252) into medicine later on If that is what you want to do. Only leave this option blank if you want to avoid the temptation to study something else instead.

▮ Your school reference

Every applicant knows their grades and personal statement are fundamental to winning a place. However, few think hard about their school reference, despite the fact that the reference presents an opportunity to set your application above the competition.

Is the reference important?

The answer to this question is that 'it depends'. It depends on your application and on the medical school. A bad reference will almost certainly have a negative impact. Although most courses require a *satisfactory* reference, there are a number of ways that a *strong* reference could help your application.

- **It may contribute to your application score** Some medical schools include the school reference as part of the overall application score, while others simply use it to filter out applicants with bad references.
- **It subjectively influences the assessor** Admissions staff are human. If they read a glowing personal reference, it will be difficult for them to separate this from the rest of your application. Even if it is not assigned points, the assessor could mark other elements higher as a consequence.
- **You are a borderline candidate** The reference could tip the balance if you are on the cusp of being invited to interview. Similarly, if you miss your offer and need to convince the school you are a strong candidate, your whole UCAS application could be reviewed a second time.

Key points

Referees almost always want to write good references but don't know what to say. They often have many to write at the same time. As a result, they sometimes produce bland, factual statements that don't tell medical schools very much beyond what they can already see from your UCAS form.

Explaining negative elements

If there is a negative element to your application that needs explaining, this should appear in your school reference. This might include unexpectedly low grades (e.g. due to illness or bereavement). Firstly, you do not have space in your personal statement to explain away potential negative aspects. Secondly, this type of explanation is more credible when written by someone other than the applicant. In this case it is particularly important that you meet with your referee so they have all the facts available and can ensure the reference is otherwise very positive.

Bad references

It is rare for applicants to receive a bad reference, but it can happen. Bad references are usually framed in vaguely positive terms but assessors can read between the lines. A bad school reference will often result in a rejected application.

What is a good reference?

Compare the following two references and remember they could have been written about the same person. Most applicants receive something closer to the first one, and you don't need to be an admissions tutor to spot the difference. The second reference is personal, enthusiastic, and unreserved. It includes specific details and provides objective evidence (e.g. the letter from St Mary's Hospice) to support its claims. The second reference also comments on qualities specific to would-be doctors.

Reference 1

Sara has been a student at John Paget's School since 2002. She achieved mostly A* grades in her GCSEs and some As. Her particular strengths are maths and science, which she is now studying at A level. I do not think she will have a problem achieving your standard offer of AAA. Sarah is a pleasant young lady who works hard and has lots of friends. She would be a very suitable candidate for your course.

Reference 2

Sara is one of the brightest students I have ever had the pleasure to teach. She consistently achieves A* grades and will almost certainly achieve straight A*s this year. Her coursework is always completed to a high standard and shows a depth of knowledge and understanding far beyond the A level curriculum. In addition, Sara is extremely mature and personable. She interacts well with her peers and teachers alike. Her academic ability and superb communication skills make her a natural candidate for medicine.

The manager of St Mary's Hospice, where Sarah has volunteered for two years, has written very strongly in support of her medical school application. I have no hesitation in joining her to commend Sara for a place at medical school. She will make a fantastic doctor.

Guaranteeing a strong reference

- **Get to know your teachers** A personal reference is more convincing than a bland, factual statement. Stay on the right side of your teachers so they can genuinely support your UCAS application. Depending on how your school is organized, it might be wise to make a point of engaging with your desired referees in a frank one-to-one conversation. Then you can explain your goals, motivation, and experience so that they can write a more informed statement than they might otherwise. This will be easier to do if you have engaged positively with your teachers throughout your time at the school, rather than leaving them feeling as if you only became interested when it suited you, towards the end.

- **Keep a portfolio** Make a note of your achievements and work experience. If someone you work alongside seems particularly impressed by you, ask for a brief reference that you can use later on. A couple of enthusiastic letters of support could be incorporated into your school reference.
- **Choose the right person** It's worth noting that enthusiastic, outgoing people are more likely to write enthusiastic, outgoing references. If you get the chance to choose a referee, then pick someone who won't hold back.
- **Provide information** Meet with your referee before they start writing. Ask out-right whether they will support your application with a good reference. Take a list of medical school qualities and explain how you meet them. It's often good to approach a potential referee by asking a question to the effect of 'Do you feel as though you can honestly write me a good reference in support of X?' as opposed to 'Would you be able to write me a reference for X?'.
- **Ask (politely) to see the reference** As already mentioned (see p. 218), references are traditionally confidential. However, it is increasingly common for applicants to be shown their reference. This provides an opportunity to correct errors and/or provide further information.

▌ The personal statement

While it is natural to feel anxious about the personal statement, you should see it as an opportunity to set yourself apart from a pool of applicants with identical grades. Indeed, your personal statement is the only voice that you have in your entire application!

Some general rules

The personal statement is extremely important. It may take multiple drafts and several weeks to perfect, but this is time well spent.

- **Don't waste space** You have 47 lines or 4,000 characters, whichever you reach first. This is ~500 words. Every word must be chosen carefully so that you can convey as much information as possible in clear and concise English.
- **Do not copy** All UCAS forms are electronically checked for plagiarism. Do not consider copying even part of a sentence because you **will** get caught.
- **What have you learned?** Listing experiences is not enough; every time you describe an experience you should communicate what you learned from that experience, what personal qualities this demonstrates (see p. 225), and why it makes you better than another candidate for the place (without saying it in as many words!).
- **Seek help** While it must be your own work, it is vital to seek advice and criticism from parents, teachers, and friends (who you trust not to copy). Act on the comments they make and do not be afraid to make major changes. Most submitted personal statements won't look anything like they did when they were first written!
- **Save your work** Write your personal statement in a Word document and save it regularly. This makes it easier to save, print, edit, and check than writing it directly into your UCAS form.
- **Think of your reader** The admissions tutor reading your personal statement may have hundreds of personal statements to go through. Make their life easy by using clear and concise English; make sure to avoid long 'waffly' sentences and vague statements.
- **Be convincing** If you make a claim that is unusual for a student finishing their A levels, you must back it up with evidence.

Key points

Start early and make multiple drafts. From start to finish it should present a clear argument about why you will make an excellent doctor, backed up by personal experiences and the ability to reflect on and learn from these experiences.

Qualities and skills of a doctor

The qualities that medical schools look for come from two documents published by the General Medical Council (GMC) called *Tomorrow's Doctors* and *Good Medical Practice*. Both are available online at www.gmc-uk.org. These qualities include:

- Honesty
- Communications skills
- Teamwork
- Ability to learn
- Awareness of limitations

- Integrity
- Dedication
- Respect for others

You could aim to highlight some of these skills in your personal statement, but only when you can evidence the statements you make. It does you no favours to say 'I am good at making decisions and communicating effectively' without providing evidence that you are indeed that person and have developed those skills. Contrast this statement with an evidenced alternative: 'I led a team of five writers as the Editor of our school newspaper, which required taking on board a range of viewpoints, making decisions about what to include, and communicating effectively with writers, school staff, and readers'. A few more words, but infinitely more valuable than a generic statement that anyone could write.

How is it marked?

While the specifics vary between medical schools, the following are consistent:

- **Fixed marking criteria** Markers are given clear instructions of what to look for and how to score it, so that marking is fair and reproducible.
- **Marking criteria are easy to predict** Although few medical schools publish their marking criteria, they will be based on finding applicants with the academic and personal abilities to complete the course. An example of a mark scheme is shown in the box.

Many mark schemes reward reflection on experiences. For example, writing 'I attended a multidisciplinary team meeting, which taught me the value of effective communication between healthcare professionals' is likely to score better than 'I attended a multidisciplinary team meeting, which included physiotherapists, occupational therapists, and community nurses'.

Example medical school UCAS scoring template

All candidates must meet minimum requirements: predicted/actual grades AAB; minimum grade A in chemistry; satisfactory school reference.

- **Commitment** (maximum 10): Valid reasons for studying medicine; relevant work experience; enthusiasm for medicine.
- **Insight** (maximum 10): Demonstrates understanding of qualities, knowledge, and attitudes required of a doctor; shows learning from personal/work experience.
- **Suitability** (maximum 10): Varied interests; achievement beyond educational work; ability to relax.
- **Academic ability** (maximum 10): A level subject choices; predicted/actual grades; number of subjects; prizes won; other academic distinctions; very strong school reference; high grades despite personal adversity and/or struggling at school.

Key points

Make the marker's life easy—clearly state what you have learned and what qualities of a doctor this demonstrates.

How is it used?

The personal statement serves two purposes:

- **Selection for interview** Personal statements are used to identify candidates who are likely to perform best at interview. UCAS applications are ranked, with applicants above a certain threshold being invited for interview.
- **Material at interview** Your personal statement will almost certainly be used to structure your interview. Make sure that you can justify every statement that you make.

Some medical schools disregard the UCAS form as soon as the interview lists are drawn up. At these schools, all candidates invited to interview have an equal chance of winning an offer. At others, the UCAS score can help balance poor performance at interview. Check the websites of medical schools you are applying to (see Chapter 8); some of them clearly state how they use this information.

What to include in a personal statement?

Your personal statement should be a clear and logical document explaining why you would make an excellent medical student and doctor. It should describe all your main achievements and experiences whilst emphasizing that you have the necessary qualities and ability to learn.

Why do you want to be a doctor?

This is a surprisingly complicated and involved question. There is no single correct answer; as you describe your reasons it is important to be aware of the implications of, or responses to, common answers:

- **To help people** This is a noble intention and it should be true for all doctors. However, it is also true of nurses, midwives, physiotherapists, and many professions outside of healthcare. If altruism is really your main objective, charity work or politics may allow you to help more people. What is it about helping people *as a doctor* that appeals to you?
- **The love of science** Most doctors do enjoy learning about science, but again so do many in other professions. If science is your main interest, why not take a science degree and become an academic? Medicine is not always as scientific as we'd like it to be; many patients leave hospital with no formal diagnosis or understanding of what caused their symptoms. Why does *medical* science in a *clinical* environment appeal to you?
- **The profession** There are many aspects of the medical profession that may appeal to you including teamwork, contact with people, making important decisions, leadership, status, daily challenges, the salary, and social responsibility. If you describe the aspects that appeal to you the most, it is important that they make you appear in a positive and non-selfish light. What are the *positive* aspects of being a doctor that are not found in other professions?
- **A logical exclusion of alternatives** Hopefully you have considered numerous careers alongside medicine. While it is important to exclude these yourself, it is not enough to say that medicine was the only career left. Medical schools want students with a burning enthusiasm for medicine and being a doctor, and this needs to come across in your personal statement. Why is *medicine* the best possible use of your skills and qualities?
- **The challenge** There are many challenges in medicine: coping with limited resources, diagnosing diseases, communicating with patients, ethical dilemmas, emotional turmoil, etc. Which challenges of the profession attract you and what evidence do you have that you will be able to cope with them? Ideally, you will be able to back this up with work experience that might have shown you some of the more difficult aspects of a medical career. This doesn't mean you have to observe a mistake with devastating consequences or watch someone break bad news. However, you should have thought about these things and possibly asked healthcare professionals you shadowed (at an appropriate moment) about them.

Your answer is likely to include a combination of these reasons, backed up by personal experience and a demonstration that you know what the job is like. Try to come up with arguments against the reasons you have written, then rewrite the section, including evidence to answer these arguments.

What experience do you have?

Along with stating why you would make a good doctor, you must also describe the extracurricular activities (see p. 46), work experience (see p. 54), voluntary work (see p. 64), employment (see p. 66), or research (see p. 68) that you have undertaken. If you are applying for deferred entry you should also outline your gap-year plans (see p. 34). Some people also include significant life events (e.g. severe illness) if this portrays them in a positive light.

Personal statements that simply list such experiences can make extremely dull reading and risk a poor score, even if the experiences are incredible. It is better to use this information to back up any claims or statements that you make (along with how the experience taught you to further your learning).

Most interesting experience If there is something about you that really makes you stand out from other applicants, then describe it in the first paragraph. Make sure you can describe why this experience is relevant to applying to medical school (e.g. 'While winning a gold medal in the Olympics was exhilarating, I became aware that I wanted more from life than simply being the fastest cyclist...').

Why you want to be a doctor While describing your personal reasons, use your work experience to demonstrate that you are aware of the role and challenges of being a doctor. Make sure you clearly state where the work experience was (hospital cardiology ward, GP clinic, etc.) and, if the length of work experience was impressive, include the duration too. What inspired you? What *exactly/specifically* did you find interesting? Take the opportunity to reflect on the situation; is there any further insight that you can demonstrate?

Academic suitability While there is no need to repeat your exam results, you should mention any other academic achievements. You can also mention particular academic interests supported by relevant experiences (e.g. reading *New Scientist*) or researching a medical topic well beyond the A level curriculum (make sure you are ready to answer challenging questions at interview on this topic!). What have these academic interests taught you?

Professional suitability You need to demonstrate that you have the qualities necessary to be a member of the medical profession (see p. 2). To do this you can use a wide range of experiences, not just those in a healthcare setting. Anything that you have done that required you to learn skills relevant to being a doctor (see p. 54) can be used to demonstrate your professional suitability.

Commitment to medicine Demonstrate your commitment to medicine using examples of long-term voluntary work or employment. Describe any challenges you faced and what you learned from these experiences. If these experiences were in a healthcare setting, use examples of where you interacted with a patient, to demonstrate your communication skills and your ability to learn from situations.

What to avoid in a personal statement?

It can be difficult to spot your own mistakes when writing a personal statement, so you should always seek the advice of others before submission (see p. 232). The following examples should help you avoid some of the most common personal statement blunders.

Key points

Your personal statement needs to be extremely concise and clear. Keep two maxims in mind: 'keep it simple' and 'less is more'. Always display yourself in a positive light and make sure you describe a range of experiences.

Inappropriate use of experiences

Poor description of experiences can lose you marks; common mistakes include:

- **Lack of reflection** Simply describing your experiences is insufficient. Admissions tutors want to know that you gained insight from experiences and have the ability to reflect on and learn from them. Highlight how your experiences increased your awareness of, and strengthened your desire for, studying medicine.
- **Exhausting one example** Breadth is crucial to demonstrating commitment. While one experience may be particularly informative, if you use it repeatedly it suggests that you have not done anything else. Try to include a variety of experiences including work experience, voluntary work, and extracurricular activities.
- **Listing experiences** There is also a risk of including too many experiences so that the personal statement reads like a list. Be selective and use the space to describe a few of the best experiences thoroughly.
- **Out-of-date examples** Avoid using experiences from many years ago unless they are especially relevant. A month in hospital as a child is worth including, but joining the Boy Scouts for a year at the age of 12 is not.
- **Inappropriate examples** Consider what experiences say about your personality. If they show a lack of honesty, good judgement, or common sense they should be left out, regardless of the outcome.
- **Keep it positive** Focus on the positive aspects of a situation (see box).

Avoid ...

'I spent a lot of time caring for my ill grandmother over the last year, which led to my lower than expected AS-level results (the time was very stressful and, whilst I tried to study, it was not always easy to do so).'

'Having cared for my grandmother, who had severe Parkinson's disease, I learned about the difficulties experienced by family carers first-hand. I have resolved to always consider the holistic support available when managing patients with chronic illness.'

N.B. If this applicant had communicated with their referees (see p. 218), the school reference could describe, at length, the difficulties faced and justify the lower than expected AS levels.

'I shadowed a GP for two weeks and this showed me that I would really enjoy the challenges of being a doctor. On several occasions I witnessed the doctor encountering difficulties. Watching him overcome these difficulties has inspired me to pursue my medical application.'

'For two weeks I shadowed a GP serving a diverse local community. I learned the importance of cultural awareness when obtaining a history, especially regarding sensitive issues (e.g. sexual health). The social dimension of medicine is a key reason for my interest in becoming a doctor.'

Other pitfalls

- **Generic statements** You will not score any points by writing your personal statement in vague terms. Be sure to include pertinent details in your descriptions of experiences, unless they detract from the experience. You should also ensure that in describing your healthcare experiences you don't breach confidentiality! Do not include patient names, hospital numbers, or excessively specific details.
- **Negative points** Your personal statement provides a relatively short space to sell yourself, so don't waste words explaining poor results or personal weaknesses. Your school reference is the correct place to explain about exam glitches or challenging personal circumstances (see p. 218).
- **Gimmicks** It can be tempting to write something extravagant to catch the reader's attention. However, writing a mature, reflective personal statement is more likely to impress than employing a literary gimmick.
- **Needless controversy** Another risky way of seeking attention is taking an extreme political or ethical position. You must be very careful if you plan to do this. Although we all have our personal beliefs, doctors should serve patients impartially and without judgement. Your application should reflect this principle.
- **An impossibly wide audience** It is impossible to write an application that will appeal to selectors at every type of medical school (see p. 102). For this reason, you should be applying to four broadly similar courses (see p. 103) and tailoring your application accordingly. For example, you could emphasize your interest in developing your communication skills or highlight your dedication to academic excellence and basic science.

- **Too many words** Long-winded descriptions are tiresome to read and waste valuable space: cut the waffle, stay away from needlessly long words, lose irrelevant details, and avoid repetition.

Key points

As you write, try to eliminate any unnecessary words. This will make the writing clearer and allow you to fit in more experiences. Be ruthless with your statement from the beginning and you'll be much happier with the finished product.

▌Finishing the personal statement

A strong conclusion is as important as a captivating introduction. It should leave the reader with a good impression of your whole application. Having invested time and effort so far, avoid a trite, over-simplistic, or exaggerated conclusion. By the end of the last sentence, the selection panel must be confident that you are a suitable candidate for their course.

How to conclude?

- **Don't repeat yourself** Your final paragraph should not be wasted repeating experiences you've already described. You have a finite amount of space and repeating examples only highlights limited experience. You may need to refer to a previously mentioned experience but leave out the details.
- **Avoid new experiences** Your conclusion should summarize what has already been written rather than adding new information.
- **Contextualize** What are the broader implications of your skills and qualities? Perhaps you've alluded to an interest in public health by describing a conversation with hospital doctors about healthcare rationing (see p. 62) or the rising incidence of diabetes. You may conclude that, having demonstrated an ability to work compassionately and impartially, your skills will be essential for practicing medicine in a resource-limited health service. In this way you are describing what you have to offer to medicine.
- **Draw themes together** You may have covered many different topics, using very discrete experiences. The conclusion should identify key 'take-home' messages for the reader.

A student's experience ...

Having discussed a range of topics in my personal statement, from browsing *BMJ* articles to shadowing a hospital doctor, I had several options for how to conclude. I felt it was best to describe how my passion for understanding science would be the driving force behind my future medical career. I also used this as an opportunity to reiterate my suitability for the traditional style of course that I was applying for.

Editing

Once you've drafted your personal statement, start editing. There is *always* room for improvement. You should aim to show your finished version to as many different people as possible and be prepared to alter your text based on their comments. Ask them explicitly to be critical—you will not be helped by 20 readers if all they do is offer reassurance. There are two broad criteria by which you need to assess your personal statement: content and style.

Content
- **Themes** Have you discussed everything you intended to? There are basic elements that you need to include (reasons for studying medicine, insights from work experience, etc.), but what about the additional topics that you wanted to cover? Do they reinforce your application or are they repetitive? Are there any contradictions? Remember, if you raise medical issues or mention a specific interest, you should be prepared to discuss these at length at interview.

- **Evidenced statements** Every claim should be supported by a personal experience. For example, anyone can list the ideal qualities of a doctor, but a good applicant will describe how they have learned and demonstrated each one.
- **Clarity** The point of each paragraph should be immediately obvious by the end of it. If there is any doubt as to its meaning, discard it and start again.
- **Representative of you** Whilst you need to remain positive, your statement must be an honest account of you, your experiences, your qualities, and what you can offer to medicine. Any attempt to mislead the selection panel will inevitably be uncovered, often at interview. Make sure you stick to the facts.

A student's experience ...

My statement focused on shadowing experiences with a district nurse, GP, and physio-therapist. I also described mentoring junior-school pupils. In my conclusion I highlighted my interpersonal and leadership skills, which are essential for a doctor working in our multidisciplinary NHS in the twenty-first century.

Style
- **Tone** Your tone should be positive and professional throughout.
- **Unique** It should be immediately obvious that you wrote your statement. Insightful reflection and thought-provoking discussion will only be remembered if they are based on personal experience. Never copy someone else's work, since UCAS auto-matically checks for this (see p. 221).
- **Consistency** This goes for all aspects of your statement, including punctuation and spelling. The use of indented versus spaced paragraphs should remain the same throughout your document.

Key points

When writing your personal statement, be sure to save your work regularly under dif-ferent filenames (which include the date) to allow you to return to older versions should you wish to.

▌ Reviewing personal statements

The following section reiterates the importance of keeping your personal statement *personal*, and describes how specific examples may be reviewed.

WARNING! Plagiarism in personal statements

UCAS now uses sophisticated software to check whether any part of your form matches material in other submitted statements. If a match is found, these applications are flagged to medical schools as containing potentially plagiarized material. In one year, UCAS found that 5% of medical school personal statements contained copied material, including 234 claiming a passion for science after 'accidentally burning holes in [their] pyjamas after experimenting with a chemistry set on their eighth birthday'. Using the internet and this book to gain advice for personal statements is essential, but there is no excuse for copying, even just a sentence. Plagiarism is a severe failure in integrity and almost guarantees immediate rejection.

Example personal statements

Example 1

Avoid ...

'Ever since I was a child I have been intrigued by how we work. I believe that there is nothing more wondrous than developing a greater understanding of the human body. This has been supported by my passion for A-level biology.'

Analysis

The student offers a reasonable reason for wanting to study medicine and tries to show evidence to support this (the passion for biology). However, they do not clearly describe how this interest will make them a good doctor and do not demonstrate how this 'passion' has affected their actions.

Instead ...

'My lifelong interest in how the human body functions has developed into a passion for human biology that has led me to read widely beyond the boundaries of the A level curriculum. Whilst I am excited about continuing these studies at medical school, it is the thought of using this interest to help people that really thrills me.'

Example 2

Avoid ...

'Last summer I spent a month designing primers for PCR amplification of single nucleotide polymorphisms (SNPs) around the Cystic Fibrosis Transmembrane Conductance Regulator (CFTR) gene to investigate the effect of these SNPs on transcription. I downloaded the surrounding sequence from the UCSC genome browser, then used Primer3 for design, followed by BLAT and BLAST to ensure they were unique.'

Analysis

The excessive use of jargon may mean that the reader cannot appreciate what the student did. There is no clinical relevance and it also focuses too much on what they did rather than why they did it or what they learned.

Instead ...

'Meeting a patient with cystic fibrosis led me to learn more about this disease. I discovered that a local research laboratory studied cystic fibrosis and, after contacting them, I was offered the chance to spend a month working with a PhD student. The research focused on the regulation of the cystic fibrosis gene, which may allow development of drugs to treat milder forms of the disease. This experience helped me appreciate the role of a doctor as the interface between patients and medical research.'

Example 3

Avoid ...

'After spending months trying to find a doctor to shadow, my hard graft paid off! I shadowed a paediatrician for three weeks, watching fairly routine jobs and playing with the children on the wards. Whilst this was amazing fun (despite a few rascals) there was a serious element to it. I learned that playgroups could be used to make developmental assessments and monitor chronic diseases. These experiences taught me a lot about the boring side to medicine, the importance of MDT, and what I want to do in life—paeds!'

Analysis

The student's writing style is too informal for a personal statement. It fails to demonstrate professionalism, which is fundamental to being a doctor. It dwells on negative aspects that make it sound like the student is complaining or uninterested. The student alludes to fairly difficult themes, but then fails to match them to the relevant experience and reflect further. While working with play therapists as part of a multidisciplinary approach is important, the applicant is applying for a role as a doctor, not a play therapist. The only comment about the paediatrician's role is negative.

Instead ...

'Part of my work experience was spent shadowing a hospital paediatrician on the children's ward. I was enthused by the patient contact and fascinated to watch how the paediatrician tailored his style of communication to suit all patients, from infants to adolescents. I later had the opportunity to practice this myself, working with a specialist who was assessing the development of children through play. I learned the importance of a team approach to medicine, and that diagnosis and management requires far more than analysing biochemistry reports.'

Example 4

Avoid ...

'Working as a head boy with my team of prefects has taught me a lot about myself and confirmed my suitability for a medical career. Beyond the obvious leadership element required for such a position, succeeding both in this role and my studies demanded expert time-management skills. I am certainly ready to take on the professional responsibilities of becoming a doctor and overseeing other hospital staff, whilst maintaining a healthy work–life balance.'

Analysis

This statement describes many skills and transferrable qualities but they are not clearly demonstrated. It exaggerates the importance of his work as head boy, claiming that this means he is ready to lead hospital staff (a situation that is many years of experience away, if ever). He does not use specific activities or experiences to justify the claims and there is no mention of the importance of teamwork, either in his position at school or within medicine.

Instead ...

'As head boy I led a team of prefects in a project to teach study skills to younger students through leaflets, revision timetables, and teaching groups of 30 or more. The project required me to assess and utilize the strengths and weaknesses of the different prefects, maintain the group's focus on our overall goals, and keep to a tight timeline. I learned the importance of teamwork and valuing every member of a group, which is as important in a multidisciplinary clinical team as in this situation.'

Key points

There is more to a personal statement than describing your experiences and listing the qualities that you think a doctor should have. Through mature reflection, your experiences should demonstrate how you already think like, and possess the important qualities of, a doctor.

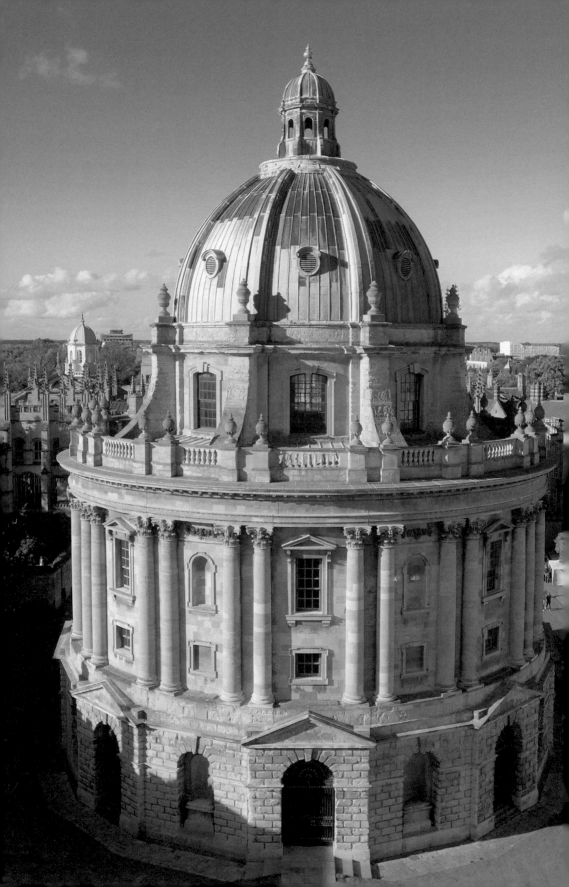

10

Getting into Oxbridge

▌Oxbridge demystified

Ancient. Wealthy. Exceptional. Inaccessible. Elitist. Intellectual. Competitive. Arrogant. The universities of Oxford and Cambridge attract many colourful descriptions, with varying degrees of truth behind each one. These institutions are often perceived as being impenetrable for all but the greatest minds. Many of the qualities essential for medical school also make you a legitimate Oxbridge candidate, including strong A level grades (see p. 98), diverse extracurricular achievements (see p. 46), and true enthusiasm for medicine. The following pages describe some of the key features that set Oxbridge applications apart, including the collegiate system (see p. 242), the courses (see p. 244), and the interview process (see p. 248).

The collective term 'Oxbridge' is used to describe Oxford and Cambridge because of features they have in common. Both were founded over 800 years ago and developed into similar collegiate institutions with reputations for academic excellence. Their similarities mean you can only apply to *either* Oxford *or* Cambridge in a single academic year, but not both (unless you're applying to the graduate-entry courses: see p. 278 and p. 271).

So what's it all about?

- **The people** The single most important advantage of Oxbridge is being surrounded by exceptional people doing exceptional work. It is a chance to learn from some of the greatest academic talent in the world—many tutors will have conducted research that defines current thinking. Consequently, the university attracts clever and hard-working undergraduates. This creates a unique working environment in which some people thrive. Others grow tired of always feeling in competition with their peers. The real opportunity here is being in a situation where you're never the biggest fish in the pond. There will always be someone (tutor or student) who will know more than you know and will push you to being better.
- **The opportunities** Unique opportunities are found through studying at Oxbridge: the supervision/tutorial system (see p. 242), many libraries, research projects (see p. 244), grants (see p. 238), and well-endowed clubs and societies. A healthy supply of benefactors ensures that Oxbridge students benefit from a wide range of opportunities that other institutions cannot always afford.
- **The reputation** Both Oxford and Cambridge are in the top five universities worldwide; everyone has heard of them, and this can only help your career. Being an Oxbridge graduate suggests you are someone who works hard and can achieve results.

What's it not about?

- **Sex, drugs, and rock and roll** While there is a good social life on offer, the balance is tipped much further towards academic work than some other medical schools. This means that not only is there less of a social life on offer but that those around you are often too busy to engage with it anyway. There are still fun, if quirky, times to be had, although often at formal hall or in a common room as opposed to a pub or club.
- **Large circles** Wherever you study, medical students have a reputation for cliquishness. This is exacerbated by the collegiate structure at Oxbridge. Medical students spend a lot of time with other medical students studying the same course at the same college. In smaller colleges this can be as few as two or three other people.

Fortunately, most colleges accommodate all students (at least in the first year) in common halls, which offers at least some chance of branching out and meeting students studying other subjects.

- **Being the best** Whilst the determination to succeed is essential to survive an Oxbridge education, unrealistic expectations can crush the aspirations of former head students and top achievers. In all likelihood, you should forget about being the best, or at least about getting to the top as easily as you did at school. The bell curve of results (once your best friend) isn't as much fun on the peak or at the tail end.

Costs and grants

A commonly held misconception is that you have to be wealthy to get into Oxbridge. Quite the opposite is true, as both universities offer a range of grants and bursaries. Basic costs such as tuition fees and books are the same as at other medical schools, with accommodation falling between London and home-county prices. Except for a formal college gown (£15–£50), there are no extras that you will be expected to pay for. Ceremonial college dinners that you are invited to are paid for by the college.

All students can benefit from book, hardship, learning, and research grants. Such financial support is available from both the college and the university itself. Means-tested bursaries are also available for students from the lowest-income backgrounds to help meet living costs. These are offered regardless of which college you attend.

Access schemes

Universities are increasingly aware that some students might have experienced more educational disadvantages than others. Some applicants come from schools and/or families with no tradition of studying in higher education. Others may have had an education disrupted by personal or medical problems.

At Oxford, all information about a candidate comes from the UCAS form. Those meeting various 'access' criteria, as well as the usual requirements for a conditional offer, are strongly recommended for interview.

Cambridge also considers this information from the UCAS form, as well as employing a separate 'Extenuating Circumstances Form' (ECF) that students complete through their school. This is used when a student's education has been seriously disadvantaged or disrupted through health or personal problems. If you perform well at interview and in the pre-admission tests, some students have occasionally been made lower-grade offers.

Both universities use contextualized results and are mindful of the different pre-university opportunities that applicants will have been able to access.

Key points

Being part of such a world-class institution like Oxbridge is a hard-earned privilege. However, when you apply for your first job as a doctor, the medical school you attended is simply not part of the application process. For this reason, Oxbridge is less of a career advantage for doctors than for other graduates. Think very carefully about what you stand to gain (and potentially lose) by applying to Oxbridge. It's not for everyone.

The Oxbridge experience

The experiences of students attending Oxford and Cambridge are defined by the environment, resources, and people. The following examples offer a glance at life as an Oxbridge medic.

A day in the life of an Oxford preclinical student ...

A typical weekday can begin at 6am for rowing practice, followed by four hours of lectures. A successful morning, falling asleep in fewer than half the lectures, is followed by a quick bike ride back to college for lunch. Afternoon dissection may last two hours, before completing a supervision essay with almost no time to spare before the deadline. The college sometimes runs talks from eminent figures, so I may pop over to the conference centre to see a Nobel Prize winner in the flesh!

A day in the life of a Cambridge clinical student ...

As a second-year clinical student at Cambridge, I am currently based at Addenbrooke's Hospital on my paediatrics rotation. There is a Special Care Baby Unit ward round that starts at 9am. I follow the clinical team for several hours on a business round, where the ST3 (junior doctor) updates the consultant on the progress of each baby under the team's care. Most of the discussion is far too specialized for me to understand, but a friendly ST2 (more junior doctor) keeps me on my toes by asking me basic clinical questions and answering any questions that I have.

At lunchtime, the clinical school holds a student grand round, where a student presents an audit from their recent orthopaedics student-selected component. There is also a *New England Journal of Medicine* Club in the afternoon, where one of the consultants discusses interesting cases in the literature that are relevant to junior doctors.

Afterwards, I make a dash for the 2pm haematological oncology clinic, where the consultant sees children with haematological malignancies. It is very specialized, but useful as the consultant allows me to examine each of the patients.

At 6pm, members of my college join me on the wards with a junior doctor who takes us on our weekly clinical supervision. For the next two hours we take histories, examine patients, and discuss management, receiving feedback at every step from our clinical supervisor. Afterwards I grab a quick bite to eat at the college canteen. I've missed a Tennis Society formal event but join the rest of my team in the college bar later on. We have a pint before escaping to the infamous 'Cindies' for some cheeky dancing.

The Union

The Oxford Union is a debating society and the second oldest University Union (second only to the Cambridge Union). Both the Oxford and Cambridge Unions are world renowned as debating forums and attract a host of international figures and celebrities. These have included Gerry Adams, Hans Blix, Pierce Brosnan, Clint Eastwood, Stephen Hawking, the Dalai Lama, Ronald Reagan, Jerry Springer, and Desmond Tutu. The Unions also hold workshops to help sharpen your debating skills and often field one of the most successful teams at the World Universities Debating Championships.

May week

After the madness of exams, May week (quintessentially for Oxbridge, in June) begins. This is the period of post-exam enjoyment, where your pigeonhole is swamped by invitations for garden parties and formal dinners from societies, colleagues, and friends. After a year of hard work, you have earned an extravagant annual college ball. Lasting from 8pm till 8am, this is a night of fine food and drink, popular live acts, funfair rides, and a spectacular fireworks display. It makes a refreshing change from the cheesy 'bops/ents' (discos) that run throughout the rest of the year.

A student's experience ... not that different!

I think going to Oxbridge is very much like attending any other medical school. The course is a little more theoretical to begin with, but outside of that, you do what appeals to you. I find I have an experience closer to my medic friends at other universities than non-medics in my own college.

A student's experience ... diversity prevails!

As a student from a 'non-traditional' background, I applied to Cambridge University with some initial hesitation. My school did not have a history of sending students to Oxbridge and I was the first in my family to study beyond high school. Although I had my own preconceptions about Oxbridge, having experienced the environment first-hand I can reassure those interested in applying that your background need not deter you. Yes, there are some very wealthy students who have attended the best public schools (as indeed there are at other universities), and who are themselves as unique and engaging as everyone else. However, despite the stereotypes, Oxford and Cambridge genuinely are diverse, multicultural institutions working hard to address any imbalances that remain in their student make-up. If you are a strong candidate, then you can compete for a place regardless of your sex, ethnicity, or personal, health, or social circumstances.

The colleges

In the UK, the collegiate system is unique to Oxford, Cambridge, and Lancaster (see p. 146) medical schools. Medical students at other institutions usually live on a campus or in a city and travel to their teaching centre or hospital each day. A centrally placed Students' Union is found at the heart of their community and most students participate in extracurricular activities at university level.

Oxford and Cambridge differ because they are each made up of over 30 independent colleges. The colleges operate independently, despite all belonging to the same university. An Oxbridge student's preclinical life outside of lectures and practical sessions is based almost entirely within their college. The college provides key amenities to its students, such as:

- **Accommodation** Some colleges offer accommodation for all three preclinical years, either within college or in college-owned properties in town.
- **Dining** There are formal and informal halls, a distinction based solely on strict serving times and whether or not a formal gown and smart dress must be worn.
- **Supervisions/tutorials** These are small teaching groups made up of students from the same college (see p. 242).
- **Facilities/financial aid** The number and quality of grants, libraries, and even gym facilities vary between colleges.
- **Clubs and societies** Almost all are duplicated at college and university level. The university sports teams play at a much higher standard and consist of the best players from across the colleges. At Oxbridge, the Students' Union is replaced by each college's Junior Common Room (JCR) and the bar.
- **Support** Pastoral and academic welfare is provided by two fellows from the college (senior academic figures, who sit on a college's governing body). Your pastoral support will sometimes come from a fellow of a discipline other than medicine.

Choosing a college

As well as choosing between Oxford and Cambridge (see p. 245) you can also apply to a specific college. Since you will spend so much time in your college this is a decision to consider carefully.

- **Exclusion criteria** First make a list of the colleges that are applicable to you. Be aware that some colleges are single-sex or for graduates only. At Oxford, Permanent Private Halls are often small foundations associated with a particular religious order. They can only award a limited number of degrees.
- **Size** Would you prefer a large college where you meet new people every term or the cosier atmosphere of a small college and familiar faces?
- **Locality** Particularly in Cambridge there can be a 'large' (in Oxbridge terms) distance between central and out-of-town colleges. Avoid the latter if you can't ride a bike and still want to make it to lectures on time.
- **Age** Colleges range from a few decades to many centuries old and most architectural tastes can be accommodated.
- **Facilities/grants** These are very dependent upon the wealth of each college and can make a big difference, including book grants worth hundreds of pounds each year, free access to the college gym, and travel grants.

- **Culture** You can only get an authentic feel for each college by visiting and speaking to current students. Avoid 'rational' decisions based on out-of-date statistics and hearsay.

The choices

Just like universities, Oxbridge colleges have their own individual characters. These are shaped by the diversity of students and the unique infrastructure that each college has developed over the years. Look at the college prospectus and the 'alternative' (i.e. student-written) prospectus for each college of interest. As well as the college website, the student JCR might provide helpful information online. If you still have questions, each college has an Undergraduate Admissions Office that will be happy to take your call.

The only real way to gain an appreciation of each college is to attend the college open days and speak to people studying medicine there. Nevertheless, the 'tasting' guide below might be helpful as an overview of the choices on offer:

- **Vintage Burgundy white wine** e.g. St John's (Cambridge), Christ Church (Oxford). Old and opulent, benefitting from its unique *terroir* in the centre of town. These money houses have a reputation for attracting the rich, croquet-loving public-school boys. Despised and envied by the other colleges for their size, wealth, and arrogance.
- **Dr Pepper®** e.g. Girton (Cambridge), St Hugh's (Oxford). Out of town and out of mind for the rest of the university. As a result, the people here have to get along very well, and they usually do. If you can find them on a map of the city, you win a place.
- **Milk** e.g. Clare (Cambridge), Corpus Christi (Oxford). These are friendly colleges; genuinely happy places filled with smiley people. Often not as cut-throat competitive as some of the other colleges.
- **Iced tea** e.g. Newnham (Cambridge), Harris Manchester (Oxford). You don't choose them, they choose you. Either single-sex or graduate colleges.

Open applications If you really can't make your mind up, you can send an open application. This means a college is allocated based on the least subscribed college at the time your application is received. However, this doesn't necessarily mean it's easier to win a place by submitting an open application. If you apply to an oversubscribed college, strong applicants at Cambridge may be 'pooled' for consideration by undersubscribed colleges. If you are applying to Oxford, you will automatically be allocated a second college, even if you stated a preference for your first choice. These mechanisms prevent strong candidates from losing out by applying to colleges of their choice.

If you dislike a particular type of college, avoid being allocated one by stating a preference. You can't change your mind once you have been allocated.

Studying medicine at Oxbridge

Wherever you study medicine, there are certain skills and certain knowledge you will be taught. Although the content of every medical school education is largely the same, information can be delivered in many different ways (see p. 92). The Oxford and Cambridge courses offer a unique style of training in terms of the depth of coverage, teaching methods, and assessments.

The course

The six-year course for undergraduates is divided into two stages. The first two years cover basic sciences, with a research project taking up the third year. The Oxbridge student then enters the second stage, 'clinicals', lasting three years.

- The initial three-year preclinical stage is when the core sciences are delivered. Students from all medical schools must learn about a vast number of subjects relevant to clinical medicine: anatomy, biochemistry, neurobiology, pathology, pharmacology, physiology, and psychology. However, whilst other courses often concentrate on the subject details directly relevant to medicine, the Oxbridge courses emphasize studying each subject in its own right and for its own sake.
- Tutorials/supervisions are incredible teaching opportunities unique to the Oxbridge medical courses. Typically, the format is that a small group of medical students (2–4) engages in a teaching session with a specialist in the relevant area.
- Very little clinical exposure (no more than a few hours a term) is provided during the preclinical stage. As a result, Oxbridge students are introduced to patients later than those studying elsewhere.
- Oxbridge students must submit an additional application during their third year before starting clinical medicine. Previously, students could apply to move to one of the medical schools in London, through a competitive application process. From 2021, both Oxford and Cambridge students will complete their clinical phase in their respective universities.

Tutorials and supervisions

In common with other medical schools, Oxbridge uses lectures to deliver core material to students. Medical students at Oxbridge also benefit from tutorials (Oxford) or supervisions (Cambridge). There are as many as four such sessions a week during the preclinical stage, each of which can require preparatory work (e.g. an essay or set of problems) to be completed beforehand. Such 'one-to-few' tuition is useful for solving any difficulties, as well as encouraging a deeper understanding of the course material.

It is crucial that candidates appreciate the demands that such a teaching method adds over and above a standard medical course. The time commitments are significant and not everyone is suited to the intense learning environment.

Assessment

At the end of each year, most medical students sit various exams (e.g. multiple-choice questions, short-answer questions) to assess their competence in the subjects covered. This ensures you have met the standards required by the GMC to be awarded your degree at the end of the course (see p. 7). At the end of each year in the preclinical stage at Oxbridge, every subject is assessed by an additional exam paper that is entirely essay-based. Essays require a different set of skills from multiple-choice or short-answer questions.

In addition to working towards a medical degree, Oxbridge medical students work towards a 'traditional' honours degree leading to a Bachelor of Arts (BA) qualification after the first three years. This is comparable to the intercalated (BSc) degree that is available at many other medical schools (see p. 91).

At the end of three years of preclinical training, Oxbridge medical students are awarded a first, 2:1, 2:2, or third-class degree, based entirely on performance in their third-year essay papers. The results of these papers do not otherwise count towards the medical qualification. Whilst the essays are fundamentally scientific, the preclinical examiners will demand a degree of literary flair. If you flinch at the mere thought of your old English literature lessons, think carefully before applying to Oxbridge.

Course differences

In short, there are very few differences between Oxford and Cambridge courses. The key thing is to decide whether you suit the more science-orientated syllabus shared by both universities. Table 10.1 shows the main course differences.

Table 10.1 Course differences between Oxford and Cambridge

Stage	Oxford	Cambridge
Preclinical course	A more integrated, systems-based approach (but still very traditional) (see p. 92)	A more traditional, core subject-based course (anatomy, physiology, etc.)
Third-year BA	Most people do the 'Final Honour School' leading to a BA in medical sciences in one of five options: neuroscience; molecular medicine; myocardial, vascular, and respiratory biology; infection and immunity; or signalling in health and disease	Greater flexibility in the Cambridge Tripos exam system, which allows students to choose from a wider range of subjects in their third year, with the possible option of extending their studies by another year to an additional subject (e.g. law)
MBPhD programme	A PhD programme can be pursued after the preclinical years, although a formal MBPhD programme, like the one at Cambridge, does not exist	An additional three years of laboratory research can lead to a PhD in any science subject; often an extension of the third-year research project
Clinical course	Modular assessments throughout the year, with finals completed by January of the sixth year; the 10-week elective is performed in the sixth year	Predominantly end-of-year exams; the seven-week elective is performed at the end of the fifth year

■ The Oxbridge interview

The infamous Oxbridge interview is surrounded by colourful myths, almost all of which you can disregard. After submitting your application form and completing the BMAT (see p. 86), you may be invited for interview, typically in December. There are usually two interviews at two different colleges (four interviews in total). Sometimes one will focus on science and another on non-science questions. Other times they might both include an element of science and non-science.

What makes the Oxbridge interview different?   Of course, almost all medical schools interview applicants (see p. 304). This is to ensure that only those with the attitude and interpersonal skills required by a doctor are accepted. However, because of the unique Oxbridge course style, interviewers also want to determine whether you will thrive in their specific environment.

Unlike interviews at other medical schools, which use the same broad questions for each candidate, Oxbridge interviews are often less scripted. Instead, interviewers are free to allow a conversation to develop. Although some candidates view this as an obstacle, it is better seen as an opportunity. The discursive style permits interviewers to see how you think, how you cope when faced with unfamiliar topics, and how you interact with adults in a relatively pressured environment. It also replicates the style of a typical tutorial/supervision (see p. 242), so it can help you determine your suitability for this style of teaching. Often, the interviewers at Oxbridge are the same people who act as tutors on the course, and so they are heavily invested in finding the applicants that will gain (and contribute) the most as students.

Why did you apply to Oxbridge?   Carefully consider your reasons for applying to Oxbridge. The last thing you need is to fumble on questions you knew would be asked. There are no 'right' answers, but you should bear in mind a few key points:

- Whilst there are plenty of attractive features, you should focus on your interest in the academically orientated medical course, which is unique to Oxbridge. The buildings may be breathtaking but you are applying to study medicine, not architecture.
- In highlighting the benefits, avoid denigrating any other university and/or its course. Firstly, you do not know where your interviewers qualified from. Secondly, you are unlikely to demonstrate your best thinking by criticizing individual medical schools. It is far better to describe how the style of Oxbridge suits your own learning style and abilities; this is important across all of your interviews, as you should always focus on the positives and why you want to be somewhere, rather than the negatives and why you don't want to be somewhere else.

Why would you be successful at Oxbridge?   Think about skills you will need to cope with the unique style of the course. For example, four tutorials/supervisions a week, on top of five full days of timetabled work, demands effective time management.

If you're thinking about Oxbridge because you're not a 'people person', think again. Although there is little clinical training in the first three years, the Oxbridge medical courses do not exist solely to produce academic doctors. In fact, less than 5% of Oxbridge medics go on to pursue an entirely academic medical career. In common with others, Oxford and Cambridge medical schools aim to produce competent and professional clinicians, and avoiding people won't be an option.

Oxford or Cambridge?   This is a topic of conversation that is worth avoiding. There are far more similarities than differences between Cambridge and Oxford.

- Usually students decide which to choose based on the type of town that would suit them best. You can only appreciate this by visiting them both.
- There are very few differences in the courses (see p. 245) and to decide based on these differences would require you to have unrealistic certainty about your future career intentions. Decisions concerning third-year projects or MBPhDs are made later on in your preclinical education. Avoid bringing up these topics unless you are unusually well informed.

Science questions at interview A medical school interview is not designed to check your knowledge of A level science. This should be implicit in your exam grades. However, science questions may still be asked for a variety of reasons. They could arise because on your UCAS form you claim an interest in a particular area of medicine. If this is the case, you need to be particularly careful that what you have mentioned truly is an interest and that you have the degree of knowledge implied in your statement. Doctors on the panel will not take long to discover whether or not you really know about a subject for which you claim a particular enthusiasm.

Alternatively, science knowledge may be used to see how you think around a problem. Oxbridge interviews, in keeping with their general teaching style (see p. 92), aim to push students beyond material they have covered as part of a set syllabus. This means you need a solid appreciation of A level material so you can approach science questions sensibly, using first principles.

A level science relevant to medicine Medicine is essentially the use of science to understand, diagnose, and treat disease. Biology, chemistry, and physics are all used to varying degrees. Sometimes the link is obvious: the study of cardiac physiology is directly applicable to medicine. Other areas are more subtly relevant. Your understanding of organic chemistry and the stereochemistry of organic molecules could be important in appreciating drug design and how compounds specifically interact with their target receptors. Physics may be tested when answering questions on the auditory system; this requires an understanding of the nature of sound waves, pressure calculations, and moments.

The style of such questions is to make you think outside of your comfort zone. Clearly, the questions you will be asked are determined by the areas studied at A level. Having said that, do not be quick to dismiss a question because you 'haven't covered it at school'. You may need to take logical steps from A level knowledge to reach a sensible answer. Stay flexible and remember to vocalize all of your steps and assumptions, once you've clearly thought about them. Interviewers are interested in how you think at least as much as what you know.

Key points

Keep your eyes open to topics relevant to medicine during your A level studies. It is not possible to prepare for every potential question but fostering an interest in clinical topics might help. A rote-learned approach to answering interview questions, including science ones, will be spotted by the panel. Instead, concentrate on making sure that you have a confident grasp of all of your A-level material (see p. 24).

Inside the Oxbridge interview

It is difficult to describe an Oxbridge interview, simply because everyone is so different. Some colleges employ a list of questions, but these only help to start a general discussion. The key to answering any question is thoughtfulness, clarity, and detail. Don't be afraid to ask for a little more time to think about your responses. When you think you have an answer, vocalize all the steps you made to get you there. You do not have to always be 'right'—there is often no right answer as such—but they do want to see you are comfortable with new ideas.

   The following are examples of questions that could be asked in an Oxbridge interview. Don't forget, you will still be asked common (see p. 308), ethical (see p. 310), and/or clinical science (see p. 316) questions.

Key points

When you read the science examples that follow, remember they are specific to a particular candidate. If you don't know the answers, don't panic, as it is unlikely your interview would have developed in this direction. Interviewers tend to follow the candidate's lead. When you answer a question correctly, they will pursue that answer to see how much you know. The result is a challenging interview that might seem impossible to another candidate. You should also remember that interviewers will coach candidates who don't know the answer but are on the right path. Bear this in mind when talking to other candidates about their interview questions.

Example I: Science questions

The following is a transcript of an interview with a student who described an interest in studying nerve conduction and action potentials at school:

Interviewer What is the refractory period for our nerves and what does this mean in terms of their frequency range?

Student The refractory period is around 1 ms. This puts an upper limit on the frequency of impulses along a nerve of around 1 kHz, since frequency is the inverse of this time period.

Interviewer So, for light entering your eye, what information about the energy is transferred by the impulse frequency along the nerve?

Student The wave-particle duality theory of light would describe the intensity of light as varying with photon frequency.

Interviewer The result of our nerves having a limit of 1 kHz to interpret light is that our eyes are relatively poor at discriminating between light intensities. Is there any way you think the eye compensates for this, to gain additional information about the intensity of light?

Student Perhaps, by possessing light receptors which react to different ranges of light intensity. Or using the iris to constrict the pupils and diminish the fraction of light reaching the retina.

Example II: Science questions

Here's an interview transcript from a student who mentioned studying oxygen–haemoglobin dissociation curves in biology:

Interviewer How does a foetus obtain oxygen from its mother?

Student Foetal haemoglobin has a higher affinity for oxygen than adult haemoglobin.

Interviewer Can you think of any other circumstances in which this principle of higher haemoglobin affinity is exploited?

Student At low oxygen pressures, such as high altitudes.

Interviewer Take a guess at what you think the maximum altitude is that we can live for a sustained period of time, without life support?

Student 5,000 m?

Interviewer Around that. The effect of altitude on haemoglobin is why the people of the Andes who first colonized the region were unable to have babies. What else happens to the human body with altitude?

Student The low oxygen saturation of the blood may increase your respiratory drive, causing you to hyperventilate.

Interviewer What is the effect on the pH of the blood?

Student Loss of acidic carbon dioxide leads to alkalosis.

Interviewer What is the other problem from hyperventilating?

Student Loss of water vapour, which can cause dehydration.

Example III: Problem solving

- If you were put in an irregularly shaped room and asked to measure the volume, how would you do it?
- When an ice cube in a glass full of water melts, what happens to the level of the water in the glass? Why? What would happen to the level if the ice cube melted in a glass of cooking oil?

Example IV: Theoretical discussion

- What is science?
- What has the biggest advance in medicine been and why?
- If you had the power to eradicate one disease, which would it be and why?

An insider's view ...

A common mistake made by students at interview is to think that the answer to a science question is our most important focus. As interviewers, we are far more interested in how applicants think and how they approach scientific problems. Sometimes we don't even know the answer ourselves.

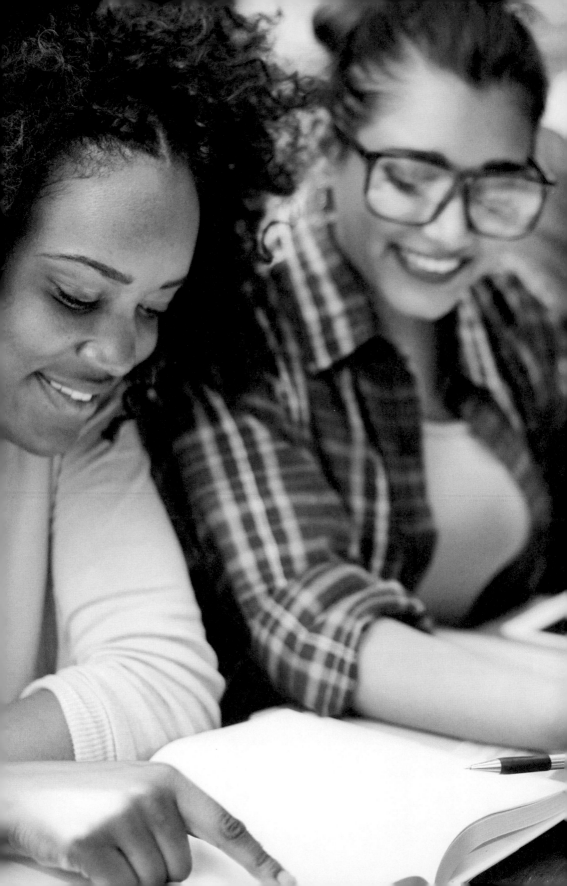

11

Graduate-entry medicine

▌ Introducing graduate medicine

Graduate-entry courses are accelerated, typically lasting four years instead of five. Although medical degrees in the UK usually take at least five years, this is different from other countries. In the USA, for example, school leavers enrol on a four-year undergraduate degree. Only when they graduate can they compete for the opportunity to spend another four years at medical school.

The graduate-entry model is now well established in the UK. A number of traditional medical schools, and some new ones, have launched courses designed for graduate applicants. These are shorter because the course designers assume that a graduate's first degree gives them knowledge or experience that overlaps with early medical school teaching. Graduate-entry medical courses vary in the types of degree they will consider for admission (see p. 254).

(see p. 254)

A student's experience ...

Studying medicine as a graduate is very different from my previous degree. The days are full and I am expected to sign a register at the start of almost every teaching session. However, studying medicine is a lot more fun because it is immediately obvious why each fact is important. It's finally an opportunity to apply my previous study of science to problems that impact on the lives of real people.

To apply or not to apply

Just because you are a graduate does not mean you *have* to apply to graduate-entry courses. You can also apply to traditional five- or six-year courses instead. In fact, there are good reasons why you might want to avoid graduate-entry programmes:

- **Limited choice of medical schools** Not all medical schools offer graduate-entry courses (see p. 265). If you want to study in a particular place, you might be unable to choose a graduate course.
- **Workload** Graduate-entry courses really are accelerated. The days are full, holidays are reduced, and there is an emphasis on 'self-directed learning'. This has been caricatured as 'do-it-yourself' medicine.
- **Environment** Some courses are very small (fewer than 25 students) and can feel claustrophobic.
- **Competition** There are lots of graduates wanting to study medicine but relatively few places. This means that accelerated courses are *much* more competitive. Applicant to place ratios vary from about 8:1 to 47:1 (see p. 261).

Of course, there are advantages to applying to these courses:

- **Money** Graduate-entry courses are much cheaper. One less year of being a student can save you between £17,000 and £25,000 (see p. 14), while the extra year on a standard course means one less year in your final employment, which may mean you lose out on about £120,000. Under the current system, those on traditional courses receive the NHS bursary (see p. 16) in their fifth and sixth year, but graduate-entry students are supported through years two, three, and four.
- **Environment** Students on graduate-entry courses are (usually) older, which creates a different environment from those dominated by school leavers. You will meet

people with a range of life experiences (and former careers), as well as many in your own age group.

- **Selection processes** Most graduate-entry courses place less emphasis on GCSEs and A levels. They are more interested in your degree. This can be an advantage if your earlier grades would score well in a game of Scrabble.
- **Time** Graduate-entry courses save a year of studying. If you already have a degree, you might be eager to start work and enter (or re-enter) the 'real world' as soon as possible.

A student's experience ...

I took the path of most graduate applicants and applied for a five-year course as a back-up choice. I was rejected by the graduate schools but offered a place on the traditional course. After doing the arithmetic, I realized I just couldn't afford five years of being a student on top of my existing student loans. It was a very sad day when I declined my offer to start medical school. If I'd thought harder at the beginning, I would have used that space for a fourth graduate course. Who knows what might have happened then?

Making a decision

Should you apply for graduate-entry courses? If you are a graduate, the answer is 'probably'. The financial and time advantages, particularly having already worked through one degree, should not be underestimated. However, graduate courses can be very competitive. For this reason, many applicants include one standard course as a 'back-up'. This is a legitimate strategy but only worth considering if you can afford to pursue a five-year course. As well as an extra year of tuition and living expenses (see p. 16), you are entitled to significantly less financial support from the NHS and the Student Loans Company (see p. 17).

If you apply to accelerated courses, you should bear in mind the applicant to place ratio. You should also remember that other applicants, your competitors, have had more time to build strong applications too. Course selectors will expect to see a good range of work experience and extracurricular achievements. Your competitors at interview will be more confident, more mature, and have a greater range of life experience to rely upon than school leavers. For these reasons, you should pay even more attention to the contents of this book than school leavers.

Key points

The NHS pays a bursary to medical students (see p. 16). This covers some tuition fees and, for many students, mileage, car parking, and a modest subsistence grant. Graduates on full-length courses are only entitled to this help in their final year. However, students on graduate-entry courses benefit from support for the last three years. This considerably alleviates the financial burden of studying medicine as a graduate.

The academic requirements

In general, staff on graduate-entry courses are more interested in your degree than your previous qualifications. GCSEs and A levels pale in significance. However, graduate courses have widely varying course entry requirements compared with undergraduate courses. They fall into three broad camps:

- **Strict courses** These have very clear criteria regarding the subjects they will accept and those they will not. In most cases they require a strong bioscience/life science background. This is true of Barts (see p. 273), Birmingham (see p. 270), Liverpool (see p. 272), King's (see p. 274), and Oxford (see p. 278).
- **Intermediate courses** These have broadly prescriptive admissions policies (e.g. Warwick (see p. 282), Birmingham (see p. 270)). If your degree is not explicitly listed, write and check before applying to these courses. The last thing you want is to waste a place applying for a course for which you are ineligible.
- **Open courses** These will consider any recognized degree. They include Cambridge (see p. 271), Newcastle (see p. 276), Nottingham (see p. 277), Southampton (see p. 280), St George's (see p. 275), and Swansea (see p. 286). One justification is that graduates will have developed transferable skills to help them meet the challenges of an accelerated course. In many cases, but not all, these schools require candidates to sit an entrance exam (e.g. GAMSAT, see p. 255) that tests basic bioscience aptitude or knowledge. Others may require experience of science at A level.

> **A student's experience ...**
>
> I was very careful to find out the admissions requirements of each school I was interested in attending. One replied to say I needed a first-class degree to win an interview. Having been predicted a first, I was encouraged and promptly applied. I was not shortlisted. When I asked for feedback, it turned out I had misunderstood their email. They required a *first-class degree*—simply being *predicted* a first was not sufficient. It was heartbreaking to have thrown away one of my four choices on a misunderstanding.

What about grades?

Almost all graduate-entry courses require an upper-second class (2:1) degree. A small number will consider 2:2 degrees but such candidates may be at a disadvantage. Nottingham (see p. 277) will consider candidates offering 2:2 degrees, as will St George's (see p. 275), Swansea (see p. 286), and Warwick (see p. 282), if the candidate also offers a Masters or PhD.

Although a 2:1 is usually the minimum standard, it is sometimes an advantage to hold a first-class degree. At the very least it will come in handy when building a career as a doctor. However, bear in mind that not all medical schools award 'points' for a first during the application process. If you scored highly in your undergraduate degree, think about which medical schools are likely to value your hard work. For example, the Birmingham (see p. 270) entry criteria are weighted so that candidates with first-class degrees (i.e. graduated with a first, not simply predicted) are strongly advantaged.

Do A levels matter?

Medical schools vary in attitudes towards pre-university qualifications. In general, they are less important, although some have requirements for biology and/or chemistry at AS or A level. In most cases this is true of courses that do not require a bioscience subject studied at university. Graduate-entry courses typically requiring chemistry at A or AS level include Cambridge (see p. 271), Kings (see p. 274), Liverpool (see p. 272), and Oxford (see p. 278). Some medical schools will accept a substantial component as part of your undergraduate degree if not offered at A level (e.g. BSc(Hons) in biochemistry without A level chemistry). Others have a biology requirement (e.g. Southampton (see p. 280) requires this to A level). A small number of graduate courses have science requirements without explicitly requiring specific subjects, although this changes year on year. Check specific entry requirements *carefully* to avoid wasting a valuable UCAS application.

What about postgraduate qualifications?

As with degree class, admissions policies vary. Some medical schools award points for an MSc/MPhil or PhD, others do not. Some schools (e.g. St George's (see p. 275), Swansea (see p. 286), and Warwick (see p. 282)) may overlook a 2:2 degree for candidates holding a postgraduate qualification. As a rule, PhDs carry more weight than Master's degrees. If you are an 'unusual' candidate in this respect, shop around to make your qualifications count. Do not be disheartened if your chosen schools do not explicitly reward your qualifications during the selection process. They may still be useful. You may well find yourself talking about your PhD thesis when asked about a 'challenging time' in interviews. In any event, your qualifications will carry plenty of weight throughout the rest of your career.

Graduate Australian Medical Admission Test (GAMSAT)

Graduate courses use a number of different admission tests. Most of these are the same as those used for selection to undergraduate courses (see p. 123). However, one exception is the GAMSAT, which is used by a handful of courses. The following should be noted:

- **A knowledge exam** Unlike the UCAT (see p. 82), the GAMSAT requires academic knowledge. This includes biology and chemistry (to first-year undergraduate level) and physics (AS level).
- **Three parts** The exam is divided into three sections: reasoning in humanities and social sciences (75 questions in 100 minutes), written communication (2 questions in 60 minutes), and reasoning in biological and physical sciences (110 questions in 170 minutes).
- **A marathon test** The GAMSAT takes five and a half hours to complete, with a one-hour break part way through.
- **Preparation** As with other admission tests, preparation is key. Sample questions and a practice GAMSAT exam are available online and from good academic bookstores.

Making the most of your time

If you have spent any time in the job market, you will be familiar with the idea that a degree is not enough. Your degree has earned you the right to apply to a graduate-entry course. That's the good news. The bad news is that, by definition, everyone else you are up against must have a degree as well. As one commentator has written: 'a degree is no longer a meal ticket to your future: it is only a licence to hunt'. Extracurricular activities mark candidates who are well rounded, interesting, and able to balance multiple commitments (see p. 46). They also give course selectors a good insight into your personality. You do not want to fall into the trap at interview of answering every question with 'During my degree…'.

One of the great advantages of being within a university environment is that your opportunities are infinite. You are only really limited by your own motivation. There are many sources of inspiration within or associated with your university:

- **Student representation groups** These usually take the form of committees within your department. They are forums for communicating student ideas to faculty members. Consider them an opportunity to improve your course and a means of interacting with academic staff. Great for winning that perfect UCAS reference (see p. 218).
- **Student media** Most universities run a student newspaper, magazine, radio station, and/or television service. Learning to write well is useful for medicine—as well as anything else you choose to do. Write about topics relevant to healthcare and kill two birds with one stone.
- **Uniformed organizations** The Armed Forces have specific reserve units for students. Although students cannot be sent to war, they can be offered trips abroad and training courses, often leading to civilian qualifications. There are also opportunities to gain leadership experience. Organizations include the Officers Training Corps (Army), University Air Squadrons (Royal Air Force), and University Royal Naval Units (Royal Navy). The Police also run a system of Special Constables which could provide a unique set of experiences.
- **Volunteering groups** Most universities run a volunteering organization of some description. If not, there will be plenty of opportunities within the local community. Opportunities could include subject tutoring, helping with day trips for disabled people, or working as a refugee caseworker. They are only really limited by the time you can commit.
- **Student societies and sports clubs** Students' unions often run hundreds of clubs and societies spanning every possible activity from knitting to paragliding. These are a great opportunity to relax and expand your range of extracurricular activities (see p. 46).
- **Part-time work** Paid employment is often the best way to gain real responsibility. There are lots of 'student jobs' (e.g. bar work) but don't feel confined to these. Consider registering with a local employment agency just to keep abreast of work in the local area. Try to develop transferable skills you can talk about later on at interview. Think about communication, teamwork, and leadership. You may need to demonstrate one or all of these at some point during the selection process. If you choose to go down this path, be careful that such work doesn't undermine your degree performance. A third-class degree framed by a well-rounded portfolio of extracurricular activities will not ease your passage into medical school.
- **Additional study** Most universities run short evening/weekend courses for adult learners. You could study something outside of your core subject (e.g. archaeology)

or pick up a language over the duration of your degree. Look up local colleges if your institution can't help.

- **Research** Approach your lecturers if you are interested in research. This can also serve as useful work experience. Do not be afraid to approach academics in other departments; fortune favours the brave. Research also looks very good on an application, particularly if you are able to demonstrate outputs (e.g. named on a conference presentation or published paper).
- **Travel** Try to make the most of your holidays. If finances allow, or you can save enough throughout the year, there are incredible experiences to be had. Think carefully about where to go and what to do. Travel can be a great way to broaden your mind whilst having fun along the way. With tickets to/from European cities starting at £10, even cash-strapped students can find themselves exploring Prague or Vienna at the weekend.

A student's experience ...

In two years of being in the Officers Training Corps, I launched helicopter raids on Jersey, sailed around the Canary Islands, dived in the Red Sea, and undertook Arctic survival training with Commandos in Norway. I also commanded a platoon of 20 cadets under what were sometimes very difficult conditions. However, these were easy compared to the massive task of articulating so many experiences within the confines of a UCAS form.

Branching out

You might be a student but you are also part of a wider local community. There is no reason why you should not stand for election as a parish, district, or even county councillor. Likewise, you could be eligible to serve as a school governor or sit as a magistrate hearing cases in your local courts (see www.gov.uk/become-magistrate). Don't feel you always have to tread ground that is already well trodden by other students. If you want to stand out, branch out.

A student's experience ...

Having developed an interest in my local community, I explored the possibility of becoming a magistrate. I spent a few days in the visitors' gallery at my local magistrates' court before applying. I now volunteer one day every week, deciding cases alongside two other magistrates. We are advised by a legally qualified clerk, but I am learning all the time. I believe (and hope) our decisions have a positive impact on the lives of victims of crime and, in many cases, on the perpetrators as well. It has certainly provided insight into what the world is like outside the university campus!

▍Work experience

Just like applicants to traditional courses, you will need to undertake some work experience. Don't skip the main work experience chapter in this book (see Chapter 5). Graduate applicants should demonstrate significantly more experience and more introspection towards their experience in contrast to the undergraduate cohort. This is for three reasons:

- **Admissions tutors expect more** You have had more time to gain work experience than students who are 16 and still at school. You also have a greater need to demonstrate a commitment to medicine—you are changing careers after all.
- **There is more competition** As emphasized ad nauseum in this chapter, winning a graduate place is particularly difficult. Your application really needs to shine to succeed.
- **The competition has significant experience** On the whole, graduates tend to have very rounded application forms. They have had time to find experience and may have been collecting opportunities for years. Graduates also come from a huge range of backgrounds—some of which are naturally well suited to the medical school selection process. It's hard to gain a better insight into healthcare than someone who worked as a nurse for 20 years. This shouldn't stop you trying though, but should spur you on to find as many experiences as you can.

The good news

Fortunately, there is some good news. It is usually much easier for graduates to arrange work experience; simplest while you are still at university. You will have long vacations and support in various forms from your institution.

- Most students' unions have volunteering societies. Get involved.
- If your institution has a medical school, don't be afraid of it. Look at the website for clinical staff who teach on the course. They might be worth contacting. Medical students in later years will also know senior doctors who might let you shadow them or at least ask questions.
- If you live away from home, spread your net of contacts wider. Write to GPs, hospitals, hospices, etc. in your home area and around the university. Ask academics in your department and medical students as and when you come across them. Campus GPs are unlikely to permit shadowing for confidentiality reasons.
- Long university vacations are ideal for exploiting meaningful work experience. A long summer could permit work as a healthcare assistant, phlebotomist, or hospital porter.
- Careers services in higher education are much larger and better organized than at school. Book an appointment and seek advice. There might also be bursaries available to cover work experience costs.
- Watch out for university first aid societies (usually supported by St John Ambulance). These are student units, based at most universities, that offer an opportunity to learn new skills and provide first aid at major public events.

More good news

Even if you have graduated and entered the 'real world', you still have trump cards left to play.

- **Use your degree** Your degree does carry weight in the job market. Graduates could find temporary work as a doctor's secretary or research assistant. A good science education could help in securing biomedical research experience (see p. 68). Many GPs need graduates familiar with scientific/biomedical vocabulary to summarize patient notes. If your degree is related in some way to medicine, you are more likely to be accepted into work experience/shadowing because of your qualifications.

- **You are older** This can work in your favour. Many jobs good for work experience (e.g. phlebotomy) have a minimum age. Graduate applicants should be eligible for some roles that are inaccessible for school leavers.
- **Transport** If you are lucky enough to own a car, or can borrow one, look for opportunities further afield.

A student's experience …

I studied biomedical science and one of my favourite lecturers was a medically qualified epidemiologist. I asked his advice after a seminar and he offered to call friends of his from medical school who worked locally. This resulted in four very different hospital placements over two years. A great start to my application!

A warning

As a graduate, you may feel as if you are in a very strong position to apply to medical school. You might be bright, confident, and successful in an established career. You might have a first-class degree, a PhD, and a string of research publications. Or you might have worked with patients in the NHS for years.

Whatever your position, you can *never* have enough work experience. A senior physiotherapist applying to medical school might learn more about the doctor's role (and perspective) by shadowing (see p. 62). A new graduate or PhD student should aim to gain insight into the NHS as well as patient contact. Whatever your experiences as a graduate, there is *always* something you can do to improve your chances. Do not fall into complacency.

Key points

Don't ever become demoralized or complacent about your application. There will always be candidates with better and worse applications than yours. The important thing is to keep working hard and learning about medicine through work experience. Persistence and diligence pay dividends eventually.

▮ Choosing a graduate-entry course

Graduate courses are similar to those designed for school leavers. The core knowledge and attitudes required to be a doctor will be covered wherever you study. In addition, most graduate courses channel graduates and school leavers into a single group for the clinical parts of the course. For example, you could receive one year of basic science teaching, then enter 'year three' alongside those who entered directly from school. However, like traditional courses, each institution has its own set of peculiarities. There are a huge range of factors, from location to course structure, which you need to consider, including:

- **Eligibility** Graduate courses vary in their academic and work experience requirements. If this is not clear, ask. The last thing you want to do is throw away one of your four choices. See Table 11.1.
- **Year size** Graduate courses vary enormously by size. They range from Oxford with around 30 places to Warwick with around 180. Some applicants prefer a small, intimate year group, others a larger, thriving cohort.
- **Composition** Some medical schools (e.g. Warwick and Swansea) only accept graduates. This creates a different environment from schools in which school leavers predominate.
- **Organization** Many graduate courses are new and still evolving, and this can impact on how much you enjoy and gain from the next few years. Try to gain an overall impression from current students and staff at open days.
- **Competition** See Table 11.2; consider choosing at least one 'safe(r) bet'.

How to choose

The same basic rules apply as for choosing any course. Leave no website or prospectus page unread. Call if you have questions and visit on open days. Try to contact current students; even those on other courses will have a view on the university itself. The Student Room (www.studentroom.co.uk) is a good resource for asking questions to specific groups of students from specific universities.

Make a list of all courses, then eliminate them one by one. First, strike out those for which you are not eligible to apply, then those you would not consider for geographical reasons, teaching styles, assessment styles, etc. Continue in this way until you are left with only four.

Eligibility criteria

Table 11.1 summarizes the academic requirements of each graduate course in the UK; for the complete profiles see Chapter 12. Courses with narrow selection requirements typically advertise a list of acceptable degrees on their websites. These lists are rarely exhaustive and, if there is any doubt, you must confirm the acceptability of your degree before applying.

Selection requirements for graduate courses vary widely. As they are so competitive, you *must* shop around to find which institutions best match your application. For example, a candidate who has already graduated with a first-class degree in biomedical science might rank Birmingham (see p. 270) over King's (see p. 274). This is because the pool of candidates with a 2:1 in any discipline will be larger than those with a first in a science or health subject. Similarly, an applicant with a 2:1 in history should not waste an application by applying to Birmingham.

Table 11.1 Academic entry requirements for graduate-entry courses

Course	Degree	Subject	AS/A level	Admission test
Barts	2:1	Science or health subject	Depend on degree	UCAT
Birmingham	2:1[1]	Life science subject	Chemistry or biology	UCAT
Cambridge	2:1	Any	2 from chemistry, biology, physics (within last 7 years)	None
King's College	2:1	Bioscience or nursing	A grade A level chemistry	UCAT
Leicester	2:1	Any	None	UCAT
Liverpool	2:1	Biomedical or health subject	Chemistry and biology, physics, or maths	GAMSAT
Newcastle	2:1	Any	None	UCAT
Nottingham	2:2	Any	None	GAMSAT
Oxford	2:1	Applied/experimental science	Chemistry and another science	BMAT
ScotGEM	2:1			GAMSAT
		Any	Minimum B in chemistry or equivalent	
Sheffield	2:1	Life science	Chemistry or biology	UCAT
Southampton	2:1	Any	Chemistry or AS chemistry with biology/human biology	UCAT
St George's	2:1	Any	None	GAMSAT
Swansea	2:1[2]	Any	None	GAMSAT
Warwick	2:1[2]	Any	None	UCAT

[1] Although the entrance requirement is a 2:1, 'strong preference' is given to candidates with first-class degrees.

[2] May accept a 2:2 together with a higher degree (e.g. MSc or PhD).

Table 11.2 Competitiveness of graduate medical schools in the UK, 2020

Medical school	Competition (applicants per offer)	Chance of interview (applicants per interview)	Success after interview (offers per interview)	Prestige (offers per place)	Competitiveness score
King's College	33.4	11.1	3.0	1.5	5
ScotGEM	30.1	18.8	1.6	1.5	5
Newcastle	27.9	7.7	3.6	1.3	5
Barts	25.0	7.5	3.3	1.5	4
Southampton	21.0	6.0	n/a	1.5	3
Birmingham	20.7	8.0	2.1	1.3	4
Oxford	11.4	5.0	3.2	1.2	5
Sheffield	11.1	5.0	2.2	1.2	3

Table 11.2 *(Continued)*

Medical school	Competition (applicants per offer)	Chance of interview (applicants per interview)	Success after interview (offers per interview)	Prestige (offers per place)	Competitiveness score
St George's	10.0	3.3	3.0	1.7	4
Liverpool	10.0	6.3	1.6	1.7	3
Swansea	8.0	3.2	2.5	1.1	4
Warwick	8.4	3.6	1.7	1.4	3
Nottingham	7.2	4.2	1.7	1.2	4
Cambridge	4.7	3.5	1.3	1.3	5

Key points

Don't simply pick four courses on the basis of familiarity or reputation. You may need to be strategic to guarantee your ambition of graduating as a doctor.

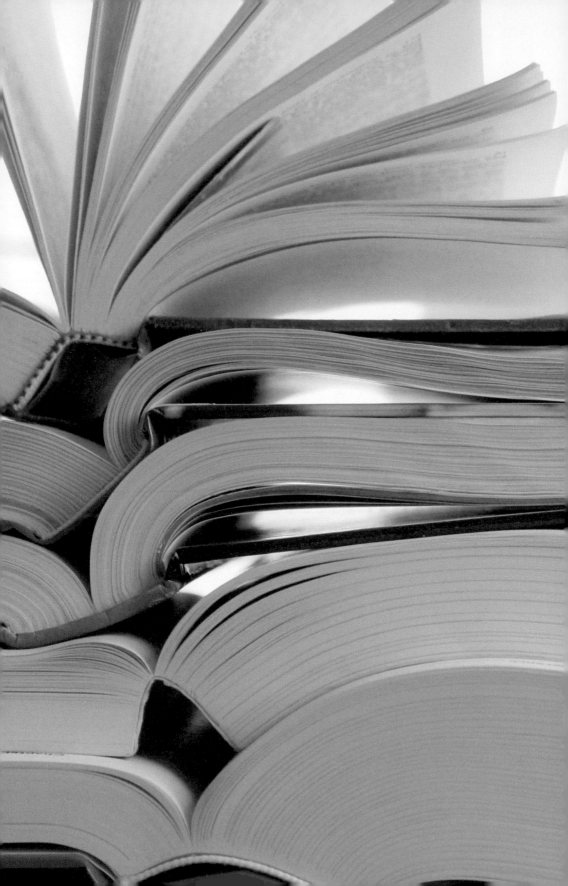

12

Graduate-entry medical schools

Understanding the profiles

Many of the graduate-entry medical schools have different facilities and buildings from the undergraduate courses and they all have different curricula (at least for the first one or two years). The following pages give descriptions of every graduate-entry medical course in the UK, except for Cardiff, which was not been included because its entry criteria are limited to graduates of only four degrees (awarded by Cardiff, Bangor, and the University of South Wales). Leicester (see p. 150) will accept graduates on the basis of their university qualifications but these applicants are then admitted to a single five-year course together with school leavers. All other UK graduate-entry courses should be represented, although it's likely that this list will change from year to year.

The profiles on these pages are designed to complement the longer profiles written for the undergraduate courses (see p. 124). Two medical schools are entirely devoted to graduate applicants (Warwick on p. 282 and Swansea on p. 286), so these medical schools have full two-page profiles.

The writers To ensure the most accurate information, the profiles were written in collaboration with medical student representatives from each graduate medical school (see p. xiv).

Warning!

While every possible step has been taken to ensure the accuracy of this information. It is possible that there are mistakes. Furthermore, medical schools are continually striving to improve their courses and methods of selecting the best students, so the details may change from year to year. Before you make an important decision based on the information shown, check the medical school website or contact its admissions team.

Key to the profiles

To make it simple to compare medical schools, the profiles have been written in a consistent format, starting with a description of each medical school followed by a table (see Table 12.1 for template).

Graduate students join their colleagues on the undergraduate course for the clinical years at the majority of medical schools. This phase of the course is described in the profiles written for the undergraduate courses (see Chapter 8) and the page reference for the relevant medical school is shown for each profile.

Entrance requirements

The entrance requirements for graduate-entry courses are extremely complicated, with some taking into account GCSE, A level, and degree results and full-time healthcare work post-qualification. Graduate schools are relatively new and many of these requirements are in a state of flux. Since there is no point in applying to a medical school when you do not meet the basic requirements, it is essential that you check the admissions website to be certain that you meet all the requirements before submitting your UCAS form.

Table 12.1 Sample profile explaining the criteria collated for each school

Best aspects	Why studying there is better than sliced bread		
Worst aspects	Why studying there can make your blood boil		
Requirements	Degree, A level, and GCSE requirements (please take into account the warning on p. 266)		
Type of course	Stone, Red brick, Plate glass, or Carbon fibre (see p. 102)	**Year size**	Medical students per year group
Course length	Total length of course	**Admission test**	UCAT, BMAT, or GAMSAT (see p. 74 and p. 255)
Applicants	Number of applicants	**Student mix:**	Proportion of international students in a year group
Interviews	Number interviewed	**% international**	
Offers	Number of offers given (see p. 261)		
Competition	All medical courses are highly competitive; this subjective scale aims to highlight how they compare to other medical schools		
Work	All medical courses have packed timetables and intense workloads (expect at least 40 hours per week); this subjective scale highlights how much free time you might get compared to other medical schools		

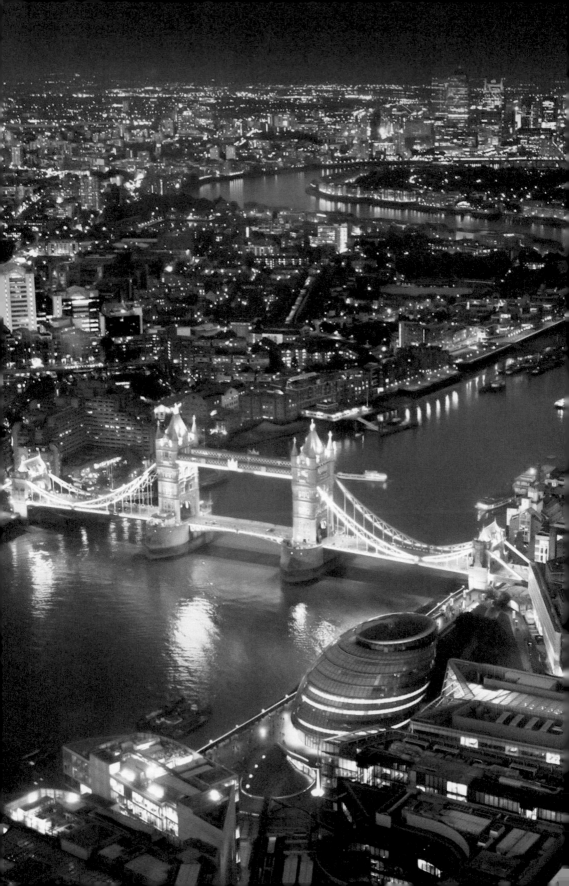

England

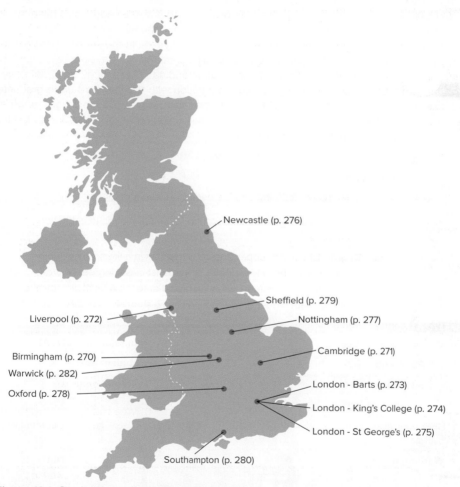

Figure 12.1 Graduate medical schools in England.

Newcastle (p. 276)

Sheffield (p. 279)

Liverpool (p. 272)

Nottingham (p. 277)

Birmingham (p. 270)

Cambridge (p. 271)

Warwick (p. 282)

Oxford (p. 278)

London - Barts (p. 273)

London - King's College (p. 274)

London - St George's (p. 275)

Southampton (p. 280)

Birmingham

The course consists of one year of problem-based learning (PBL) and case studies, followed by three clinically focused years integrated with the standard undergraduate course. In the first year, students work in groups of eight on seven themed modules covering basic science, anatomy (including prosection), ethics, and medicine in society, with all these aspects integrated into each of the case studies. PBL teaching is supported by weekly anatomy sessions and tutorials with experts in the field being studied. There are weekly GP practice visits to help develop clinical skills.

During the first year, each group has their own room to use at all hours as a base that is supplied with IT facilities, textbooks, anatomy models, and the all-important kettle.

The pressure eases over the three remaining clinical years. In the second year, graduates join the third-year undergraduates in hospital placements four days a week, changing hospitals between semesters. Students continue attending GP practices on certain days to maintain a connection with primary care. Integration with the standard undergraduate course during the clinical years provides an opportunity to widen your social group, whilst enjoying the challenge and excitement that the clinical setting has to offer. See p. 130 for details of the clinical course. See Table 12.2.

Table 12.2 Birmingham

Best aspects	Self-directed learning and the dedicated teaching rooms
Worst aspects	Working with the same small group for so long leads to cabin fever at exam time
Requirements	**Degree** 1st-class or upper 2nd-class honours in a life science subject: scoring criteria heavily weighted towards 1st-class degrees and/or completed degrees (not simply predicted grades); **A level** biology and chemistry with higher grades scoring more shortlisting points.

Type of course	Red brick	Year size	40
Course length	4 years	Admission test	UCAT
Applicants	827	Student mix:	
Interviews	104	% international	0%
Offers	50		

Uncompetitive ... Competitive

Working really hard ... Not working/chilling out

Cambridge

The course was established in 2001 and takes four years to complete (compared to the usual six years). There is a choice of four Cambridge colleges: Wolfson, Hughes Hall, Lucy Cavendish, and St Edmund's. The college provides accommodation and small-group teaching (see p. 242). All preclinical and clinical teaching is bolstered by small-group supervisions, which provide a forum for detailed discussion and prevent students from falling behind unnoticed.

In the preclinical years, graduates are mixed with the standard course students and taught in a mixture of lectures, practical sessions, and supervisions. In parallel, graduate students receive 'level one' clinical training during the university holidays at West Suffolk Hospital (WSH) in Bury St Edmunds, 30 miles from Cambridge. The parallel structure provides an opportunity to immediately apply preclinical knowledge to clinical scenarios at the WSH. At the start of Year 3, having completed two preclinical years and level one training, graduate students join the Year 5 standard course students for 'level two'. This entails specialty placements at Addenbrooke's Hospital (Cambridge) and regional hospitals throughout East Anglia. Final-year 'level three training' is spent exclusively back at WSH, where accommodation is provided free of charge (as it is during level one too).

The graduate programme offers the same style and high standard of teaching as the standard course (see p. 136). The workload is extraordinarily tough in level one as you must keep up with the standard course students without the advantage of 26 weeks' holiday a year, but it eases as soon as level two begins. See Table 12.3.

Table 12.3 Cambridge

Best aspects	Very thorough teaching and clinical exposure; spending time in Bury together fosters very close lifelong friendships
Worst aspects	A very competitive, anxious atmosphere with fellow students very good at creating mass panic in the lead-up to exams
Requirements	**Degree** upper 2nd-class honours in any subject; **A level** chemistry (in the previous seven years) plus at least one of physics, biology, or maths. At least AAA preferred.

Type of course	Stone	**Year size**	43
Course length	4 years	**Admission test**	n/a
Applicants	258	**Student mix:**	
Interviews	73	**% international**	0%
Offers	55		

Uncompetitive ⸻ Competitive

Working really hard ⸻ Not working/chilling out

Liverpool

The course provides students with the opportunity to embark on the journey into clinical practice while being supported with teaching delivered on campus. You also needn't worry about being ill-prepared for immediate clinical exposure—there is an intense course in essential clinical and communication skills before you join the five-year course students who are entering into their second year of study.

Teaching includes extensive case-based learning, anatomy sessions, and lectures, which form the core of the spiral curriculum. Students familiar with self-directed learning will rapidly augment their prior knowledge but still feel a strong connection to the medical school throughout their first year. All of the resources of the undergraduate course are at the disposal of graduate students, including prosections in the Human Anatomy Resource Centre (HARC) and lecture recordings.

Clinical experience in the first year is based at one of five hospitals in Liverpool and the surrounding area. Approximately every six weeks you will spend a week on a medical or surgical ward, exposing you to the clinical environment and providing you with time to practice history taking and examinations.

At the end of their first year, graduate students sit the same examinations as the second-year students on the undergraduate course, which includes MCQ written papers and an OSCE. The rest of the clinical course is described on p. 152. See Table 12.4.

Table 12.4 Liverpool

Best aspects	The intense 'catch up' clinical course before starting clinical placement ensures you are prepared for clinical placement		
Worst aspects	It can still be daunting to join a cohort of second-year undergraduates who have all received the same teaching at medical school		
Requirements	**Degree** upper 2nd-class in a biological, biomedical, or health science subject, **A level** DDD, chemistry and either biology, physics, or maths; **GCSE** C in English and maths		
Type of course	Carbon fibre	**Year size**	30
Course length	4 years	**Admission test**	GAMSAT
Applicants	500	**Student mix:**	
Interviews	80	**% international**	0%
Offers	50		
Uncompetitive			**Competitive**
Working really hard			**Not working/ chilling out**

London—Barts

Graduate students at Barts follow a tailored curriculum whereby their first year of study covers all undergraduate preclinical content (years 1 and 2). The syllabus takes a 'systems-based approach', with each module covering a different body system over the course of four to eight weeks. First-year graduate students spend most of their time at Barts' East End campus sites in Whitechapel and Mile End. Thanks to Barts' close ties with the Royal London and surrounding hospitals, there's ample opportunity for first-year graduate students to kick-start their portfolios with research projects, mentorship schemes, and clinical audits.

With around 20 hours of contact time per week, students are expected to supplement lectures and practical sessions in their own time with dedicated online resources and recommended reading lists. The medical school's dedicated libraries, IT labs, and study rooms provide ample space for students to find a spot and hunker down. Further, weekly student-led PBL sessions serve as an invaluable tool for revising taught content through discussion of clinical cases, and weekly placements in general practice or hospital wards provide students with valuable clinical experience. Following their first year, graduate students are placed on clinical rotations at a choice of Barts Health hospitals (either within or outside of London). Accommodation is provided for any placements outside of London and all relevant teaching is carried out on-site. See Table 12.5.

Table **12.5** London—Barts

Best aspects	Early clinical exposure in world-leading hospitals, and research opportunities		
Worst aspects	Cost of living in London can be exorbitant		
Requirements	**Degree** upper 2nd-class honours in a science or health-related subject; **A level** none for bioscience degrees, grade C at A2 or AS in chemistry or biology if missing from another science degree, B in chemistry or biology plus one other science if applying with a non-science degree.		
Type of course	Carbon fibre	**Year size**	40
Course length	4 years	**Admission test**	UCAT
Applicants	1,500	**Student mix:**	
Interviews	200	**% international**	10%
Offers	60		
Uncompetitive			**Competitive**
Working really hard			**Not working/ chilling out**

London—King's College

The graduate and professional entry (GPEP) course at KCL starts with a transition month in August. This is composed of two weeks of clinical skills and two weeks of anatomy (including full dissection). This is intense, with around seven hours of lectures per day. The transition month is designed to get you up to speed for year two, and assumes you have prior knowledge from your life sciences-related undergraduate degree. The reward for surviving the epic first month is to join year two of the regular MBBS, and the remainder of the course (see p. 158) is completed in a standard (non-accelerated!) fashion. Years two to five work like any other medical degree, but you skip the intercalated BSc. Throughout the rest of the course you complete progress tests, with the aim of improving your score with each subsequent test. The 'fifth' year (your fourth) kicks off with an enjoyable eight-week long elective to anywhere in the world (plus two weeks of summer holiday).

The graduate route is tough but certainly not impossible—indeed, the requirement of a life sciences degree was only introduced recently, with previous graduates being from any background and mostly graduating successfully. See p. 158 for further details of the clinical course. See Table 12.6.

Table 12.6 London—King's College

Best aspects	Well-established course; dissection; being taught at the internationally renowned hospitals of Guy's, King's, and St Thomas'; diverse patient mix; long elective period		
Worst aspects	Relatively tough, lecture-heavy first year; frequent exams		
Requirements	**Degree** upper 2nd-class honours in biosciences subject or nursing (covering life sciences); **A level** chemistry (A) for nursing graduates		
Type of course	Red brick	**Year size**	28
Course length	4 years	**Admission test**	UCAT
Applicants	1,404	**Student mix:**	
Interviews	127	**% international**	7%
Offers	42		
Uncompetitive	🏆 🏆 🏆 🏆 🏆🏆🏆🏆		**Competitive**
Working really hard			**Not working/ chilling out**

London—St George's

The course is based on a scheme developed at Flinder's University in South Australia. It is founded upon PBL and there is a heavy emphasis on independent learning. In the first year, students rotate through six overarching themes which cover all the clinical science, statistics, and ethics modules that the traditional five-year course covers in the first two years. Each week starts and finishes with a case-based learning session. Areas of focus are outlined in learning objective lists (known as LOBS) which are released on a weekly basis. The learning is supplemented with weekly lectures, clinical skill sessions, and anatomy sessions in the dissecting lab. The style of learning can be tough for students arriving from non-scientific disciplines, but experience has shown that they perform just as well. The teaching style is varied: a typical week includes two days of PBL, two days of lectures, and a day of clinical skills. Exams are frequent, meaning everyone stays on top of their work and few fall behind.

After the first year, students in the graduate programme join those on the traditional five-year course (at the beginning of their third year). Each year builds on the year before; so-called 'spiral' learning. See p. 160 for more details of the clinical course. See Table 12.7.

Table 12.7 London—St George's

Best aspects	Friendly, modern course in a truly multidisciplinary environment; teaching within tertiary hospital where some of the most complex patients are treated
Worst aspects	GAMSAT; over-reliance on students' own resourcefulness; the administration can feel disorganized
Requirements	**Degree** upper 2nd-class honours in any subject or a higher degree (Master's or PhD)

Type of course	Plate glass	Year size	60
Course length	4 years	Admission test	GAMSAT
Applicants	1,000	Student mix:	
Interviews	300	% international	0%
Offers	100		

Uncompetitive		Competitive
Working really hard		Not working/ chilling out

■ Newcastle

Newcastle welcomes a wide range of graduates and health professionals onto its accelerated course. Its students have come from backgrounds as diverse as film studies, history, PPE (philosophy, politics, and economics), and psychology. Graduate students cover two years of undergraduate medicine in a single year before joining the undergraduate course in its third year. The course attracts highly motivated students who are able to organize their time effectively.

Learning is case-led, problem-based, group-learning hybrid. Over the course of the first year, students work through 25 cases in seminar groups, with each case centring around a patient with a particular clinical condition. These case-led seminars are fortified with lectures and (prosection-based) anatomy sessions, with a large portion of self-directed learning via Newcastle's online bespoke Medical Learning Environment (MLE).

One of the best aspects of the course is the support provided by tutors and course leaders, with frequent opportunities to give feedback on all aspects of the course as well as to improve aspects based on the cohort's requirements. Integrated history taking, clinical skills, and clinical reasoning sessions help to prepare you for clinical placements, where you are able to practice the skills you have developed as well as build on communication skills.

The small-year cohort makes for a tight-knit group; many students appreciate studying alongside highly motivated colleagues from different backgrounds. After the first year, graduates join the third year of the undergraduate course to develop their clinical and knowledge skills further. See p. 166 for more details of the undergraduate course. See Table 12.8.

Table 12.8 Newcastle

Best aspects	Great support from all your tutors and colleagues		
Worst aspects	The pure intensity of the course; you don't know what self-directed study is until you have a go at the accelerated programme!		
Requirements	**Degree** upper 2nd-class honours in any discipline; or a practicing healthcare professional with a post-registration qualification		
Type of course	Carbon fibre	**Year size**	25
Course length	4 years	**Admission test**	UCAT
Applicants	920	**Student mix:**	
Interviews	120	**% international**	0%
Offers	33		

Uncompetitive — Competitive

Working really hard — Not working/chilling out

Nottingham

The broad entry requirements promote diversity in terms of age and background. Around a third of students come from non-science backgrounds, including English, classics, arts, music, and economics.

The first 18 months is based at the Royal Derby Hospital campus, distinct from the undergraduate course (see p. 168). It utilizes PBL, with students arranged into groups of eight to ten, and taught by other students. Four and a half hours every week are dedicated to working through a PBL case, from initial presentation to diagnosis and definitive management. The PBL sessions are supported by lectures, anatomy and pathology workshops, GP practice attachments, and clinical skills sessions to ensure all learning types are catered for. There is a strong emphasis on clinical relevance and rote learning is discouraged. Teaching is well adapted to the mature intake and is relaxed and friendly, aided by an approachable teaching staff.

Formative assessments follow the completion of each system-based module, while summative assessments occur at the end of year one (July) and the end of the 18 months' preclinical course (February). After the first 18 months, the GEM (graduate-entry medical) students join the third-year undergraduates to begin a 17-week clinical practice course, before completing the final two years' clinical placements at hospitals around the Trent region. Many GEM students move to Nottingham during the clinical phase, as it is more convenient for teaching and placement sites (e.g. Hopper Bus, Medilink), campus facilities, and the Nottingham city centre for shopping and nightlife. See p. 168 for more details of the clinical phase. See Table 12.9.

Table 12.9 Nottingham

Best aspects	Clinical placements from the start; learning in a friendly environment		
Worst aspects	Formative assessments every six weeks; learning at a brisk pace!		
Requirements	**Degree** lower 2nd-class honours degree in any subject; significant healthcare work experience		
Type of course	Red brick	**Year size**	118
Course length	4 years	**Admission test**	GAMSAT
Applicants	1,074	**Student mix:**	
Interviews	250	**% international**	4%
Offers	149		
Uncompetitive			**Competitive**
Working really hard			**Not working/ chilling out**

Oxford

The first year of the graduate course is taught completely independently from the undergraduate course and focuses heavily on the scientific basis of medicine, with teaching via lectures and college-based tutorials, and much of the content covered by self-study. Clinical skills are developed through one clinical day a week, which alternates between district general hospitals and GP practices, with the medical school providing transport there and back. Anatomy is taught with the use of prosections, although there are opportunities for enthusiastic students to learn via dissection. The second year continues with more basic science teaching but integrates with the fourth year of the undergraduate course for a nine-week clinical pathology course and clinical placements in medicine and surgery.

The final two years are completely integrated with the undergraduate clinical course. The majority of the clinical teaching is done in Oxford, based at the John Radcliffe Hospital, as well as at surrounding district general hospitals, with a series of attachments to different clinical specialties. The fourth year provides special study blocks, allowing you to pursue areas of interest, as well as a 10-week elective that most students take overseas.

Given its small size, the graduate entry programme tends to produce a fairly cohesive group with lots of socializing. Most students live in college accommodation that is spread throughout Oxford for their first year, and there are typically two to four graduate-entry students at each college. Graduates traditionally perform well in the final exams—practical evidence that the first couple of years are worth so much hard work! See p. 170 for more details of the clinical course. See Table 12.10.

Table 12.10 Oxford

Best aspects	Tutorials and lots of clinical contact
Worst aspects	High expectations; and one of the heaviest workloads of any course at Oxford
Requirements	**Degree** upper 2nd-class in applied and experimental sciences; **A level** two sciences, including chemistry; **GCSE** biology/double science if degree is in a non-bioscience subject

Type of course	Stone	Year size	30
Course length	4 years	Admission test	BMAT
Applicants	400	Student mix:	
Interviews	80	% international	7%
Offers	35		

Uncompetitive					🏆🏆🏆🏆🏆	Competitive

Working really hard						Not working/ chilling out

278 Graduate-entry medical schools

▌Sheffield

The GEM course at Sheffield is open exclusively to graduates from a 'widening access' background who also have a degree in a relevant life science. Students accepted on to the GEM course are able to bypass the first year of the undergraduate degree; however, the remainder of the degree is exactly as for the normal undergraduate programme. Having skipped the first year of the course, your first taste of medical school is predominantly clinical and relatively free of book learning.

As the GEM curriculum maps the undergraduate one exactly, it is well established and so more resistant to some of the ups and downs that are sometimes associated with new course designs. Anatomy is a particular highlight at Sheffield, with the use of real human cadavers in teaching, along with a fantastic support staff and excellent dissecting space. One of the unique benefits of the Sheffield course is that it offers two seven-week blocks for students' own elective work, a welcome break from rigidly structured didactic learning.

Sheffield is a city that seems to keep hold of its new medical graduates, with one of the highest retention rates in the UK. This is less hard to believe when you look at the perks of living here: a phenomenal bar scene, the peak district only 20 minutes away, a fantastic shopping centre, and a world-leading theatre all on your doorstep. See Table 12.11.

Table 12.11 Sheffield

Best aspects	For the 2020 cohort, thanks to a generous donation from an alumnus, the £3,700 shortfall in funding that all other grads are expected to pay was waived!		
Worst aspects	Same degree as the undergraduate one just without the initial year to get everyone to the same level		
Requirements	**Degree** upper 2nd-class in life sciences; **A level** at least BBB with chemistry or biology		
Type of course	Red brick	Year size	15 places for UK students
Course length	4 years	Admission test	UCAT
Applicants	200	Student mix:	
Interviews	40	% international	0%
Offers	18		
Uncompetitive	🏆 🏆 🏆🏆🏆 🏆🏆🏆 🏆🏆🏆🏆		**Competitive**
Working really hard			**Not working/ chilling out**

▌Southampton

Students on the graduate course are treated as adults from the outset; there's a dedicated staff team and a strong emphasis on self-directed learning. During the first two (largely preclinical) years, teaching is based around systems and diseases. The course is taught through a variety of lectures, facilitated problem-based learning (PBL) tutorials, anatomy tutorials, and bedside teaching.

PBL forms the foundation of the weekly structure and is initiated by trigger material on a Monday, leading into a week of lectures and bedside teaching at Southampton General Hospital and the Royal Hampshire County hospital. PBL concludes every week on a Friday, when each student presents their material, and the sessions are normally followed by a plenary with a consultant in the relevant field. Case material helps identify key learning points for the group. In addition, once every two weeks a group of four students attend a GP practice for an afternoon. In total, one and a half days a week are spent in clinical environments during the first two years.

In year three, the graduates join fourth-year students on the traditional course for clinical rotations. See p. 176 for more details of the parts of the course shared with the undergraduates. See Table 12.12.

Table 12.12 Southampton

Best aspects	Dedicated graduate-entry medicine staff team for the first two years; good pastoral support; long summer holidays; small cohesive group		
Worst aspects	Self-directed learning: opportunity for some, or nightmare for others		
Requirements	**Degree** upper 2nd-class honours in any subject; **A level** chemistry (at least grade C) or **AS-level** chemistry and biology/human biology (both at least grade C).; **GCSE** minimum grade C in maths, English, and double-award science (or equivalent)		
Type of course	Plate glass	**Year size**	48
Course length	4 years	**Admission test**	UCAT
Applicants	1,250	**Student mix:**	
Interviews	-	**% international**	7.5%
Offers	60		
Uncompetitive	🏆 🏆 🏆🏆🏆 🏆🏆🏆 🏆🏆🏆🏆		**Competitive**
Working really hard			**Not working/ chilling out**

Warwick

Warwick is unusual in only accepting applications from graduates (of any subject); there are no school leavers. This means there is an adult atmosphere about the whole course, which is designed with the graduate learner firmly in mind.

University The medical school was purpose-built in 2000, including a lecture theatre, common room, clinic facilities, seminar rooms, and a computer suite. These facilities are available 24 hours a day, which is great for night owls, and everyone else at exam time! There is also a Bio Med Grid, which incorporates technology, leather couches, and a bio-medical reference library, for those who prefer to spend as little time as possible in the physical library. Local hospitals are up to 15 miles away but most students work at the £500-million University Hospital in Coventry. The hospital includes a Clinical Sciences Building for members of the university, including students, to gain respite from patient areas. Car parking is a problem but few are brave enough to rely on public transport in the clinical years.

Course The first 12 months of the programme are particularly intensive, condensing the preclinical phases of an undergraduate medical degree into one academic year. Students cover core anatomy, pharmacology, and physiology of all body systems, plus all the medico-legal and ethical underpinnings of clinical practice. Clinical skills teaching begins immediately. Case-based learning (CBL) takes place twice a week during which students work through patient scenarios as a group, to revise and cement knowledge from the lectures.

Clinical placements begin full-time in the second year with rotations in surgery and general internal medicine, with further specialized rotations seeing you through to the final year. There is plenty of opportunity to gain exposure to specialties of interest during placements across the three main teaching hospitals in the area (Warwick Hospital, George Eliot Hospital, University Hospital Coventry & Warwickshire). Beyond these, you'll spend time with some of the many GP practices that support your clinical learning.

The summative exams (i.e. the ones that count) take place at the end of the academic year and cover everything you've studied up to that point, so it's not a course where you can 'forget and move on'!

Lifestyle Owing to the slightly odd location of Warwick University (i.e. located in Coventry, not Warwick), most medical students live in Coventry, Leamington Spa, or Kenilworth. There are a huge range of societies on offer representing nearly every medical specialty, as well as sports clubs, music groups, and the opportunity to freely mingle with other non-medic societies on main campus as well. Should you wish to be part of it, you'll also be assigned medic 'parents'—older students who will look after you during your first year and introduce you to members of the wider medic family.

Factoid Peer teaching is an enormous part of being a Warwick medical student—there are evening seminars running every night of the week, with societies leading revision days covering all aspects of the curriculum. See Table 12.13.

Table 12.13 Warwick

Myth	Full of biomedical science students who didn't make it first time			
Reality	Students from almost every discipline with an unrivalled passion to learn and succeed			
Personality	World-class musicians, scientists, sportspeople, and immensely talented allied health professionals can all be found at Warwick.			
Best aspects	Incredibly high-standard anatomy teaching in first year from international experts using a collection of exceptional plastinated specimens			
Worst aspects	First year can feel enormously daunting, especially approaching exam season, owing to the sheer volume of content			
Requirements	**Degree** upper 2nd-class honours in any subject; a lower 2nd-class degree candidate must hold a Master's or PhD			
Course length	4 years		Structure	Campus
Type of course	Plate glass		Year size	192
Typical offer	2:1		Admission test	UCAT
Applicants	1,600		Student mix:	
Interviews	450		% international	2%
Offers	270			
Uncompetitive				Competitive
Low living costs				High living costs
Working really hard				Not working/ chilling out
Contact details	Warwick Medical School, The University of Warwick, Coventry, CV4 7AL Tel: +44 (0) 2476 574 880, Web: https://warwick.ac.uk/fac/sci/med/			

An insider's view ...

At Warwick there is an excellent ratio of students to consultant doctors in the clinical years. This means students often receive one-on-one teaching and are assigned a different specialist to oversee their progress throughout each clinical rotation. Each consultant has a team of junior doctors, so there are always plenty of clinical teachers available. This model is ideal for graduate students, who develop strong professional relationships with their senior colleagues and make the most of time on the wards.

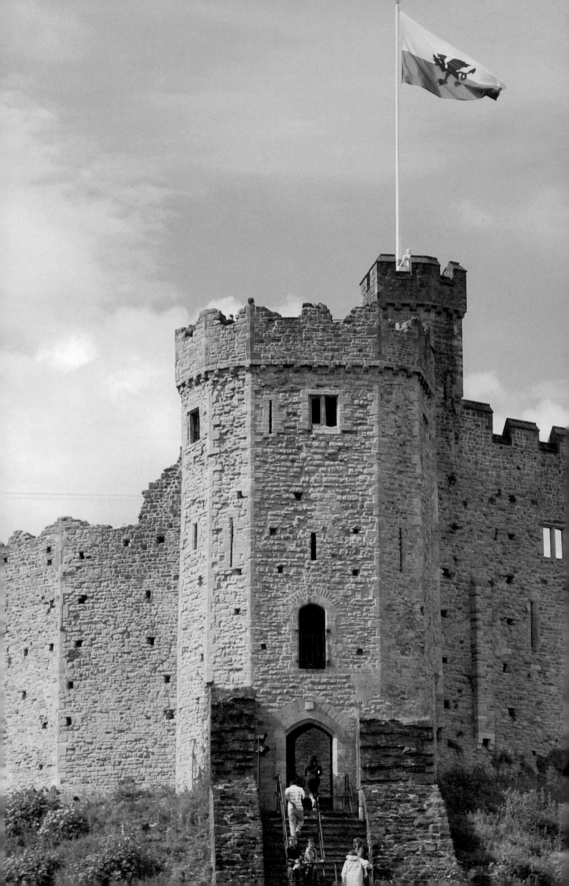

Wales

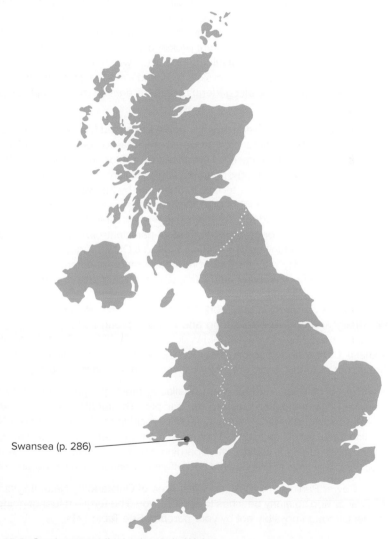

Swansea (p. 286)

Figure 12.2 Graduate medical schools in Wales.

Swansea

Swansea and Warwick (see p. 282) are the only two graduate-only medical schools in the UK. The course at Swansea was established in 2004 and aims to reduce the acute shortage of doctors in Wales. Swansea University Medical School is one of the UK's fastest-growing medical schools, specially designed to help graduates of any discipline achieve the core knowledge required for work as a doctor.

University Swansea University became an independent degree-awarding institution in 2007 when it devolved from the University of Wales. In 2017, Swansea opened a second campus, Bay Campus, which is located on the beach on the eastern approach into Swansea. Swansea Medical School and all teaching facilities remain based at the Singleton Park Campus which is set in mature parkland and botanical gardens, overlooking Swansea Bay beach and adjacent to Singleton Hospital. Swansea Medical School contains lecture theatres, an anatomy suite, clinical skills labs, and a medical student common room. Singleton Hospital, a 550-bed district general hospital, is right on the edge of campus and contains a clinical skills lab and a 24-hour library.

Course The first two years are predominantly university-based but there is still significant clinical exposure. Teaching is organized around a case-based 'learning week' format. At the start of each week, a patient case is introduced by a tutor and, throughout the week, clinical sciences (anatomy, physiology, pharmacology, etc.) are taught in a way that is relevant to the case. On Fridays there is a clinical forum, run by the week's leader, to consolidate the knowledge learned throughout the week.

During the first two years, students have three five-week clinical apprenticeships based in hospitals around Wales. Alongside this, students participate in Swansea's unique and innovative Learning Opportunities in a Clinical Setting (LOCS) programme, in which they are able to choose half-day experiences from a huge range of different clinical settings. Popular examples include observing autopsies, psychiatry in a prison, cardiothoracic surgery, and shadowing a midwife.

The final two years are spent largely working in hospitals and GP practices. These placements are usually around five weeks long and can be spread across South West Wales (Swansea, Carmarthen, Haverfordwest), Mid-Wales (Aberystwyth), and North Wales (Bangor, Rhyl, Wrexham). Commuting to some placements is very difficult with limited public transport. Although not essential, a car is a major asset to students on this course.

Lifestyle Although halls of residence are available, most graduate medics live in affordable private accommodation close to the campus. The medical school is extremely outdoors- and sports-orientated. University facilities include the 50-metre Wales National Pool, a running track, tennis and squash courts, and a newly refurbished gymnasium. The Gower beaches are ideal for surfing, kite-boarding, and other water sports. The medical school itself has close links to the Gambia and offers a short-term exchange programme.

Factoid The Gower Peninsula was Britain's first Area of Outstanding Natural Beauty. With world-class waves and so many beaches to explore, you'd be forgiven for not going home in the summer (although possibly not by your parents). See Table 12.14.

Table 12.14 Swansea

Myth	Cardiff's poor younger brother
Reality	A modern perspective on the age-old tradition of teaching medicine; the result is competent, knowledgeable, and dedicated doctors
Personality	Make things happen; the common saying 'Swansea is a graveyard of ambition' refers to the phenomenon that when strangers visit Swansea they never want to leave!
Best aspects	A 'hands-on' course with very early clinical exposure; multiple beaches along the Gower peninsula and stunning walks in the Brecon Beacons; free parking in all hospitals
Worst aspects	Small cohort may breed cabin fever; little holiday due to intensity of course; lots of rain
Requirements	**Degree** upper 2nd-class in any subject, or lower 2nd-class with a higher degree (MSc or PhD); **GCSE** C in maths and English or Welsh

Course length	4 years	Structure	Campus
Type of course	Plate glass	Year size	90
Typical offer	2:1	Admission test	GAMSAT
Applicants	800	Student mix:	
Interviews	250	% international	5%
Offers	100		

Uncompetitive		**Competitive**
Low living costs		**High living costs**
Working really hard		**Not working/ chilling out**

Contact details	School of Medicine, Swansea University, Singleton Park, Swansea, SA2 8PP Tel: +44 (0) 1792 602 618, Web: www.swan.ac.uk/medicine

An insider's view ...

In Swansea we welcome graduates with a first or upper second degree in any subject and at any one time we may have up to a third of the class qualified in non-science subjects—history, languages, philosophy, etc. This enriches both the staff and the student experience. Students with non-science degrees are not disadvantaged. Indeed, many of them are among our academic 'high flyers'. Part of our success is due to the individual attention that we can give students in a school that is 'small but perfectly formed' and many of our students take leadership roles across Wales and beyond, e.g. in Wilderness medicine, the Surgical Society, the Rural and Remote Health Track, and the Swansea–Gambia link.

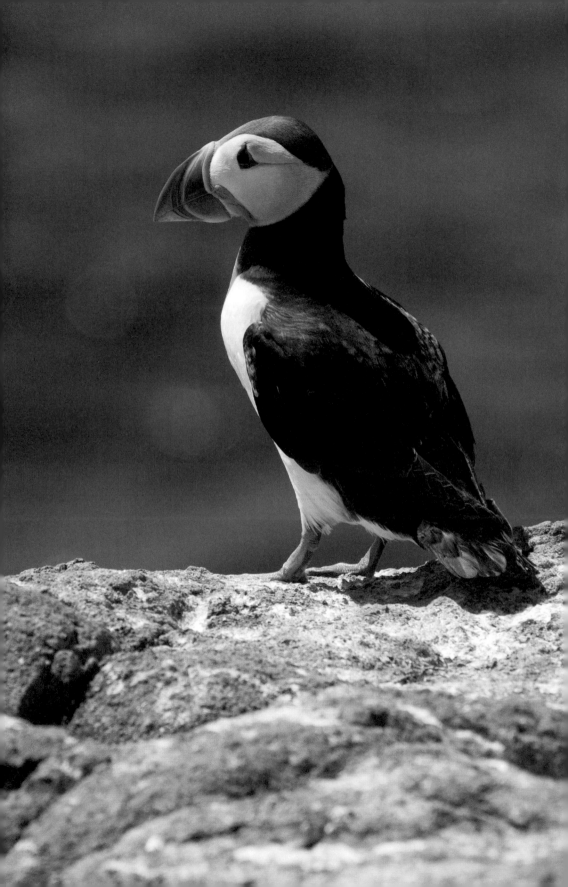

Scotland

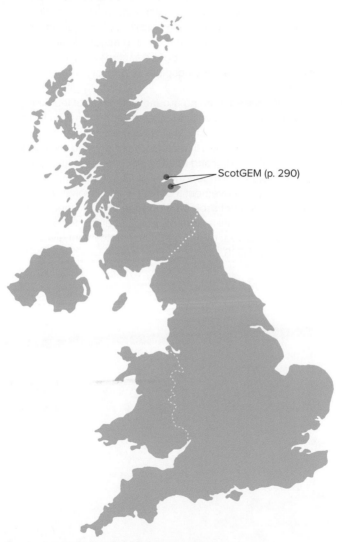

ScotGEM (p. 290)

Figure 12.3 Graduate medical schools in Scotland.

Scottish Graduate-Entry Medicine (ScotGEM)

Scotland's first ever graduate-entry medical course only opened in 2018, as a joint venture between St Andrews, Dundee, and a range of NHS organizations. There is a heavy emphasis on remote and rural and primary care.

Much of the course is delivered in and around Inverness and Dumfries in the second year (with accommodation provided), as well as in St Andrews and other parts of Fife, which is where all students are based throughout the first year. In the third year, all students complete a longitudinal integrated clerkship—basically a placement in a single location (in primary care in a remote or rural setting) for the entire academic year—where they learn and work alongside GPs. Final exams follow, before all students spend their fourth and final year working traditional rotations across hospitals of one of the four health boards (and completing an elective).

A new curriculum of case-based learning around a clear set of learning outcomes dominates the first two years, based first around systems and then life cycles. From the beginning, students spend time at least one day a week in primary care, so that they can immediately apply what they've learned in lectures, anatomy, and clinical skills sessions. In year two, a diverse series of half-day and full-day placements in secondary care are built into the programme. ScotGEM's unique 'Agents of Change' component trains students across all four years in quality improvement techniques and involves carrying out research, audits, and healthcare improvement projects alongside clinical work.

Tuition fees are covered for Scottish students only, but all students can access a unique annual £4,000 NHS bursary per year of postgraduate employment given back to the health service in Scotland. See Table 12.15.

Table 12.15 ScotGEM

Best aspects	Strong and early clinical focus; dedicated staff; good pastoral support; return-of-service bursary		
Worst aspects	Self-directed learning; remote and rural may be ideal for some but a problem for others		
Requirements	**Degree** 1st-class or upper 2nd-class honours in any subject; **A level** minimum B in chemistry or equivalent; **GCSE** minimum B in maths or equivalent		
Course length	4 years	Structure	Campus
Type of course	Carbon fibre	Year size	54
Typical offer	2:1	Admission test	GAMSAT
Applicants	2,431	Student mix:	
Interviews	129	% international	0%
Offers	80		
Uncompetitive			Competitive
Low living costs			High living costs
Working really hard			Not working/ chilling out
Contact details	University of St Andrews, College Gate, St Andrews, KY16 9AJ Tel: +44 (0) 1334 463619, Web: www.st-andrews.ac.uk/subjects/medicine/ scotgem-mbchb		

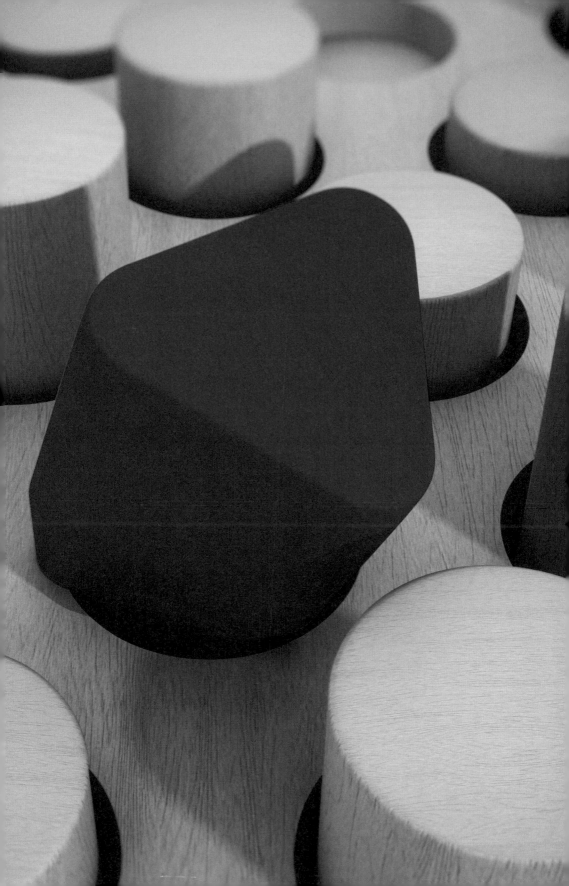

13

Non-traditional applications

▌ Non-traditional qualifications

It's a common complaint of admissions tutors that all medical school applications look the same. Most applicants are predicted straight A grades, play sport for their school, and play a musical instrument to a high standard. Of course, medical school applications do not always look this way; successful applicants may have a wide range of grades, qualifications, and social backgrounds. It is important to be aware of how such diversity will affect your chances and be handled by medical schools, so this chapter explores how applicants with different qualifications (see p. 294), non-traditional backgrounds (see p. 296), health problems, and criminal records (see p. 298) should approach their applications.

Academic challenges

Neither medical students nor doctors have to be geniuses. However, medical school is competitive and applications need evidence of high academic achievement and commitment to learning. Medical schools want to know that applicants are able to cope with the equivalent of three rigorous A levels over two years.

Resitting entire A levels Many medical schools take a dim view of resitting A levels or taking longer than two years to complete them. Attitudes vary between different medical schools; some simply refuse to take applicants with resits while others will only consider them when there were extreme and well-documented mitigating circumstances (and typically straight As on the resits).

Missing your offer This is dealt with on p. 322.

> ### Key points
>
> Having to resit A levels or taking longer than two years to complete them means your chances of getting into medical school are low. If you are in this situation you can either apply to the more lenient medical schools, using the school reference (see p. 218) to document the mitigating circumstances (which need to be extreme), or study another degree and apply as a graduate (see p. 252).

Equivalent qualifications

Most British applicants to UK medical schools will base their applications around A levels or Scottish Highers. One common alternative is the International Baccalaureate (IB). Medical schools often have a standard offer for IB students, just as they do for those sitting A levels, and this can usually be found on the medical school website. Many schools also require chemistry (and sometimes biology) to be taken at a higher level.

Medical schools accept many other equivalent qualifications. Admissions teams are advised by their university international office as to what grade or score is required from such applicants. You must contact universities in advance of applying through UCAS to confirm this information and get their response in writing. Although your school, government, or exam board advise that a given score is equivalent to A*AA at A level, British universities might not share this view. Do not waste a UCAS space on an institution that does not fully recognize your qualifications.

Breaks from education

There are many reasons why applicants might have taken time away from education. Although there is nothing wrong with taking time out (e.g. for employment or through illness), medical schools will often require evidence of recent academic success and an explanation of breaks in education.

- **Graduates** Graduates in employment will usually apply to graduate-entry courses (see p. 252). These courses expect applicants to have breaks from education, although evidence of recent study benefits applicants too.
- **Mature non-graduates** Although mature candidates bring additional life experience, they need to demonstrate that they are as academically capable as students fresh out of A levels. Evidence of achievement in recent study is very important for these applicants.
- **Illness** If illness has meant time away from education, this must be documented carefully. Your circumstances should also be supported by strong references. Illness can mean additional insight into healthcare and be turned to your advantage (see p. 224).

There are many ways to provide evidence of recent academic success:

- **Local colleges** These institutions offer a range of courses, from vocational qualifications to A levels. They are a good place to start if you do not meet the necessary grade requirements. If you already have strong A levels, consider taking another one (maybe chemistry) to re-establish former studying habits.
- **Short university courses** Most universities run short courses aimed at the public. These sometimes lead to qualifications (e.g. certificates and diplomas).
- **Distance learning** If you want to delay sitting in classes until after receiving a medical school offer, you might consider distance learning. The Open University (www.open.ac.uk) runs lots of courses in natural sciences and healthcare (among others), leading to certificates, diplomas, and degrees. As these are formally accredited, they serve as strong evidence of current academic ability. Similarly, constituent colleges of the University of London run accredited and respectable distance-learning programmes (www.londoninternational.ac.uk).
- **Access courses** These are aimed primarily at applicants without the right qualifications to get a medical school offer. They offer good evidence of recent study but do not guarantee you a place at medical school.
- **Massive open online courses (MOOCs)** These are online modules or programmes of tuition that are often provided by a large university. Many courses are available free. Those that facilitate an assessment and then provide a certificate of completion usually charge a small fee. There are lots of MOOCs available but some of the most popular include edX (www.edx.org) and Coursera (www.coursera.org).

▌Non-traditional backgrounds

Medicine attracts a huge range of different people. There is a growing understanding that patients are best served by a diverse medical profession. This means diverse strengths, backgrounds, and experiences.

EU students Students from European Union (EU) countries outside of the UK may be treated differently to international students applying from non-EU countries. This may depend on the precise terms of the agreement of the withdrawal of the UK from the EU.

International students Medical schools may only permit a quota of international applicants each year. As the number of international students is limited, these applications are often dealt with differently and may be even more competitive than those from UK candidates. International students have traditionally been charged higher fees than applicants within the EU. These fees increase during the clinical years. It is not unusual for tuition fees (excluding transport, accommodation, etc.) to be around £25,000 per year, rising to £50,000 per year during the clinical course.

Mature students The term 'mature students' refers to three different groups:

- **Graduates** See p. 252 for guidance on graduate applications.
- **Non-graduates with suitable qualifications/grades** If you fall into this group, see p. 100 before beginning your application.
- **Mature applicants without suitable qualifications** These applicants will either need to sit A levels through a further education college or complete an access course.

Access courses

These are courses run by institutions that do not have a medical school (e.g. further education colleges) and aim to help mature students applying for medicine to demonstrate recent academic study. The courses usually involve one year of full-time study. It is very important to do your research before embarking on an access course. Many medical schools do not recognize courses in place of formal qualifications and some only accept applications from students at specific institutions. In all cases, medical schools require an access course pass at a predetermined level, usually 'distinction' or above 70%. Access courses may also have specific admission requirements (e.g. some only accept candidates from their local area). Table 13.1 introduces some of the major access courses available in the UK; some courses have already had students accepted to certain medical schools, while others have not been tested. It is best to check with medical schools before starting the access course.

Table 13.1 A selection of access courses available in the UK

Institution	Location	Partnerships
City and Islington College	London	Students have been accepted by at least five medical schools
College of West Anglia	King's Lynn, Norfolk	Former students accepted by 20 medical schools, including some graduate-entry courses
Sussex Downs College	Lewes, East Sussex	All students guaranteed an interview at Brighton and Sussex Medical School but students have also been accepted by a number of other medical schools

Foundation courses

These are usually run by a medical school or its partner institution, and are sometimes now called 'gateway courses'. Like access courses, they require one year of full-time study and are aimed at applicants without the qualifications necessary for medical school; however, students are guaranteed a place at a specific medical school afterwards. There are two broad types of foundation course:

- Those designed for highly achieving applicants without the necessary science A levels, such as those run at Cardiff (see p. 198) and Manchester (see p. 164).
- Those designed for applicants who did not perform as well as they might otherwise have done due to defined barriers to learning. These courses are run by Aberdeen (see p. 186), Bristol (see p. 134), Dundee (see p. 188), East Anglia (see p. 178), Edge Hill (see p. 202), Glasgow (see p. 192), Hull (see p. 142), King's (see p. 158), Lancaster (see p. 146), Leicester (see p. 150), Lincoln (see p. 203), Liverpool (see p. 152), Nottingham (see p. 168), Plymouth (see p. 172), Southampton (see p. 176), St Andrew's (see p. 194), and York (see p. 142).

As these courses are aimed at people from varied and complex backgrounds, it would be overly complicated to summarize their entry requirements and key features in this book. See the individual organization websites for up-to-date details.

Transferring between courses

It is not usually possible to transfer into medical school from a non-medicine university course. Transfers between medical schools are only permitted in exceptional circumstances. In general, transferring is not a viable route into medical school.

A student's experience ...

I left school at 16 with average GCSEs and worked with my uncle as a bricklayer. When work dried up, I took a job in a nursing home. I must have mentioned to someone that I'd have liked to study medicine because one of the staff nurses gave me a college prospectus advertising access to medicine. I had no idea this was an option for someone with my skills and qualifications. The college provided huge amounts of support (including advice and mock interviews) and a year later I embarked on a new career at a London medical school.

Fitness to practice

There is no shortage of hurdles to jump over before winning a place at medical school. For some applicants the biggest of these is determining whether they are 'fit' to work as a doctor.

What is fitness to practice?

Fitness to practice refers to the suitability of students and doctors to work within the medical profession. Each medical school has its own Fitness to Practice Committee whose job it is to ensure all students meet minimum professional standards. Committees are independent but act under guidance from the General Medical Council. They convene whenever concerns are raised about an applicant's fitness to practice. Common areas of concern include:

- **Criminal activity** Particularly those relating to fraud, offences against property (e.g. theft), violence, and sex offences.
- **Drug or alcohol abuse** Including driving under the influence of alcohol/drugs, supplying drugs, and drunkenness affecting daily life.
- **Dishonesty** Concerns may be raised about cheating in school exams, plagiarizing coursework or UCAS personal statement, or lying on the UCAS form.
- **Health concerns** Any student with long-term disability or chronic illness may need to declare this.

You must contact medical schools in advance of applying if any of these apply. Withholding information will be interpreted as further dishonesty and is likely to attract severe sanctions (e.g. expulsion). The fitness to practice procedure at a typical medical school is as follows:

- **Applicant enquiry** Applicants make a confidential enquiry to the admissions office stating their personal circumstances. Although a decision cannot be made at this stage, the admissions tutor may know from experience how certain problems are dealt with by the Fitness to Practice Committee. Details in writing may be required before an application is submitted.
- **Application** The UCAS application process proceeds independently.
- **Fitness to practice process** If your application has been successful, the Fitness to Practice Committee convenes to consider your particular case. You may be allowed to proceed, subject to certain conditions, or have your offer withdrawn if you are not considered fit to practice.

As fitness to practice is usually considered after the admissions process, declarations made beforehand should not influence whether you receive an offer. However, this may vary between institutions, so ask if uncertain.

Physical disabilities

Disability is not a bar to studying medicine. Its definition (under the Equality Act 2010) includes any 'physical or mental impairment which has a substantial and long-term adverse effect on your ability to carry out normal day-to-day activities'. This includes mobility problems, hearing and visual impairments, epilepsy, and chronic disease (e.g. diabetes). Almost 13% of UK medical students have a disability falling under this definition.

Medical schools need to establish that candidates are likely to complete the course and be fit to practice medicine afterwards. This does not mean students can be turned away simply because they would be difficult to support. The Equality Act requires employers (and academic institutions) to make 'reasonable adjustments' to accommodate disabilities. An applicant's fitness to practice should only be in doubt where there is a high risk that the applicant could not finish the course, or work as a doctor, despite reasonable adjustments.

Mental health problems

As with physical impairments, mental health problems can be declared through UCAS. Although a history of mental health problems is not itself incompatible with medicine, it could raise two key questions that the Fitness to Practice Committees may consider as part of their duty of care both to you, the potential student, and to the general public:

- **Risk to patients** Some uncontrolled mental illnesses could pose a risk to vulnerable patients.
- **Risk to mental health** Medicine is a physically and mentally demanding discipline—there is lots of pressure and a heavy exam load during and after medical school. This could aggravate some mental health problems.

Medical school policies on mental health vary. Decisions will depend on the condition, severity, response to treatment, insight, and interference with day-to-day professional life. Mild to moderate mental health conditions affect 15–25% of the general population and are no less prevalent amongst medical students.

Learning impairments

Although all medical students have achieved good grades, learning impairments such as dyslexia still feature for many. Fitness to Practice Committees must establish whether an applicant with dyslexia will be safe to practice as a doctor. In most cases, applicants performing highly in previous academic work have learned to compensate for their impairment. However, medical schools may be interested in whether affected applicants have insight into problems they could potentially face in the future (e.g. safe prescribing).

Key points

Applicants must raise potential fitness to practice issues in advance (or at the time of) applying. Fitness to Practice Committees will not be sympathetic to applicants hiding health problems or criminal records.

Serious communicable diseases

All medical students (and doctors) perform procedures that carry a risk of exposing the patient to blood (e.g. blood tests). For this reason, successful applicants are subject to blood tests for blood-borne viral infections (HIV, hepatitis B, and hepatitis C). Infection is not an absolute barrier to medical school entry but the course may need to be modified to avoid some exposure-prone procedures. New medical students are also screened for other infections (e.g. tuberculosis) and immunity to rubella and chicken pox.

Criminal records

New medical students must apply for an enhanced Disclosure and Barring Service (DBS) check. Regular DBS checks include all convictions, cautions, reprimands, and final warnings, regardless of how long has passed since they were incurred. Enhanced disclosure includes checking with local police forces that can add any additional information (e.g. about ongoing investigations or cases not leading to conviction). Fitness to Practice Committees will consider the nature and time of offences before deciding whether fitness is impaired. They will also consider whether allowing a candidate with a criminal past to work as a doctor could pose a risk to patients or bring the profession into disrepute.

Key points

Minor traffic offences (e.g. speeding) do not have to be declared unless they resulted in a court summons or criminal proceedings.

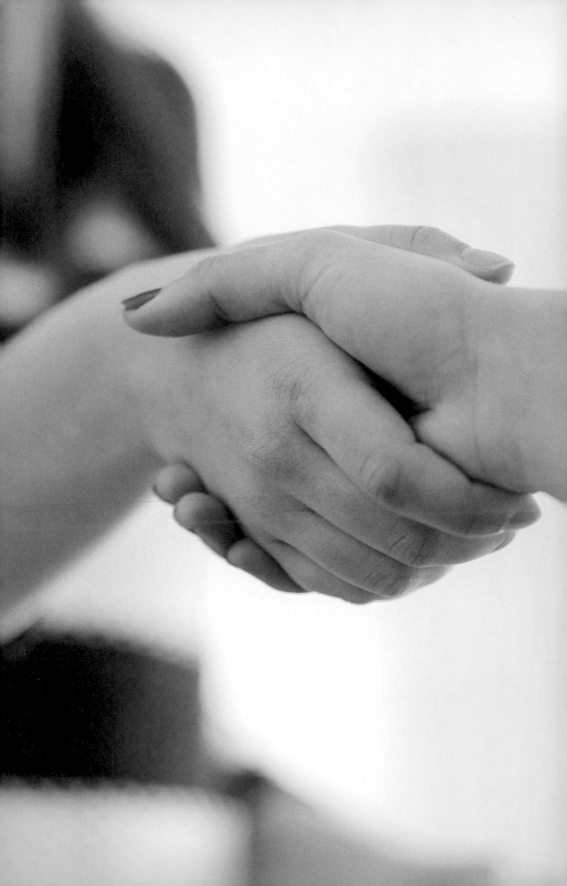

14

How to succeed at interview

▌The medical school interview

The vast majority of medical schools choose to interview potential medical students, and the interview is a common source of anxiety. This chapter takes you through how to prepare (see p. 306), questions to expect (see p. 308), and answering ethical questions (see p. 310). It also has some useful background information on medicine (see p. 316) and healthcare (see p. 318).

Importance of the interview

Medical schools choose to interview for three reasons:

- **To select the best students** With as many as 20 applicants for each place, medical schools do not have an easy time choosing who to accept. Most applicants have at least A*AA predictions, a plethora of work experience, and a range of extracurricular activities. The interview helps selectors make this difficult decision.
- **To select the best doctors** All medical graduates are guaranteed a job as a doctor. You are not just applying for a course; you are being considered for an entire career. Few jobs with such responsibility and a training budget of £250,000 have such short interviews.
- **To assess communication** Medicine is all about people, so doctors need to communicate well. It's important that medical schools select those people who are best able to understand and articulate challenging concepts This is easier to assess at interview than on a form.

Who is the ideal candidate?

There is no such thing as a 'typical' medical student; medicine welcomes all genders, races, religions, and sexualities. Interviewers are looking for evidence of your potential to become a good doctor. This can include everything from commitment to medicine to your attitudes, values, and personal qualities. However, medical school selectors cannot see into the future, so judgements are based solely on your UCAS application, admission test results, and behaviour within the interview room.

How does the interview usually work?

Interviews vary enormously between different medical schools. Often there are two interviewers and sometimes a small panel. The interviewers may be doctors and/or other people teaching at the medical school, such as scientists and social scientists. Some medical schools also invite current medical students and lay representatives (i.e. people not involved with the medical school) to join selection panels.

If you are faced with a panel, don't panic. In most cases, one or two people will ask questions while the others watch and make notes. Don't be thrown by this: all applicants will have the same experience. The panel interview aims to gain a more balanced view of your suitability by allowing people with a variety of different life experiences to weigh in on your performance.

Interviewers usually score your performance against set criteria. These are the same for all applicants to ensure fairness and consistency. To get an idea of what the criteria are likely to be, you should read *Good Medical Practice* and *Tomorrow's Doctors* (see p. 221). These lay out the qualities necessary for a successful doctor. The exact criteria used will, however, vary between medical schools. Interviewers may use a mark scheme that incorporates these qualities and helps provide consistency throughout the process. An example score sheet is included on p. 305.

In many cases, applicants are each given a score during the interview and ranked against each other, with the top interviewees receiving an offer. When ranking applicants, some schools include other factors such as UCAS form score and performance on admission tests. Others go solely on performance at interview. Some schools are open about these details and provide an admissions statement on their website. If they do not, it cannot hurt to call and ask.

How to find out more

Once you are invited to interview, do lots of research to avoid surprises on the day.

- Read the interview letter very carefully. This should provide most of the information you need, including a time, date, and interview location.
- Check the medical school website for any information on what style of interview will be used.
- Telephone or email the medical school admissions office. Ask about the status of the interviewers (e.g. doctors, lay people) and the length and format of the interview. Consider asking for the interviewers' names too.
- If you do manage to get the names of your interviewers, then do some internet research. Where do they work? What department are they based in? Do they have a special interest in teaching or research? What kind of research do they spend their time doing? All this information can help gain an idea of each interviewer's perspective.
- Use open days or personal contacts (including those made at open days) to ask about interview questions, though be careful when doing this that you're not trying to gain an unfair advantage (otherwise called 'cheating').
- Use medical school entrance forums (see p. 382) to find out what other candidates were asked. Use this information with caution as questions and interviewers frequently change. However, it can give a good idea of the types of question you are likely to be asked.

▍Preparing for the interview

Being an ace at interviews requires long-term and short-term preparation. You have been preparing for this moment ever since you decided to apply. The harder you have worked to build a strong application, the easier it will be to sell yourself at interview. However, the next couple of pages are about short-term preparation. This means going into the interview with a good idea of what you are going to say and how you will conduct yourself.

Gaining medical knowledge There is an assumption that really interested candidates will know something about medicine. This doesn't mean you have to understand the pathophysiology of pseudopseudohypoparathyroidism (in fact, most final-year medical students won't), but you should know some basic details about common medical conditions (see p. 316 for examples). This can simply mean reading about conditions you discover during A levels and work experience or reading useful publications (e.g. *British Medical Journal* and *New Scientist*, see p. 381). Take especially close interest in any medical conditions that have been in the news recently as these are often interview question fodder.

Keeping up to date If there has been a widely publicized medical news story in recent weeks or months, you must know about it. This should not require much effort; for example, just looking at the 'Health' section of the BBC News website every few days should be sufficient. There are many other sources of useful information including websites, podcasts, newspapers, and magazines. Make sure you pick a respected and reliable source rather than just the most readable. Candidates who are up to date on interesting or controversial medical news really stand out. This can be in an area of special interest for you, for example understanding the basics behind a new drug that's set to change the medical landscape.

Content of a medical interview After greeting you, interviewers will often start with one or two predictable questions (see p. 308), followed by discussion about your application form, and then ethics (see p. 310) and/or science (see p. 316) questions. Most schools (essentially all other than Oxbridge) employ stand-alone questioning techniques. This means questions will not always flow from one another and are unlikely to change regardless of how you answered earlier questions. Put any 'bad' answers behind you and move on.

Practising for interview Even the most confident applicant can be unnerved by an interview panel. For this reason, practice is the best way to avoid wasting all of your preparative efforts. The ideal scenario for mock interviews is to have an older person with some knowledge about the course interview you; schoolteachers can be very useful here. If you know a doctor (or even a current medical student), ask them to help too. Your aim should be to try to recreate as much of the experience of a real interview as possible; that includes the introduction, types of questions, duration, and formal closures. Your 'interviewer' will help put you on the spot, challenge your responses, and, hopefully, provide feedback afterwards.

Keep up to date with current medical issues

- Check the health pages on the BBC News website regularly.
- Most newspapers run a health supplement during the week; find one you like and follow a few topics.
- Don't forget to keep abreast of non-medical current affairs as well; there are health implications of almost every news story. *The Economist* provides a good weekly summary of the world's news in a single magazine.
- Most publications have accessible websites, RSS feeds, or regularly updated podcasts

available on iTunes to help you keep up to date with their content. Occasionally you may need to subscribe (and occasionally pay) for some content.
- Radio 4 runs informative medical programmes—use BBC iPlayer to find these.

Before the interview As soon as you are invited to interview, find out as much as you can about the process. Make sure you have clothes suitable for interview. Whatever you choose to wear, you should look smart to make the best possible impression. Remember, you are applying to join the medical *profession* and should look professional.

- Men should ideally wear a suit, but at least a shirt and tie. Shirts should be tucked in and ties kept an appropriate length.
- Women should wear a skirt/trouser suit/trousers and blouse. Clothes should not be too revealing.
- Both sexes should consider removing any piercings (besides simple ear piercings for women).

Interviewers are not assessing your appearance but they do have to gauge each candidate's personality in just 30 minutes. Medicine is a conservative profession and your interview is not the time to push boundaries.

The day of the interview Arriving in good time is vital. This gives you plenty of time to overcome unexpected obstacles en route and prevents you feeling rushed or flustered. Plan well ahead and have maps ready to locate the interview room when you reach the university. If possible, get someone to drive you as this will reduce stress associated with public transport and connecting journeys. If it is at all viable to spend the night before your interview in a local hotel, doing so will reduce transport-related stress dramatically. Read any notes you have prepared to jog your memory of responses to predictable questions and flick through a newspaper for any important medical stories that the interviewers simply could not ignore. You should arrive for the interview at least 15 minutes before it is due to start, but similarly avoid arriving three hours before and camping in reception.

The interview Interviewers' decisions are not finalized within the first 30 seconds, but first impressions really do matter. Follow the interviewers' lead; usually you will be introduced and offered the chance to greet and shake hands with each of them. Avoid vice-like or weak handshakes and try to appear confident (the best handshake is one that's of the same strength as the person shaking your hand—tough to navigate but worth the practice). After a greeting you will probably be offered a seat, which is likely to be across a table from the interviewers. Sit in a comfortable position, but ideally upright or leaning slightly forward. Avoid slouching or leaning back (and definitely don't put your feet on the table!). Try to make eye contact with the person talking to you (without staring) and smile when appropriate.

If you have tics, or know you respond in a particular way when nervous, try to overcome the temptation. Interviewers expect a degree of nervousness but they will become impatient after 30 minutes of spinning a pen or tapping your leg. Keeping still makes you seem more confident.

Always make sure you answer the specific question asked and do not be afraid to take the time you need to consider a response. Applicants often grow anxious about sitting in silence but, contrary to popular belief, you do not have to fill every quiet moment with sound. Take a glass of water if it is offered. Not only will it prevent you drying out but also it can offer you a suitable pause to think a little longer about questions. Preparation is important but the panel do not want to hear you acting out a carefully rehearsed script. Ideas should be fresh in your mind and you should expect to do some mental work while you're in the interview room.

Predictable questions

Whilst it is impossible to anticipate all the questions you will be asked at interview, there are some you should expect. This is because the interview panel are looking for specific knowledge or qualities, some of which can only be elicited in a limited number of ways. Use the following examples as a guide but be prepared to answer questions on similar topics that are worded differently. Remember, every answer you give is an opportunity to highlight important values that might be on the mark scheme.

Tell us about yourself This question is supposed to 'break the ice' but can fluster any candidate. Very often the idea is simply to help you relax—the interviewers are not expecting a biographical account of your entire life up to the present day. Briefly describe the subjects you study, the school you attend, and what you do with your spare time. Include an interesting (but not outrageous) fact, if possible, but you should keep your answer relatively brief. Don't be afraid to repeat information on your UCAS form—there is a good chance the interviewers have not read it thoroughly. There is no excuse for not answering this question well as it is an early opportunity to make a strong first impression.

Why do you want to be a doctor? Think very carefully about this question, as it *will* come up in one form or another. There is no 'correct' answer and you should be honest when articulating your own motivations for studying medicine (see p. 4). However, do not under any circumstances go to interview thinking the answer is 'obvious' and one you can articulate on the spot. Most applicants find it very difficult to articulate their reasons, and those without a confident and fluent response to this question risk disaster at interview.

It is worth remembering that interviewers may not always accept your answer and move on; they may challenge anything you say. If your greatest desire is to help people, why not become a nurse? If you like science so much, surely a chemistry degree would be more appropriate? Think carefully about these questions beforehand. Use this book and your work experience (see p. 54) to prepare appropriate responses.

How do you relax? This is another question that almost always appears in some form. It is asking how you unwind, but do not let your guard down. This is a serious question and the panel are not interested in how you like to lie-in at the weekends or take long bubble baths. Medicine can be a stressful career and interviewers want to see that you have durable coping mechanisms. Try to focus on anything you do that functions as 'active relaxation' (i.e. something that proactively improves your well-being, as opposed to sitting doing nothing). Use this as an opportunity to demonstrate your extracurricular achievements (see p. 46) and transferable skills (e.g. teamwork, time management skills). Like all interview questions, this one offers the opportunity to make a good impression, if you are well prepared.

An insider's view ...

I began the interview like every other, by asking the candidate why he wanted to become a doctor. He replied—whilst ticking off three fingers—'money, status, power'. Quite taken aback, I asked him to explain his reasoning. He started to talk about when his grandma was ill and how he had had a lot of contact with her GP. Thinking he might yet redeem himself, I encouraged him to continue. He had met her GP on a number of occasions and was particularly impressed by...his car.

Even the most predictable interview question can be answered badly!

What was the most challenging thing you faced during your work experience? Your answer will clearly depend on your personal experiences but this should not stop you brainstorming answers in advance. Related questions could ask about the most 'interesting' experience, whether anything concerned you, and whether there was anything you thought could have been dealt with differently. Ideally you should have noted important events in a reflective diary during (or shortly after) each placement (see p. 62). This is an opportunity to talk about your work experience, show you learned something, and demonstrate that you can reflect on experiences.

'According to your personal statement...' Questions based on your UCAS form (see p. 216) may be asked for several reasons. The form could raise a topic of particular interest to the interviewer or there might be a discrepancy with something you said at interview that they want to clarify. Alternatively, the interviewer may just be filling time. Regardless of the motive, try to anticipate these questions before you get to the interview. If you've written that you read every issue of *New Scientist*, be prepared to discuss articles that you have read recently. You should be able to talk around topics described in your personal statement without simply repeating what you've written. These questions are designed to probe the things that you internalized from the things you mentioned in your personal statement but didn't have the space to comment on extensively.

Do you have any questions for us? Most interviews will end with the selectors asking if you have any questions for them. There are two ways to approach this. If you genuinely have a sensible question, then ask. Perhaps it is unclear from the website and prospectus how many students can pursue an intercalated degree (see p. 91). If the course is split between preclinical and clinical phases, you might want to know how much clinical exposure there is in the first couple of years. Such questions can show you have thought hard about how the course is structured. However, be careful not to ask questions that are answered elsewhere: you will come across as wasting time and having not prepared adequately. For the same reason, do not make up questions just to appear interested. It is perfectly acceptable to say all your questions were answered by the prospectus/website/open day.

Once you have dealt with this final question, you are usually free to thank the interviewers and say goodbye before heading for the door.

An insider's view...

Perhaps the most important advice for the interview day is to be yourself. If you have thoroughly prepared, then your enthusiasm and suitability for medicine will come through.

Key points

There is no excuse for answering predictable questions poorly. Every applicant who prepares properly should answer these questions well. However, many candidates become flustered as the obvious questions are often difficult to answer convincingly on the spot. Don't throw away a medical school offer because you didn't prepare.

▌Ethical principles

It is useful to think through some ethical dilemmas before arriving at your interview; a number of these are found on p. 312. While you are unlikely to guess what questions you will be asked, these pages will allow you to practise the thought process necessary to answer them. The following pages describe the principles that medical students and doctors are taught to apply to such issues.

Core principles

Ethical thinking in medicine is governed by a number of fundamental principles. Think about each of these when answering ethical questions.

Autonomy This principle recognizes that individuals have a right to control their own lives. In medicine this means that, where possible, patients should be helped to make decisions about their *own* care. Instead of deciding on a course of treatment, doctors should try to discuss the pros and cons of each available option, allowing the patient to give informed consent (see p. 313). This approach can increase patient satisfaction and ensure they comply with the agreed course of treatment. However, it can be time-consuming and difficult to negotiate well when clinicians feel pressured for time.

Beneficence This really just means 'do good'. Of course, if ethical dilemmas could be resolved by simply doing 'good', there wouldn't be a need for these pages. Beneficence usually means doing what is in the interests of the patient. However, as you will see from the scenarios on p. 313, this can be difficult to determine when doctors and patients have different ideas about what is in the patient's 'best interests'.

Non-maleficence Similar to the principle of beneficence, non-maleficence simply means avoiding harm. In fact, 'first, do no harm' has been a principle of medicine since ancient times. For example, doctors should take care not to use treatments that inadvertently cause harm to patients, even if the aim is to cure disease. However, in some instances, short term harm (or the risk of long term harm) may be acceptable in order to achieve a longer-term good.

Justice This principle means treating all patients fairly and equally, for example without prejudice in relation to factors such as ethnicity and religion. It can also refer to fair distribution of healthcare resources. For example, in the UK, it is generally accepted that patients in one area should have access to the same treatments as those living elsewhere.

Dignity All patients have the right to respect from healthcare professionals. For example, doctors should avoid judging individual patients and should be courteous at all times. The duty of confidentiality is closely related to protecting patients' dignity.

Integrity and honesty Integrity means acting according to a consistent set of values and principles and with a sense of 'honesty'. In most cases, doctors should be honest to protect the trust patients have in the medical profession. Honesty is also important to facilitate autonomy—without honest information, patients cannot make decisions about their illness and treatment.

Practical use of ethical principles

These principles guide daily medical decisions. For example, most people accept that doctors should keep their patients' personal details confidential. You could just accept confidentiality, but it can also be justified according to the core principles described previously:

- **Autonomy** Patients have a right to choose who knows about their medical problems.
- **Beneficence** Failing to preserve confidentiality rarely results in a benefit, although there are exceptions to this (e.g. the patient with HIV who has not told their partner)
- **Non-maleficence** Sharing personal information can cause great harm to patients (e.g. embarrassment or discrimination).
- **Justice** All patients have an equal right to confidentiality.
- **Dignity** Disclosure of sensitive medical details could cause a loss of patient dignity.
- **Integrity** Doctors are expected to maintain patient confidentiality at all times, even when talking to friends or publishing research.

Although ethical dilemmas posed in interviews are often about 'big issues' (see p. 312), doctors have a duty to act ethically in their day-to-day work as well. Interviewers could well ask 'Why should patient records be kept confidential?' or 'Should doctors always tell patients what is wrong with them?'. In all cases try to keep the core principles in the back of your mind.

Conflicting principles

It is also important to recognize that ethical principles often conflict with one another. Should patients be allowed to make decisions (autonomy) that will cause them harm (non-maleficence)? Should the NHS provide fertility treatment (autonomy and beneficence) if this means there is less money available for cancer treatments (justice)? It is when these principles conflict that an ethical 'dilemma' arises. Although you will be expected to have an opinion, you should recognize that there is rarely a single correct answer. Try to understand all sides of the argument and reach a balanced answer. The interviewers are trying to understand how you think, not expecting you to solve an age-old ethical problem in five minutes.

A few ethical dilemmas

Although ethical dilemmas rarely have clear, definite answers, a logical approach should always be employed when considering them. Consider each option available in terms of the core ethical principles (see p. 311). Try to retain a degree of impartiality and consider both sides of the argument. If you have strong personal beliefs, carefully consider how you might present them in an interview situation. As there is no 'right' answer, you are unlikely to impress course selectors by dogmatically clinging to one point of view at the expense of others. Doctors often have to tread through difficult ethical territory and interviewers will want to assess your ability to develop a balanced understanding of complicated issues. This is not to say that you should not have (or even express) a view. Doctors have to make decisions as well so, after considering all sides, do not be afraid of suggesting your pre-ferred solution. In many cases, this might even be preferable to clinging tightly to the fence and refusing to reach a conclusion.

Abortion

This debate typically occurs between 'pro-life' and 'pro-choice' groups. Pro-life groups claim that a fetus is a human being who should not be killed, whereas pro-choice groups emphasize a woman's right to choose what happens to her body. The debate is often said to hinge on when life begins. Is it at the moment of conception, when the nervous system forms, when the heart first beats, or at birth? There are also other issues at stake: whether terminations are justifiable when the child would be born with profound disabilities, and where the line is drawn between 'abortion' and 'murder'.

In the UK, legal abortions occur up to the twenty-fourth week of pregnancy, or later if there is serious medical risk to the mother's health or gross fetal abnormality. Abortion requires the signed agreement of two doctors that there is a greater risk to the woman's physical or mental health (or to that of her current children) if the pregnancy is allowed to continue. However, this is true of all pregnancies (the risk of childbirth is higher than that of abortion), so the Abortion Act 1967 effectively allows any woman to have an abortion before the 24-week limit.

Stem cells

Before cells differentiate into skin, bone, liver, or another tissue type in the body, they are known as undifferentiated precursor cells. At this stage they have the potential to become some (or even all) of these 'differentiated' cell types. Embryos are a rich source of stem cells that, once recovered, can be used to grow tissues in laboratories to create accurate disease models, improve understanding, and, potentially, find cures for disease. Stem cells can also be transplanted into patients and have been tested in conditions such as Parkinson's disease; in theory whole new organs can be grown from them without the risk of transplant rejection. The cells are taken from surplus embryos created during in vitro fertilization treatments. Again, those who believe life starts at conception sometimes con-sider the process of obtaining stem cells to be 'murder'. In the future it might be possible to use stem cells induced from adult cells (induced pluripotent stem cells) or to collect the sparse population of stem cells still present in adults.

A similar topic involves putting a human cell nucleus into an animal cell to form a chi-mera or hybrid for research. In UK law hybrids are not allowed to grow beyond a small cluster of cells before they are destroyed. CRISPR-Cas9 technology is now enabling high-fidelity gene editing of cells; somatic cell applications could cure diseases (e.g. hereditary blindness, sickle cell disease) but germline applications have wider implications by being potentially transmissible (look up the 'He Jiankui affair' of 2018). Some groups describe such techniques as 'playing God' and worry about fully-grown human hybrids and novel diseases.

Euthanasia

This describes deliberately ending a person's life for their 'benefit'. Some argue that this need arises when a person's quality of life has deteriorated to such an extent that dying 'with dignity' is a better option than continuing to live an unbearable life. This issue may arise in patients suffering severe pain or those who have lost all motor functions and so are unable to speak or move (e.g. advanced motor neurone disease).

Opponents often fall into two camps: those who believe in the sanctity of human life and the immorality of taking life in this way, and those who argue that euthanasia might be misused by relatives or devalue populations (e.g. the elderly) who feel pressured to relieve their burden on friends and family. Euthanasia currently amounts to murder in the UK, although assisted suicide is lawful in nearby countries such as the Netherlands and Switzerland (such as through the organization Dignitas, which has attracted much media interest). Supporters of euthanasia describe its illegality as a violation of personal freedoms and human rights. Opponents argue that although everyone has a 'right to life', there is no 'right to death'.

Key points

Note the important difference between euthanasia and assisted suicide. In the former, the patient's life is ended by another person. For example, some criminals in the USA are executed by lethal injection. Euthanasia can be voluntary or involuntary. Assisted suicide is different. In this case the patient ends their own life, but with help from a third party. For example, a doctor might prescribe drugs that the patient chooses to take themselves. Both euthanasia and assisted suicide are illegal under UK law as it currently stands.

Consent and capacity

In order to carry out a test, operate, or examine a patient, it is necessary to obtain consent. Touching a patient without consent may amount to battery. For consent to be valid, it must be informed (i.e. the patient must know the potential benefits and risks), given voluntarily, and given by a patient with *capacity* to consent. Capacity is the ability to understand, retain, and use information relevant to the decision. It may be lacking due to, for example, mental illness, brain damage, or intoxication.

When a patient lacks capacity, the medical team must make any decisions in their best interests. The team should take into account many factors, such as the patient's previously expressed wishes (when they had capacity), their personal beliefs, and the thoughts of their family. Ethical dilemmas often arise when the various contributors disagree but, ultimately, doctors (or a court) make the final decision.

The question of capacity is more complicated when dealing with children. This area of law is informed by an important case from 1985: *Gillick v West Norfolk Health Authority*. Mrs Gillick sought a declaration that GPs should not prescribe contraception to her daughters, who were aged under 16. She argued that this encouraged minors to have sex. However, the court found that children can have capacity to request contraception if they possess sufficient intelligence, comprehension, and maturity. A similar principle is applied to other dilemmas involving children.

∎ Ethics in modern healthcare

You probably encountered ethical dilemmas during your work experience, perhaps without even realizing it. If you haven't yet finished your work experience, keep an eye out for ethical issues—they are pervasive. Some commonly encountered dilemmas are introduced below; try to think about these, identify the issues raised, and develop a personal view where possible. Again, this is not a complete list so keep abreast of the news, read articles online, and discuss what you read with other people.

Access to resources

The National Health Service (NHS) is a massive organization paid for by the taxpayer. It costs over £140 billion every year. Although taxation can be increased, most people appreciate that the NHS has a limited budget. One inevitable consequence of limited resources is that the NHS cannot pay for all treatments all the time.

- **Luxury treatments** Should the NHS pay for potentially 'non-health-related' issues such as in vitro fertilization (IVF) and gender reassignment? In a budget-limited system, some people believe funds should be allocated to patients with diseases instead. Others argue that psychological well-being is an NHS responsibility because it is an important part of health.
- **Expensive drugs** Should the NHS pay for very expensive drugs? One drug used for breast cancer (Herceptin) costs around £22,000 per patient every year. What about expensive drugs that only work occasionally or increase life expectancy by only a few weeks?
- **The 'postcode lottery'** One aspect of the NHS is that it is broken into individual NHS trusts. This is so that healthcare resources can be tailored to the needs of particular populations living within each area. However, one consequence of allowing local trusts a degree of independence is that resources may be available to people living in one area and not those living elsewhere. This is called the 'postcode lottery'. For example, some NHS trusts refuse to pay for Herceptin. Some allow three cycles of IVF on the NHS whereas others only permit one. This has important implications for principles of fairness and equal treatment (see 'Justice', p. 311).

Private healthcare

Although most patients are treated by the NHS, some pay for treatment through private hospitals. These often employ doctors who also work for the NHS. Those supporting private healthcare argue that patients should have choice about where they are treated. If patients want to pay extra, why should anyone stop them? They also argue that by seeing a private doctor, patients do not clog up NHS appointment times and waiting lists. It is also worth remembering that private patients essentially pay twice for healthcare since they still pay for the NHS through taxes.

However, others argue that NHS doctors should not support private healthcare. This is for two reasons. The first is to do with fairness. Why should people with money receive 'better' treatment and in less time than those treated in the NHS? The second argument maintains that private healthcare undermines the NHS. Since NHS waiting lists are often long, it is claimed that doctors should be spending more time in the NHS rather than in private practice. However, doctors working privately could argue that work done in their free time is no-one else's business.

Nurse practitioners (NPs)

These are registered nurses who see new patients with undiagnosed conditions. They are responsible for ordering appropriate investigations, reaching a diagnosis, and treating patients. Some people believe this is a natural extension of the nursing role. It also allows individual nurses to take on more responsibility as they develop their careers. However, others fear NPs are encroaching on the perceived role of doctors. This is followed by concerns over whether NPs are adequately trained to diagnose and treat patients safely.

Screening

This is the process of looking at a great number of people to identify those with disease who do not yet have symptoms. The idea is that early diagnoses will improve health outcomes. One of the best-known screening programmes in the UK is for breast cancer. Women between the ages of 50 and 70 are invited for a breast X-ray (mammogram) every three years.

   Although it sounds like a great idea, there are a number of downsides. Screening can lead to overdiagnosis, misdiagnosis, worry, and a false sense of security when screening suggests there is no disease. It is expensive, and some screening tests also carry risks of their own. For example, mammography is used to screen for breast cancer but carries a (minute) risk of causing cancer by exposing women to radiation. These reasons explain why there are only screening programmes for a small number of diseases.

Medical students

As a medical student you will be expected to spend a lot of time with patients. In many cases, you will learn personal details about patients, examine them, and see them in a state of undress. Of course, doctors do these things, but only when necessary to help diagnosis and/or treat patients. Medical students do not contribute to patient care directly and so it is harder to justify why they should risk causing discomfort or embarrassment to patients. However, on the other hand, medical students must see patients if they are to become competent, safe doctors. Do you think patients have a moral obligation to help with this process even if it causes them discomfort?

Key points

Keep a diary of everything you see during your work experience that makes you think. These issues will almost always have an ethical dimension. Consider each aspect of the situation in the light of the core ethical principles on p. 311. Wherever possible, follow up the case and find out what decisions were actually made. Try to understand the perspectives of everyone involved (e.g. doctor, patient, relatives). Talk through everyday ethical dilemmas with the staff you are working with. This will help you understand the system of ethics that is (or should be) applied within the NHS.

▌ Science in the medical interview

As a doctor, you will diagnose and treat patients with many diseases. Medical schools ideally want to select applicants with more than a passing interest in health and illness. Some diseases are of particular importance (or public interest) and it is a good idea to be prepared to discuss these at interview.

Diabetes

This is caused by a deficiency or failure of the hormone 'insulin', which normally instructs cells to absorb and convert sugar (glucose) into its stored form, glycogen. Diabetes is characterized by excessive volumes of urine because glucose goes into the urine and causes large amounts of water to be retained in the urine by osmosis. There are two types of diabetes: type 1 in which insulin is not produced and type 2 in which it has a reduced effect. For this reason, insulin must be injected to treat type 1 but may not be needed to treat type 2. High levels of glucose in the blood can cause complications over time, including damage to the blood vessels (heart attack, stroke), eyes (retinopathy), and nerves (neuropathy, altered sensation or movement). Type 2 diabetes is more common with obesity and so, as the average waistline expands, it is becoming an increasingly common problem.

Key points

Some medical schools will expect a greater degree of scientific/healthcare knowledge than others. For example, Oxbridge interviews are likely to travel in this direction (see p. 246). Ask each individual medical school, or people who have previously been interviewed there, whether there is a scientific element to the interview.

Myocardial infarction

This is more commonly known as a 'heart attack'. Cholesterol is deposited in the walls of arteries, producing a plaque that can impair the flow of blood to cells. Like all organs, the heart needs a blood supply and this comes from the coronary arteries that bring oxygen to the muscle (myo-) of the heart (cardio-). When these arteries become blocked the myocardium can die, potentially resulting in death of the patient.

A similar process also causes strokes. If a fatty plaque/clot in an artery in the neck breaks off, it can travel through the circulation and block an artery in the brain. This may cause infarction of brain tissue. Other strokes are caused by bleeding into the brain.

Cancer

Most cells in the body divide to replace themselves. Very few individual cells survive from birth to old age without becoming replaced. This process is tightly controlled by signals within and between cells, which ensure that they divide appropriately. However, like any process, it can go wrong. When cells begin dividing uncontrollably, they can start invading adjacent tissues and even spread to distant sites in the body (for example, via the blood), and this is called cancer.

Cancer can affect any cell in the body at any age. However, a number of factors can make it more likely. For example, chemicals in tobacco smoke can lead to lung cancer, some inherited genes can increase the likelihood of developing bowel cancer, and ultraviolet light can cause genetic defects that lead to skin cancers. Age is also an important factor. For a cell to become cancerous it must accumulate a number of genetic 'errors'. With increasing age there is more time for these errors to occur, and this is why cancers are more common in the elderly. This is important as people now live to an older age and so many cancers are becoming more frequent.

HIV/AIDS

Human immunodeficiency virus (HIV) is spread horizontally (through sexual intercourse or blood-to-blood exchange) or vertically (from mother to child). The virus replicates in white blood cells, which are part of the normal immune system. The infection can have a long incubation phase in which the patient can infect others but lacks any symptoms. When the white cells are depleted, the patient begins to contract unusual infections. This is known as acquired immunodeficiency syndrome (AIDS). Although anti-retroviral drugs are very effective at treating the disease, they are expensive and not always available in the developing world.

Pandemics

This describes an infectious disease that spreads across continents or even worldwide. Recent pandemic scares include severe acute respiratory syndrome (SARS), avian influenza, swine flu, and SARS-CoV-2 causing coronavirus disease 2019 (COVID-19).

Every disease has a certain level at which it is expected in a certain population. This is usually quite low, because the population possesses collective immunity (i.e. most people are immune and so the infection is unable to spread quickly). However, such immunity may not exist when a completely new infection is introduced. New infections have the potential to infect an entire population before individuals become immune.

Viruses are particularly adept at changing as a result of antigenic shift. Every year, changes in the surface proteins (antigens) of the influenza virus mean that a new 'flu' jab has to be designed. Occasionally an antigen on one virus is swapped (or recombined) with those from a completely different virus. The result is a dramatic shift in virus surface proteins and an entire population whose immune systems can no longer react quickly to the novel virus. If these infections are not identified and quarantined early, they can spread throughout the whole world.

Although the entire population is susceptible, the new infection does not have to be particularly severe. The mortality rate might even be similar to the virus from which the newly recombined one was derived but, because such a large population is affected, pandemics can result in many deaths. Population-based preventive measures including social distancing, self-isolation, containment, and suppression aim to decrease the epidemic peak and 'flatten the epidemic curve', as occurred across various countries in 2020 with COVID-19.

Key points

Your goal should not be to learn all about health and disease. There will be plenty of time for that later once you are at medical school. Instead, take opportunities to pay attention when anything is mentioned about health. This will show interviewers that you are interested in healthcare and understand issues from outside your A level syllabus, and will stop you making naïve mistakes at interview.

Also, you never know when something learned now will win you valuable marks during an exam in a couple of years' time!

▌Useful things to look up

This is not an exhaustive list of things you must know before interview. However, knowing about important issues and institutions in medicine could demonstrate insight to the course selectors. Don't be caught out though. If you use one of the phrases below, an interviewer is likely to ask you what it means. Whether you consider this a risk or an opportunity depends on how well prepared you are.

General Medical Council (GMC) The GMC is the organization responsible for registering and regulating doctors within the UK. It also ensures that medical schools meet a minimum standard. Any doctor in the UK can be 'referred' to the GMC if their 'fitness to practice' is in doubt. This could be because of poor health or concerns about their ability and/or behaviour. The GMC is often criticized by the public for protecting doctors, and by doctors for being too harsh.

Good Medical Practice This is a document published by the GMC that sets out the values and standards expected of registered medical practitioners. It is very short and worth reading before your interview. Search the GMC website for it (www.gmc-uk.org).

Tomorrow's Doctors Another document from the GMC that describes the knowledge, skills, and attitudes that must be learned at medical school. This document and *Good Medical Practice* help inform mark schemes for UCAS forms and interviews; use the GMC website (www.gmc-uk.org) to find *Tomorrow's Doctors*.

British Medical Association (BMA) Unlike the GMC, which regulates doctors, the BMA represents them. It is the registered trade union for all doctors and medical students in the UK. The BMA provides a number of services but a key role is negotiating with the government over issues such as doctors' pay and working conditions. It also speaks for the medical profession, often providing opinions on important health issues.

Royal Colleges Most specialties within medicine are organized into specific professional bodies, known collectively as the Royal Colleges. These aim to improve the standards and training of each group of doctors. There are many Royal Colleges, including the Royal College of Surgeons and the Royal College of General Practitioners. These organizations also set postgraduate exams, which must be passed before a doctor can become a GP or specialist trainee (see p. 7).

Evidence-based medicine (EBM) This is an important move in medicine towards applying science to clinical practice. It requires treatments to be supported by evidence, not simply by 'expert' opinion, and for every treatment to be thoroughly evaluated by clinical trials before it is recommended for use by doctors.

National Institute for Health and Care Excellence (NICE) This organization was set up to standardize the treatments available in different parts of the country. NICE publishes reports considering the evidence of each new treatment, then makes a recommendation based on its cost effectiveness. As a result, NICE decisions are often controversial, as national priorities that consider cost do not always please doctors, patients, or the public. The NICE website is at www.nice.org.uk.

Multidisciplinary team (MDT) Modern healthcare is a team effort, and the team is growing! You will already be familiar with doctors and nurses, but there are also physiotherapists, speech and language therapists, clinical psychologists, physician associates, and operating department practitioners, to name only a few. Even experienced doctors struggle with the number of different uniforms seen in a single hospital. During work experience, you may have attended an MDT meeting in which different healthcare professionals come together to discuss patients. A good understanding of how the MDT works (or perhaps should work, depending on your experience of one) can show that you have the right attitude to become a doctor.

Patient-centred care This is all about putting the patient first in healthcare. For example, patient welfare should be placed above other considerations when deciding upon a course of investigation or treatment. One aspect of patient-centred care is to involve patients, wherever possible, in their own care.

Clinical governance This is a system by which NHS organizations are expected to foster an environment of clinical excellence to ensure patients receive the best possible standard of care. This includes teaching, research, audit, and handling complaints.

Professionalism Although difficult to define, this word is used frequently to describe how doctors should act. It can refer to many different things, often at the same time, including maintaining skills and knowledge, keeping an appropriate relationship with patients, teamworking, taking responsibility, and honesty.

Key points

Health is important to people. This means there is a lot written about it—far more than you could ever hope to read in a lifetime. However, the more you read, the more insight you will have into the NHS and the medical profession.

An insider's view …

Candidates with genuine insight into the NHS really stand out. Most candidates will know something about medicine and/or the NHS. This might be because of family connections or because they keep abreast of the news. Just occasionally, you come across a candidate who has a fundamental grasp of what it is like to be a doctor and to work within a state-funded healthcare system. There is no 'one thing' these candidates say to identify themselves—the panel can just sense that they really understand.

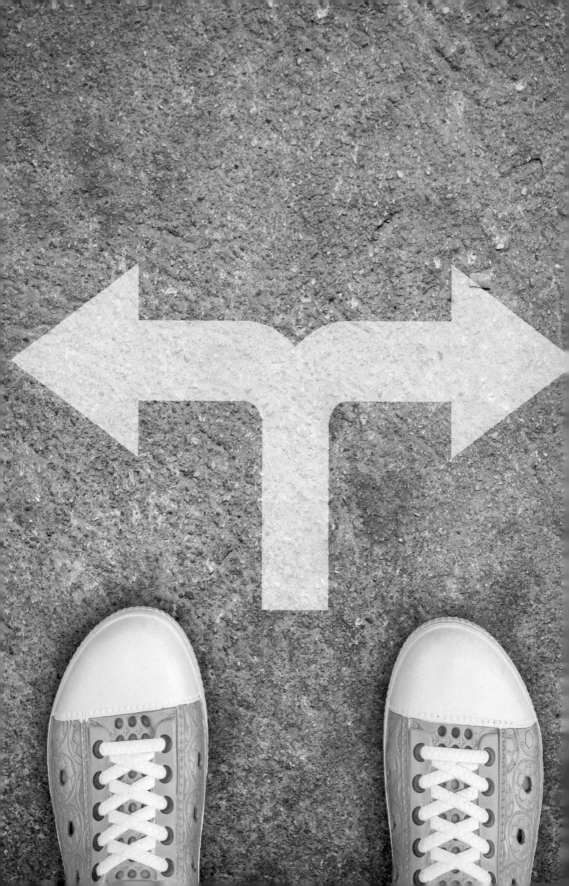

15

If things don't work out

If you don't win an offer

The number of applicants to British medical schools far exceeds the number of places. This means that many applicants (even those with a string of A/A* grades and work experience) will not be successful on their first attempt. This section takes you through how to react if you are faced with four rejections through UCAS. If you did receive an offer but didn't achieve your grades, jump ahead to p. 325.

Everyone responds differently to a final UCAS rejection. Anything from numbness to earth-shattering disappointment is completely normal. Some applicants view this as a personal rejection; however, many who would have made great doctors are rejected every year—there are simply not enough places to train everyone.

- **Take a break** For many applicants this is their first-ever taste of failure. It is normal to feel disappointed, lost, and even angry. Don't do anything rash; take a few days to come to terms with the situation. Consider catching up with any friends or hobbies that were neglected during the application process.
- **Speak to other people** Most unsuccessful applicants find it helps to talk about their experience. Friends, family, and teachers are often good sources of support. For a more anonymous sounding board consider online forums (see p. 383)—these also offer information and support from other applicants.
- **Reflect** Talking to others is therapeutic but also helps with reflection and future planning. Once you feel ready, you need to address some big questions. Do you still want to study medicine? Why were you unsuccessful? What are you going to do now? These are discussed in more detail below.

A student's experience ...

I was rejected without interview by all four medical schools. When I sat down with the careers advisor she pointed out that I'd applied to four of the most competitive institutions. I didn't even meet the minimum GCSE requirement for one of them. I had spent so much time studying and organizing work experience that I hadn't researched the courses well enough.

Do you still want to study medicine?

A rejection at this stage does *not* mean you cannot win a place at medical school and become an excellent doctor. Many current medical students (and senior doctors) got in on their second, third, or even fourth attempt. However, it is also true that not everyone is suited, or even wants, to be a doctor. This can come across to admissions staff when they read an application and can result in four rejections. Other applicants become disillusioned with medicine, talk themselves out of applying, or become interested in something else during the UCAS process. There are a number of questions you should ask yourself at this stage:

- **Why do you want to study medicine?** Your reasons for studying medicine need revisiting (see p. 2). Are they still relevant to you? Would other careers satisfy your requirements at least as well, if not better?
- **Are you being realistic?** Although many applicants win a place on the second attempt, you don't want to spend years fruitlessly applying to medical school. You

must undertake an honest appraisal of your application and abilities. Most people are bad at doing this—they either *under*estimate or *over*estimate their position. Try to recruit someone else to the process, ideally someone whom you trust to be completely honest. A teacher or school careers advisor could help identify whether you are willing to invest the time needed to make a successful reapplication. Although you should take advice, remember that the final decision is yours alone.

Why were you unsuccessful this time?

Understanding why you were unsuccessful is vital if you intend to reapply. Some factors (e.g. A level grades) are difficult to change, whereas others (e.g. work experience) are more amenable to improvement. Things to consider include:

- **Invitations to interview** A strong indication comes from whether you were invited to interviews. If four medical schools sent rejections without interview, there is a problem with your UCAS application or admission test result. Review your grades, school reference, and personal statement. If your reference is glowing and grades all read A/A*, there is probably something wrong with your statement. Similarly, if you were invited to interview four times but didn't win a place, you need to work on this aspect of your application. Or you could apply to an institution that does not routinely interview candidates (e.g. Edinburgh, see p. 190).
- **Admissions requirements** Did you meet all the necessary admissions requirements? This includes apparently 'unimportant' things such as a minimum grade in GCSE English.
- **Feedback from medical schools** Institutions vary in their willingness to provide feedback. Although most send a standard reply with advice for unsuccessful applicants, others provide specific feedback if approached. Don't come across as challenging or in disagreement with their decision. Instead, emphasize that you want to learn from the experience of applying. If necessary, wait a week to cool down after receiving their decision.

Your options

If you didn't receive an offer, you have four broad options. Think carefully and talk to other people about where you are going to go from here.

- **Keep trying this year** It's very unusual for medical schools to enter clearing but they do occasionally. Check the clearing lists on the UCAS website as soon as you get your A level results. Alternatively, it's sometimes worth a telephone call a few days after A level grades are released and before the start of term. Medical schools have been known to reconsider borderline applications if they have spaces unfilled. This is only really an option if you were rejected after interview; candidates who weren't shortlisted are unlikely to be considered borderline.
- **Reapply** Learn as much as you can from this experience, take a gap year (see p. 34), and start planning your reapplication. You might also think about less common routes (e.g. University of Buckingham (see p. 201), studying abroad (see p. 208)). This *could* be the best thing that ever happened to you, although you won't know it yet.

- **Graduate entry** Take up one of your non-medicine options and consider applying to medical school as a graduate. This needs careful thought, so read p. 252 before choosing this option.
- **Make other plans** Think about alternative science or healthcare careers (see p. 308).

Key points

You are making important career decisions. Although you should listen to other people and seek advice where possible, the final decision is yours alone.

If you miss your offer

Most successful applicants are made a conditional offer based on exam grades. The medical school will set a threshold (e.g. AAAb) that guarantees the applicant a place if they achieve the necessary results. Some medical schools stipulate additional requirements (e.g. A* in chemistry). This means another hurdle for applicants to trip over, and many do not achieve the required grades.

Trying your luck

Medical school offers are not set in stone. If you just missed your offer, call and explain your situation. Admissions teams tread a fine line between making too many and too few offers for the number of places they have available. It is only on results day that they find out whether they under- or oversold their course. If they have places left, you might just call at the right time.

> **Key points**
>
> Keep a list of telephone numbers for the admissions staff at medical schools at which you hold offers. If you miss your grades, call straight away for advice. There might still be a chance if you are proactive and don't give up at the first obstacle.

Extenuating circumstances

If your exam performance was adversely affected (e.g. by illness or bereavement) this should ideally have been recorded at the time of the exam. If not:

- **Evidence** Collect all available evidence attesting to the circumstances and their potential impact on your exam performance. A death certificate, doctor's note, or letter from another appropriate professional is a good place to start.
- **Support** To ensure your claim sounds plausible you will need support from your school. Ideally your referee will write an additional letter and/or contact medical schools on your behalf. Talk to them early if this is a possibility.

This route is only for those genuinely affected during their exams. Medical schools are unlikely to be impressed by a complaint based on minor circumstances. Similarly, while extenuating circumstances could result in sympathy for a narrowly missed A grade, they are unlikely to account for a string of D's.

Challenging your grades

Every year around 20,000 exam candidates (GCSE and A level) have their grades changed after re-marking. If your results were considerably less than expected or you were very close to meeting your offer, there is little to lose from querying your results. Candidates cannot usually liaise directly with exam boards, so you must contact your school in the first instance. Around 20% of all grades challenged are changed. Do this quickly as there are deadlines to meet for re-marking and medical schools need to know as soon as possible. It normally takes about 15 days for a priority re-mark (i.e. if a university place depends on the result) or 20 days otherwise.

The process varies between exam boards but costs range from £15 (for a clerical check) to £50 for a full re-mark. Your school can also request to see your marked exam script. The full process for appealing A level grades is as follows:

- School submits an enquiry to the exam board, which re-marks or re-moderates the necessary papers.
- If you (and your school) are dissatisfied with the result, you can appeal. The result will be considered under the exam board appeals procedure.
- The final stage is an external appeal to the Office of Qualifications and Examinations Regulations (Ofqual).

At every stage, keep medical schools for which you hold an offer informed so they don't prematurely give away your place.

A student's experience ...

I was devastated on results day when I scored ABB instead of the AAB needed to meet my offer. On calling the medical school I learned that they did not have any last-minute vacancies. I appealed both B grades and my history mark was revised to an A. Fortunately the medical school was sympathetic and took me as an 'extra' onto their course. Exam boards are not infallible after all.

Resitting

One option is to resit A level modules. Although AS-module resits are well tolerated, medical schools are suspicious about A levels taking longer than two years (see p. 23). For medical schools to permit resits usually requires extensively documented mitigating circumstances and A grades in all subjects retaken.

- Medical schools that will accept resit candidates without disadvantage: Aston (see p. 128), Exeter (see p. 140), Sheffield (see p. 174), and Southampton (see p. 176).
- Medical schools that will accept resit candidates under some circumstances, with special conditions, or may consider these qualifications to be of lower value: Anglia Ruskin (see p. 201), Brighton (see p. 132), Bristol (see p. 134), East Anglia (see p. 178), Hull York (see p. 142), Keele (see p. 144), Lancaster (see p. 146), Leicester (see p. 150), Liverpool (see p. 152), Manchester (see p. 164), Nottingham (see p. 168), Plymouth (see p. 172), Queen's (see p. 182), and Sunderland (see p. 203).
- Medical schools that will generally not consider resit candidates or at least not without significant extenuating circumstances: Aberdeen (see p. 186), Barts (see p. 154), Birmingham (see p. 130), Buckingham (see p. 201), Cambridge (see p. 136), Cardiff (see p. 198), Dundee (see p. 188), Edge Hill (see p. 202), Edinburgh (see p. 190), Glasgow (see p. 192), Imperial (see p. 156), Leeds (see p. 148), Lincoln (see p. 203), Newcastle (see p. 166), Oxford (see p. 170), St Andrew's (see p. 194), St George's (see p. 160), University of Central Lancashire (see p. 138), and University College London (see p. 162).

Key points

Be realistic about your grades. If you worked hard but scored CCC, take advice about whether you could achieve the grades required for your resit application.

Dealing with poor grades

If resitting is not an option, your poor grades will make it much harder to win a place. Access courses (see p. 295) are not substitutes for poor A level grades. If you do still want to pursue medicine, your best option may be to do so as a graduate. This means starting a degree in another subject (e.g. anatomy, biomedical science) and then applying to graduate-entry courses (see p. 252). An upper second-class honours degree may be considered in lieu of strong A levels. However, this is a long (and potentially expensive) option that requires careful thought.

If things still aren't working out

Commitment and persistence are important qualities. However, there is a point at which every unsuccessful applicant should reconsider their career options. Applicants falling into this category include those with:

- Surprisingly poor results without mitigating circumstances.
- Four rejections who are unwilling to take a year out.
- Unsuccessful UCAS applications for a second or third time.

Most UCAS applications to medical school include two other (often bioscience-related) courses. Applicants not receiving offers to study medicine may be tempted to pursue one of these instead. The ultimate aim might be to find a career outside medicine or to apply for graduate-entry courses three years later.

Graduate-entry medicine

These courses are accelerated (i.e. four years' duration) and aimed at graduates. Although most require a degree in a related field (e.g. biomedical science), others consider graduates in any subject. Most require an upper second-class honours (2:1) degree, which is achieved by over 55% of UK graduates. More details about graduate-entry courses can be found on p. 251.

> **Key points**
>
> Don't panic if you're unsuccessful first time. Avoid studying another course just for the sake of going to university. If you are considering a non-medicine degree, make this a deliberate choice after carefully considering your options.

Many unsuccessful applicants begin another degree with the intention of studying medicine later on. This is a legitimate route but requires careful thought.

- **Time** An honours degree followed by four years at medical school is a total of seven years. This is two years longer than a regular medical course.
- **Money** Home (and EU) students pay over £9,000 per year tuition for degrees at British universities (see p. 15). This is without considering accommodation, food, and other expenses for the extra two years. Two years' lost earning power can amount to more than £260,000.
- **Competition** Graduate courses attract between 10 and 55 applications for every place. This compares to between four and ten applicants for traditional courses. Many graduate applicants will have first-class degrees, PhDs, and many years of work experience. This means accelerated courses can be much less accessible than their traditional counterparts. Sometimes it's worth taking a year out (see p. 34) and re-applying for a five-year course instead.

That's not to say you shouldn't pursue the graduate route. There are many advantages to completing another degree first.

- **Better qualified** The graduate route means another degree on your CV. This can score additional points when choosing a specialty and applying for work as a doctor in years to come. However, many traditional courses permit medical students to complete an intercalated degree in just one year.

- **More experience** A first degree means three additional years to arrange work experience. It will also mean you are more experienced, more confident, and more mature when applying to medical school again.
- **Alternative careers** Many students find new interests at university. You may develop an interest outside of clinical medicine, perhaps in research.

A student's experience ...

I started a BSc(Hons) in Microbiology with a view to joining a graduate medicine course. I was swept onto a law conversion course and into a City law firm—working the same hours as many junior doctors but with an office, company BMW, shared secretary, and £60,000 per year for my trouble. The work is exciting and I haven't looked back. Medicine would have been great but other careers have their advantages as well.

Thinking outside of medicine

The future is bright for any university applicant with strong A levels. If you are thinking about alternatives to medical school, consider again what it was that made you want to be a doctor. If you lean towards knowledge and discovery, there are options within science you should explore further. If your motivations were based on helping or working with people, look at other careers within healthcare. Of course, science A levels do not confine you to these fields. The UCAS website (www.ucas.ac.uk) lists courses from aerospace engineering to zoology. It's important to remember that, however fixated you have become on medicine, there are many careers in the world. Take time to think about them properly.

Careers in science Table 15.1 gives an idea of what science (specifically bioscience) graduates do after graduating. Almost half spend three or four years working towards a research degree (e.g. PhD) which is usually funded by a stipend (~£15,000 per year), which in addition covers tuition fees and some research expenses. Depending on the field of interest, researchers work in a laboratory on graduation. They are responsible for many of the discoveries that change the diagnosis and treatment of disease in medicine.

Other relevant careers include research in the pharmaceutical industry, teaching, patent law (e.g. protecting intellectual property rights), marketing of new products (e.g. to doctors), and public understanding of science.

Careers in healthcare You will have come across many different healthcare professionals during your work experience. Most healthcare professions are accessible through degree courses, some of which are extremely competitive. Graduate healthcare careers include nursing, physiotherapy, radiography, and occupational therapy; use a similar strategy to get relevant work experience for these professions (see p. 54).

Table 15.1 Destination of bioscience graduates

Employment	42%	
Further study	44%	Usually taught MSc or research degrees (e.g. MRes, PhD)
Unemployed	9%	Including those travelling post-graduation
Unknown	5%	

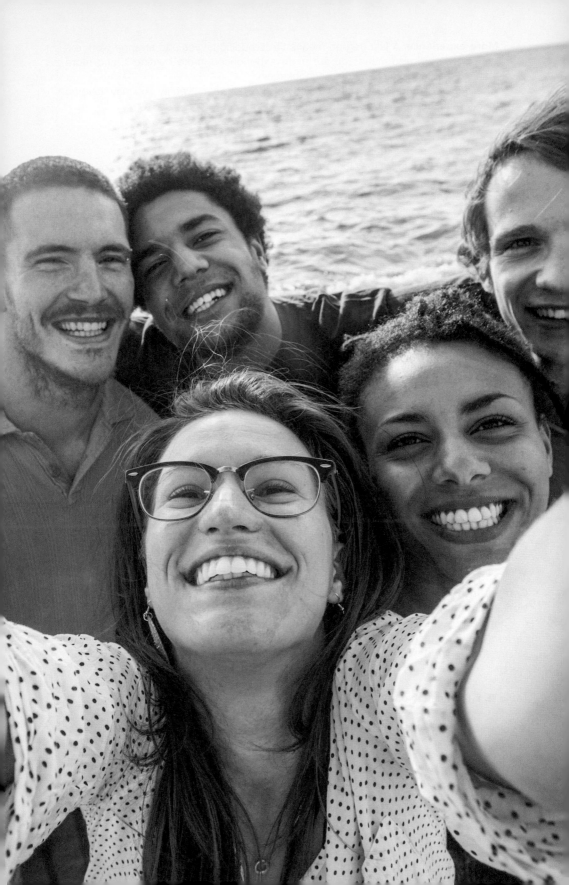

16

Making the most of medical school

■ So you're going to be a doctor...

Congratulations—you've made it! Having achieved the difficult task of getting in, you can now look forward to spending the next few years living, studying, and socializing at university. University can, and should, be one of the greatest experiences of your life, provided you get off to a good start. Unfortunately, many new undergraduates are ill-prepared for the realities of university life and enter with a mindset that is uninformed and unsustainable. There can also be practical hurdles to catch out unsuspecting 'freshers', from mix-ups with the Student Loans Company to sitting degree-level exams for the first time.

This chapter offers an insight into university life, as well as advice on how best to settle in (see p. 334). There are some tips for learning (see p. 336) and living (see p. 340) as a university student, which can be different from even the most independent A level student experience. These pages will also be relevant to medical school applicants who have not yet secured a place, as they paint a picture of life as a medical student. Finally, the importance of early career decisions will be covered—taking a step towards your possible future medical career as a doctor (see p. 344).

There's a lot to learn about medicine at medical school. However, there's also a lot to learn about how to be an effective medical student. The *Oxford Handbook for Medical School* (published by Oxford University Press) provides everything you need to get off to the best possible start at medical school.

What will university be like?

Everyone has a different opinion about what university is like and you will hear various descriptions of students, from being lazy and hung-over to studious and nerdy. The accounts will depend on the storyteller's own personal experiences and prejudices. Of course, the truth is somewhere in between.

University life will probably be different from your student experiences so far. Not only is the material delivered in a different format (see p. 336), but you are likely to be one of the many students who are living away from their parents for the first time (see p. 341). It is worth remembering that you will not only be a university student studying for their degree but also are a doctor in training. This adds an additional dimension to your learning experience and one that is different from students in other disciplines. With all this change happening at once, starting university can be a daunting time. The key to success is finding your feet early on (see p. 337) and knowing what to look out for and what to avoid.

What can I look forward to?

- **Making friends** If you look past the horrible cliché, you may begin to appreciate the fantastic opportunity that starting university offers. This is the largest and most diverse group of people you will ever meet. Starting university is a great opportunity to expand your horizons and form a new group of interesting friends, some of whom you will stay close to for the rest of your life.
- **Joining the profession** You're not only a medical student, you are a student *doctor*. This is reflected in your course content, which includes both professional and academic content (see p. 338). With the status of joining the medical profession comes significant responsibility for you as a student doctor, even at this early stage (see p. 342).

- **Life skills** Although this is likely to be your first experience of living away from home for a long period of time, you should seize the opportunity to gain independence. University is a time for maturity and developing a sense of personal identity.
- **New beginnings** One of the best things about university is the genuine opportunity to *be yourself*. The cohort of students are less likely to be judgemental than your school colleagues—so if you've held back in your academic, social, or personal life, this is your chance to show your true colours.

What should I avoid?

- **Solitude** Homesickness is common when starting university, as is the fear of not fitting in or finding any close friends. Often this is something you can get through together with the friends you make during Freshers' Week (who will inevitably feel the same).
- **Excessive debt** With the amount of financial support in place for university students, you shouldn't struggle to live comfortably, provided you are sensible with your finances (see p. 14). Debt is inevitable after completing a medical degree, but careful spending can limit the final bill.
- **Alcohol** Students are not exempt from the excessive drinking culture of 'Binge Britain'. It is worth remembering that doctors suffer one of the highest rates of alcoholism of all the professions. Medical school is a time to form a *healthy* relationship with alcohol. At best, a heavy night risks wasting the next day through the haze of a hangover. At worst it can result in death or severe injury (spend any Friday night in A&E to witness this first-hand). Drunken misdemeanours can also bring students to the attention of their institution's Fitness to Practice Committee. You do not want a written warning on record for the rest of your professional career. So, if you are partial to an alcoholic beverage, learn self-restraint early.
- **Sex** Freshers' Week is all too often the source of regretful one-night stands, fuelled by the excitement of independence and cheap alcohol. It is worth bearing this in mind when you start university.
- **Recreational drugs** The GMC (not to mention the law) looks very dimly on drug abuse and you risk ending your career before you've even qualified. Being a student does not absolve you from your responsibilities as a citizen or as a professional in training.
- **Resits** Exams are an inevitable part of any university course and provide an opportunity to assess how well you are learning the subject. They represent another milestone and a step closer to becoming a doctor. However, you do need to prepare early to avoid resits. There is a limit to the number of times you can repeat medical school exams: usually once unless there are exceptional circumstances, after which you may be asked to repeat the year or leave the course.

Starting university

There are often mixed emotions when starting university. Parents may be upset about re-leasing their 'child' alone into the world for the first time. Students themselves may experi-ence a mixture of excitement at the prospect of new experiences and anxiety that it will fail to 'work out'. In fact, you will probably find yourself looking back fondly on the emotional rollercoaster of starting university only weeks after arriving, having happily settled in and dispelled any misconceptions that you had formed. The following will hopefully help you to reach this sense of nostalgia more quickly.

Arriving at university

You should receive specific instructions by post, telling you where to go and what to do on your first day. Most first-year students arrive a week before academic term begins, which provides an opportunity to participate in a week of activities (Freshers' Week) organized solely for them.

You will probably need to exchange paperwork with the university authorities when you first arrive. Successful completion of these administrative challenges is rewarded by a room key, map, and timetable. The timetable will be useful for finding out when and where you need to be for various academic introductions and social gatherings. You can then begin the arduous task of unloading a car full of belongings into your new room (if you have been successful in persuading your parents to offer their services—highly recommended!).

Settling in

You will find it a lot easier to settle in if you are well prepared with all of your everyday necessities.

- **Bedding** It's best to check what will be included with your accommodation before you arrive, but most students prefer to bring their own pillows and duvet covers.
- **Home decor** Student rooms aren't renowned for their palatial furnishings, so it is worth bringing a few home comforts: pictures, cushions, throws, and beanbags. There are often poster sales that run during Freshers' Week too.
- **Entertainment** Remember that you will be spending a fair amount of time in your halls of residence, so it's worth bringing along something to keep yourself enter-tained when you have a moment to relax. Books, speakers, tablets, headphones, mu-sical instruments, and sport accessories can offer useful respite (if used judiciously).
- **Documents** Remember to bring important documents that the university/medical school will need to see prior to you starting the course. This may include student finance/Local Education Authority letters, criminal record (DBS) checks, and vaccin-ation forms. Photo ID (driving licence/passport) is often necessary for banking matters and has a role in proceeding past doormen at local bars and clubs.
- **Computers** All universities have significant computing resources for their students, but it is helpful to have access to a computer in your own room. A laptop has the added benefit of portability, which will be useful for clinical attachments. You won't need anything too advanced—most medical students use their computers for cre-ating documents and slide presentations, checking their email, and browsing the internet. Don't forget to look for student deals on computers and software, and uni-versity grants can help to contribute towards the cost (see p. 16).
- **Clothes** As a medical student you will need a smart wardrobe for working on the wards and in general practice, as well as day-to-day clothes. The NHS has a 'bare

below the elbow' dress code, meaning that sleeves must be rolled up (or short-sleeved shirts worn). If you choose to wear a tie, it needs to be tucked into the shirt or worn with a tie-clip so as not to hang loose. Also bear in mind that your wardrobe needs to (ideally) see you through the entire term at university. You may require a lounge suit/cocktail dress or black-tie outfit/ball gown at some point, but this decision can be deferred to a time when your social calendar has become clearer after the start of term.

- **Bike** At some universities, cycling is a common mode of transport. Visiting on an open day will have helped to determine whether a bike would be useful. If you do take one, remember to bring a heavy-duty bike lock, helmet, and lights.
- **Don't forget...** Towels, coat hangers, lamps, extension cables, kettle, crockery, cutlery, cookware, washing-up cloth, tea towels, Blu-Tack®/drawing pins, stationery, and tea/coffee. A 16–25 Railcard is an immensely valuable investment, offering one-third off rail journeys for £30 a year, and all students are eligible. If you have to wait for your bank account to be activated, bring enough cash to last a couple of weeks.
- **Storage space** Storage can be limited so you should avoid bringing too many needless extras before you know how much space is available. Find out whether you have to move the contents out of your room between terms.

Fresher's week

Every year around the middle of September, freshers (another word for first-year university students) across the UK begin a week of activities, organized by the university and student committees (e.g. JCR, MedSoc). Whilst most activities are voluntary, they are often great ways to get to know your colleagues as well as your surroundings, and are definitely worth attending. You will also gain a better idea of the services and facilities that are available. Look out for the societies fair, where you can join one of the hundreds of societies covering every conceivable interest. You may also get university 'parents': students in the years above who will be able to dispense their advice (of variable quality). Rumours about medic initiations can often run rife during Freshers' Week and it is common for students to feel anxious about what they may be asked to do. Suffice to say, you should only take part in what you feel comfortable with, whilst not forgetting your professional responsibilities. Your first visit to hospital as a medical student shouldn't be for intoxication.

Learning at university

There are fundamental differences between the teaching at sixth form and in higher education. The uniqueness of higher education requires a new approach to learning.

How is university education different from A levels?

- **Content** It goes without saying that the material you will cover at university will be different. In fact, it's not just the details of each subject that will be new to you but the way in which subjects are pursued. Lectures offer a starting point to help you read around the subject, so the learning is more *self-directed*. You will develop a deep understanding across a wide range of topics relevant to medicine. Such breadth and depth can seem daunting at first.
- **Resources** Unlike your sixth-form education, you will spend a great deal of time reading material from textbooks, journals, and websites.
- **Teachers** There will be 'teachers' at university but their role is less obvious than at sixth form. They may deliver lectures, lead practical classes, or oversee problem-based learning (PBL) presentations but, unlike high school, they will have other commitments in their area of expertise. This might include leading a research team or working full-time as a doctor. As a result, they are better seen as a resource for clarifying uncertainties than a source of spoon-feeding. Textbooks and online resources are your new best friends.
- **Dynamic curriculum** Medicine is constantly changing, from the understanding of the basic sciences (e.g. how the brain works or the pathophysiology of heart failure) to clinical developments (e.g. chemotherapies in cancer treatment or the indications for a particular operation). This information comes from ongoing research, so your lecture material is only ever a snapshot of current knowledge. Students must be aware of new research findings and gaps in medical knowledge, as well as the details that are understood.
- **Professional dimension** Unique to medical students are the legal and ethical elements of your role as a future doctor. These require additional teaching to reflect the social implications of implementing biomedical knowledge.
- **Exams** The exams you will take during your preclinical and clinical years will depend on the university at which you study. They are likely to include the following: multiple choice, short answer, essay, and practical questions (based on lab data, histology slides, and pathology specimens) and prosections (anatomical specimens from which you are asked questions). Clinical exams include mock interviews with actors, clinical examinations of patients with diseases, and practical clinical skills (e.g. taking blood from a plastic model). You may also be exposed to oral examinations (vivas).

An insider's view ...

Perhaps the biggest difference between medical school and high school is the human element. Medicine is a pragmatic application of scientific principles, requiring effective communication with each patient in view of their psychosocial context. This requires a professional awareness and emotional maturity that medical schools must impart to students before they graduate.

What will I learn?

Medicine is a broad subject, which is taught in a variety of ways (see p. 92).

- **Basic clinical sciences** Traditional courses focus their preclinical teaching on the individual subjects upon which medicine is based. This includes everything from biochemistry to psychology.
- **Systems-based courses** These teach the important principles of each subject in a series of lectures that are linked by a common set of organs. For example, studying the renal system will involve understanding the physiology of the normal kidney, visualizing the anatomy of the urinary tract in the dissecting lab, gaining an appreciation of the congenital and acquired diseases that affect the kidney (via pathology and genetics), and learning the pharmacology of drugs that act on the kidneys.

As you can see, by the end of the preclinical years, students from all types of course will have a similar understanding of how the body works and what can go wrong. This enables them to focus entirely on its pragmatic application on the wards in the clinical years.

- **Clinical attachments** After a few years of book learning, medical students begin their full-time clinical attachments. Up until this point your clinical exposure could have been anything from once a week to bi-annual patient contact, depending on your type of course (see p. 92). In the clinical years most students are assigned to medical or surgical teams in hospital, for four to eight weeks at a time.

A student's experience ...

I found it quite difficult to immerse myself in the esoteric detail of my preclinical course, which was taught as basic clinical sciences. It is difficult to see the immediate relevance of lectures when you are learning about the intricate molecular interaction between oxygen and haemoglobin. I found this depth of study made it particularly challenging to stay focused during my revision. Fortunately, I am now in the clinical stage of my medical course, studying the subject I originally signed up for. It is a lot more enjoyable when there is a clear purpose to your efforts.

How will I learn preclinical medicine?

The following teaching methods are used to different extents, depending on your course type (see p. 92). However, most courses include at least some of each type.

- **Lectures** One speaker usually teaches the entire cohort of medical students for 50 minutes. The size of the audience therefore depends on the medical school, but it can be over 300. The format is often a slideshow presentation and, if a handout is provided, this may be a printout of the slides or notes to accompany the lecture content. Your decision to take notes will depend on the quality of the notes you receive and how well the textbooks cover the same material. Remember, lectures are fantastic for grasping principles for the first time, but the minutiae can often be found elsewhere, so don't worry about catching every word.
- **Seminars** Smaller groups, usually between 10 and 30 students, are taught by one tutor. There is usually an element of participation, either through small-group exercises or direct discussion between the teacher and the group. Seminars are often used to reinforce important topics or teach discursive subjects such as law and ethics.
- **Problem-based learning (PBL) cases** The number of PBL cases you will complete will greatly depend on the type of course (see p. 92). PBL cases usually take place

over a week in which a small group (eight to ten students) are given a problem/clinical scenario to learn about independently. The group reconvenes at the end of the week to share their findings.

- **Dissection** Human cadaveric dissection is increasingly being replaced with the use of pre-prepared prosections (professionally dissected specimens) to teach anatomy to medical students. However, full cadaveric dissection is still found at many medical schools. Others use prosections, plastinates (prosections that are solidified), plastic models, or electronic methods of teaching anatomy.
- **Practical classes** During your preclinical education you are likely to encounter various practical classes in order to further understand physiology, biochemistry, pharmacology, and histology. Practical skills are often neglected by medical students, who see them as an enjoyable escape from intense lectures. Whilst they are often enjoyable, they are also examinable and offer easy marks at exam time provided the material is well understood and time is invested in producing a complete workbook.

Key points

Every subject has a list of aims and objectives that you are expected to complete by the end of the course. It is useful to familiarize yourself with these before beginning the relevant lectures or laboratory classes. This can help you concentrate on the material that is examinable (i.e. the aims/objectives) and focus your attention on 'high-yield' information.

How will I learn clinical medicine?

In many ways, clinical attachments are like apprenticeships. Groups of medical students (usually between two and eight) are assigned a clinical 'firm' to 'shadow'. You may follow a ward round and even write in the patient notes. Your firm's doctors will run clinics in which they assess outpatients and determine their management (e.g. considering a patient for surgery or altering their drug treatment), which you can also attend.

- **Good manners** You must always remain polite, *especially* towards patients. Your kindness towards them will often be reciprocated by their permission to allow you to examine them or perform procedures.
- **Lend a hand** Don't be afraid to get stuck in. Practical tasks on the wards always need doing and you will be actively contributing to the running of the ward. Ask if you need help, only do what you are comfortable with, and *never* expose yourself or a patient to risk.
- **Attending theatre** You should receive an introduction to surgery and theatre etiquette before beginning your first surgical attachment. There is a strict hierarchy within the operating room, with the scrub nurse placed squarely at the top! Introduce yourself to the whole team as soon as you enter an operating theatre. Ensure that everyone is happy with your attendance, and not just the consultant. Ask where they would like you to stand and be careful not to touch anything within the 'sterile field'.
- **Scrubbing in** This can be a useful experience if the surgeon is willing to teach in theatre. However, be warned: surgery might look exciting but it soon loses its appeal after the fifth hour of holding a retractor in position. Although you must experience assisting (especially if your consultant says you should), your time could often be better spent elsewhere. Ask your consultant if you feel you could learn more from seeing patients on the ward or in clinics instead.
- **Attention to detail** Good students soon learn that there is a wealth of detail they can never hope to master if they want to pass their exams. You won't face a question in

finals on dosing regimens of anti-retrovirals, so learning them is not a good use of time. Learn what interests you but remember it is a *strong* grasp of *basic* knowledge and underlying principles that will get you through the exams.

- **Books or patients?** It's difficult to achieve the right balance between clerking patients and learning theory. Clinicians will encourage you to take histories, examine patients, and consider their management. The ability to diagnose patients cannot be achieved from books alone. That said, it is easy to overlook the quantity of information you will need to know for your clinical exams, so it is important that you strike the right balance.
- **Asking for help** Don't be afraid to ask. You can do almost anything with appropriate supervision—ask someone to teach you. You are there to learn.

An insider's view ...

He who studies medicine without books, sails an uncharted sea, but he who studies medicine without patients, does not go to sea at all.
Sir William Osler, a Father of Modern Medicine

Living at university

If the different style of learning at university wasn't enough for you to get used to, living as a student will definitely require pause for thought. Many students find themselves having to manage finances, maintain a work–life balance, and look after themselves for the first time. Hopefully this transition to independence hasn't come all at once but, if it has, you are certainly not alone. The advice in this section should make this transition easier and point you in the right direction should you come across any difficulties.

Money

Pages 14–16 covers the cost of medical school in detail. Suffice to say you will be spending in the region of £160–£300 a week on tuition fees, rent, and living costs. The first two are fixed, but the estimate of living costs is very dependent upon your lifestyle as a student. The lower boundary doesn't prevent you from socializing, nor does the upper estimate guarantee you stardom within the upper echelons of the university high life. You will need to determine your weekly budget early on. Every so often, it is worth checking that your 'books balance', to ensure you are not overspending.

Should you run into financial difficulties, you have several options to consider after parental contributions have run dry. You could seek a larger loan through the Student Loans Company if you are not already claiming the maximum amount. If your circumstances have changed, you may be eligible for reassessment or perhaps a grant/bursary from the university. You could consider a part-time job, but beware that this does not interfere with your education. Professional trainee loans of up to £25,000 are another option, but the interest rates are often high and should be avoided if possible. Credit cards should be avoided at all costs as these debts can increase dangerously due to the high interest rates.

Key points

Should you find yourself in excessive debt, you need to reassess your current expenditure to avoid making the situation worse, as well as prioritize any debts you have to pay. Do not ignore the issue. Seek advice from pastoral tutors, students' union services, and/or the Citizens Advice Bureau.

Health

Whilst learning about the ills of others and how to treat them, it's often easy to overlook your own health. University offers a bewildering array of hazards, from fresher's flu to alcohol intoxication. Moreover, the intensity of the course makes it easy to become run down, and it is therefore important that you register with a local GP.

Make sure you inform someone if you are feeling particularly unwell and be alert to any signs of danger (in yourself and your peers). For meningitis, these may include headache, fever, vomiting, stiff neck, drowsiness, avoidance of bright lights, and non-blanching bruises.

Central to your health is your mental well-being. Whilst the overall incidence is low, doctors have one of the highest rates of depression, alcoholism, and suicide of any profession. There are various services on hand including your GP, welfare tutor, and university pastoral support services. The Samaritans can be contacted 24 hours a day on 116 123.

Work–life balance

Maintaining a work–life balance is an issue that arises for every student and medics are no exception. With so much to condense into a short period of time, you quickly risk being overrun with lecture handouts and an ever-growing reading list. Two extremes of students can materialize. One stays up until the early hours in a vicious state of catch-up, trying, often with limited success, to cover *everything*. The second stacks their workload for the coming holidays, admits defeat, and concentrates on socializing. Neither is an ideal strategy for success.

It is nearly impossible to be familiar with all of your course materials at any one time during term. More importantly, it is not necessary. If you are examined regularly (via modular tests), then there is a limited amount of information you must know for each test. Otherwise, simply concentrate on having a good understanding of the principles of your subjects and addressing the difficult concepts whilst the material is fresh in your mind. It would be foolish to begin learning esoteric details for an exam that is nine months away.

Adopting such a strategy should give you enough time in the day for personal respite. How you choose to utilize this is entirely up to you, but free time need not be unproductive. It is possible, even at this stage, to take up enjoyable activities that can be directed towards your medical CV later on (see p. 345).

Hobbies and interests

Application forms for medicine are teeming with extracurricular activities and voluntary services that are often impossible to continue to the same extent at university. Medical schools look for this breadth to ensure students can deal with demands beyond the A-level syllabus and have coping mechanisms that are adequate for the pressures of medical school.

Finding a life outside of medicine is essential to the health and well-being of student doctors. Whether it is a morning run, working for a student newspaper, or being a committee member for the medical society, you will find it difficult to cope without some type of outlet. You may wish to continue a hobby from your school days or pursue a completely novel interest that has caught your eye during Freshers' Week (see p. 335). Just make sure you have something that you can regularly participate in, which takes your mind off the workload.

A day in the life of a student doctor

The following entries give you an idea of the day-to-day life of a preclinical and clinical student. Note there will be some differences between course types (see p. 92) and the exact content of the lectures will obviously depend upon how far you are into the course.

A day in the life of a preclinical student ...

08:20 Get out of bed after hitting the snooze button for the fifth and final time. No time for breakfast. Run for the bus to the hospital. Just miss it...

09:05 Creep into the back of the first lecture, the third of six lectures on the hypothalamic–pituitary axis. Need to read about this later, as it goes completely over my head!

10:00 The next lecture is on pregnancy. The online handouts are a little sparse so it's worth getting out a notepad and taking some notes.

11:05 Grab a quick coffee before attending a PBL session on genetics and development. I am assigned to a group of seven medics (four of whom I've never met before). Our presentation is on epigenetic disorders and I have to research Prader–Willi syndrome.

12:30 Chat to friends, then grab a quick bite at the canteen.

13:30 Neuroanatomy teaching in the dissection laboratory: this session is on the motor system, looking at prosections of the cerebellum and spinal cord. I spend the hour receiving informal teaching from demonstrators and reading posters that accompany the anatomical specimens.

15:00 Pharmacology practical, investigating the effect of drugs on the neuromuscular junction. We apply various drugs like acetylcholine to a guinea pig ileum and measure its response using an electrical transducer. The experiment is a complete failure but it's an enjoyable exercise nonetheless.

16:30 Meet up with my 'student-selected component' tutor to discuss my upcoming project in the Department of Psychiatry. I will be writing a 4,000-word dissertation on the neurodevelopment of obsessive compulsive disorder (OCD)—an area I found fascinating when it was briefly covered in our lectures last year.

17:15 Get to the sports pitches for lacrosse training—an intense session in preparation for the inter-university competition later on in the month.

18:30 Stop by the library to pick up books on genetics for the PBL presentation and on endocrinology to fill in the gaps from the morning lecture.

19:00 Get home and cook myself a student special—pasta with pesto—then finish off some pharmacokinetics calculations for a seminar tomorrow.

20:45 Watch a bit of TV before getting ready to go out.

22:00 Meet up with friends at the union bar, play a few games of pool, and catch up on the latest gossip.

00:30 Check the alarm is on for 7:30 and hit the sack.

07:45 Wake up; shower and breakfast before leaving the house.

08:15 Arrive at a friend's house who is driving four of us to our current cardiothoracic placement 10 miles away.

09:00 Wait for the doctor to arrive for a cystic fibrosis clinic.

09:30 The Specialist Registrar (SpR) arrives half an hour later, after attending to emergencies on the ward. Thankfully I brought along my *Oxford Handbook of Clinical Medicine* and so managed to refresh my knowledge about the condition beforehand.

09:45 See the first patient, a 15-year-old girl recovering from pneumonia whose symptoms have worsened. The patient is given an additional course of oral antibiotics and is told to return in a fortnight for a trial of nebulized saline.

10:30 The second patient fails to turn up so the SpR uses the opportunity to teach me about cystic fibrosis; this morning's reading proves particularly useful.

11:00 The next appointment is a routine follow-up reviewing a patient's drugs. There is an interesting discussion on the risks and benefits of long-term antibiotics and the patient decides to 'watch and wait' regarding her chest symptoms.

11:30 Final patient is particularly tearful and prefers that a student doctor is not present during his assessment. I attach myself to the physiotherapist and dietician and sit in on a few of their consultations.

12:30 Grab lunch at the hospital canteen, then go to a clinical lecture on asthma and its management.

14:00 Change into scrubs and ask the scrub nurse if I can observe the scheduled lobectomy. I had previously clerked this surgical patient a few days ago on the ward. He had been diagnosed with lung cancer after smoking for 25 years.

14:20 The surgeon arrives and offers me the chance to scrub in. I spend the next two and a half hours assisting with the lobectomy—holding retractors, 'following through' with sutures, and providing suction.

17:00 Head home, but get stuck in rush-hour traffic.

18:00 Cook dinner, then head to the medical school where there is a guest speaker at the Surgical Society talking about the history of plastic surgery and offering advice for students interested in pursuing this specialty.

20:30 Return home and attempt to complete a poster presentation I am producing with a registrar. We hope to send it off to be considered for a conference.

22:45 Admin: send out an email in my capacity as vice president for the Jazz Society, arranging the next rehearsal and confirming the location for the weekend's gig.

23:30 Skim a few pages of a non-medical book before falling asleep.

The importance of early career decisions

Only 10 years ago, the career path of medical students was vastly different from what it is today. The longer hours meant that junior doctors were exposed to more clinical medicine, and the job application system allowed student and junior doctors to develop a wealth of experience before selecting their chosen specialty. However, medicine is becoming increasingly competitive, with doctors having to make career decisions earlier in their training. Applicants have had less time to distinguish themselves and demonstrate an interest in their career of choice. This section explains why making career decisions early is important, and how to pursue them.

Why is it necessary?

With increasing competition, reduced working hours, and the new job application programmes (foundation, core training, and specialist training; see p. 9), student and junior doctors now have to demonstrate their clinical interests at an early stage. This is difficult because final-year medical students and junior doctors have very similar CVs with which they need to distinguish themselves in order to win their choice of positions. The inflexibility of the new training programmes also makes it difficult to change career once you have committed to a particular specialty. So not only does your choice of specialty have to come after less clinical experience but also you need to be absolutely sure early on.

However, it isn't all bad. The process of trying to identify your chosen specialty early on allows you to engage more closely with medicine and actively identify, or dismiss, future career options.

How do I decide?

- **Clinical attachments** Student doctors are in a fantastic position to determine their future careers. The apprenticeship style of teaching means that you have the opportunity to shadow many specialties as a student doctor. Unfortunately, most students fail to exploit their placements for this purpose and instead focus entirely on training to become junior doctors. Whilst this *is* important, it does not exclude the possibility of considering each specialty as a potential career destination.
- **Asking the right questions** There are many factors to consider when making a career decision: working hours, on-call work, salary, competition, and so on. Pick the SpR and consultant's brains, and ask them as much about the lifestyle of their specialty as about the work itself.
- **Student groups** There are often student special interest groups around each specialty that are established in medical schools. These groups tend to arrange regular events/workshops and often receive lectures from guest speakers about the subject.

Key points

You may find the junior doctor's teaching to be more relevant than the SpR's and consultant's when it comes to nailing down the basics for finals. However, if you find yourself interested in a particular specialty, there is no substitute for shadowing the senior members of a clinical team and exploring their roles.

- **Student-selected modules** Every medical course includes components where the students themselves decide on an area to study. The student's efforts could be expressed in the form of a dissertation, poster, or presentation. They can be great ways to learn about an area of medicine in greater depth.
- **Outside the box** The majority of medical students enter a career in hospital medicine or general practice. However, a small minority choose to step outside these traditional confines to use their expertise in less common environments…military medicine, medical law, forensic psychiatry, tropical medicine, aid work, medical management consultancy, expedition medicine, and prison medicine to name but a few. Keep your eyes (and options) open!

How to direct your medical CV

Once you've made a decision about an area you want to specialize in, you need to demonstrate an interest. Consider some of the following:

- **Student-selected modules** Use this opportunity to pursue a project under supervision from a consultant within your specialty of interest.
- **Audits** An audit refers to a process of review and implementation of change to improve the quality of patient care and outcomes. You start by collecting data on whether *set standards* are being met (e.g. measuring whether pulse oximetry is being recorded for all chronic obstructive pulmonary disease (COPD) patients in a GP clinic). You may then identify *areas of change* based on your data (e.g. investing in more pulse oximeters, which you have found to be shared between consulting rooms). If a *change is implemented* (e.g. purchasing more oximeters for the practice), then you can *reaudit* after a certain time in order to see whether your results have improved.
- **Research** The importance of research in your medical career cannot be overstated—it not only offers extra CV points but also provides an experience of how science and medicine develop. Intercalated degrees offer a fantastic opportunity in your preclinical career for getting published (see p. 68).
- **Medical press** Publications do not necessarily have to come from scientific or clinical research. Writing for the medical press, such as a student journal, can highlight your interest and enthusiasm. Note that peer-reviewed articles are of much higher status than those published in other forms (e.g. student magazines).
- **Prizes** These can be useful in demonstrating your success in clinical exams. The application process for your first job ranks students by quartiles within their universities (top 25%, second 25%, third 25%, and bottom 25% are each assigned a different number of points). Prizes can highlight additional success. The Royal Colleges also offer prizes for essays written by medical students. These are often undersubscribed and so worth trying for if you have a talent for writing.

Key points

Medical school is the beginning of a career, so begin thinking about the direction of your career from the very first day. Invest in a medical careers guide early, such as *So You Want To Be A Brain Surgeon?* (published by Oxford University Press) It is in the same series as this book and covers all the available careers in medicine (not just brain surgery).

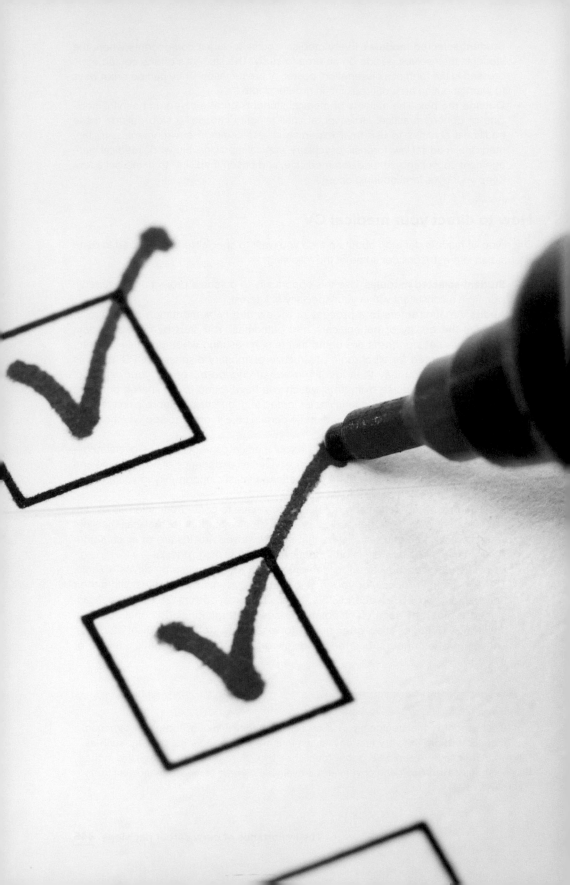

Appendix 1
UCAT and BMAT questions

▌UCAT section 1 questions

Time allowed 2 minutes

In September 1997, Scotland held a referendum on the question of devolution. Over 60% of eligible voters went to the polls, and they voted in favour of both questions on the ballot paper. On the first question, asking whether there should be a Scottish Parliament, 74.3% of voters agreed, including a majority in favour in every Scottish local authority area. On the second question, asking whether that Parliament should have tax-varying powers, 63.5% of voters agreed, including a majority in favour in every Scottish local authority area except Orkney, and Dumfries and Galloway. In response to the results of this referendum, the UK Parliament passed the 1998 Scotland Act, which was given Royal Assent on 19 November 1998. The first members of the Scottish Parliament (MSPs) were elected on 6 May 1999, and the Queen formally opened the Scottish Parliament on 1 July 1999, at which time it took up its full powers.

Under the terms of the 1998 Scotland Act, the Scottish Parliament has the authority to pass laws that affect Scotland on a range of issues. These issues are known as 'devolved matters', as power in these matters has been transferred (or 'devolved') from a national body (the UK Parliament at Westminster) to regional bodies (the Scottish Parliament, the National Assembly for Wales, and the Northern Ireland Assembly). Education, Agriculture, Justice, and Health (including NHS issues in Scotland) are among the issues devolved to the Scottish Parliament. The Scottish Parliament also has the power to set the basic rate of income tax, as high as three pence in the pound.

The 1998 Scotland Act also provides for 'reserved matters', which Scots must take up through their MPs at Westminster rather than through their MSPs. Such reserved matters, on which the Scottish Parliament cannot pass legislation, include Foreign Affairs, Defence, and National Security.

In Scottish parliamentary elections, each voter has two votes: one vote for the MSP for their local constituency, and one vote for the candidate or party to represent their Scottish Parliamentary Region. There are 73 local constituencies, and eight Scottish Parliamentary Regions; each local constituency is represented by one local MSP, and each region is represented by seven regional MSPs. These local and regional MSPs account for the total membership of the Scottish Parliament. Thus, every Scotsman or Scotswoman is represented by a total of eight MSPs (one local and seven regional).

Based on the text on p. 348, answer the following four questions:

1 In the 1997 referendum, more voters in Dumfries and Galloway were in favour of a Scottish Parliament than were in favour of the tax-varying powers for a Scottish Parliament.
   A True
   B False
   C Can't tell

2 The Scottish Parliament can raise the basic rate of income tax by three pence in the pound.
   A True
   B False
   C Can't tell

3 NHS issues in Wales are among the issues devolved to the National Assembly for Wales.
   A True
   B False
   C Can't tell

4 There are a total of 129 MSPs in the Scottish Parliament.
   A True
   B False
   C Can't tell

▌UCAT section 2 questions

Time allowed 2 minutes
Linden Grove School is designated a Specialist Language College. All students at Linden Grove must study at least one language to GCSE level and many students take GCSEs in two languages. All students in Year 11 at Linden Grove take at least one of three languages:

61 students in Year 11 study French
35 students in Year 11 study German
47 students in Year 11 study Spanish

These numbers include students who take a single language, as shown in the first chart, as well as students taking more than one language, as shown in the second, third, and fourth charts.

No student in Year 11 studies more than two languages.

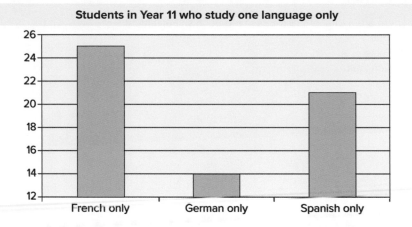

Students in Year 11 who study one language only

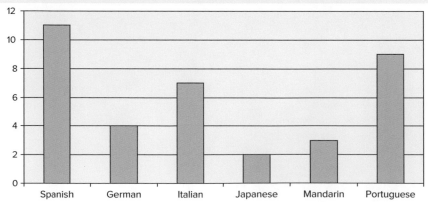

Second languages of students in Year 11 who study French

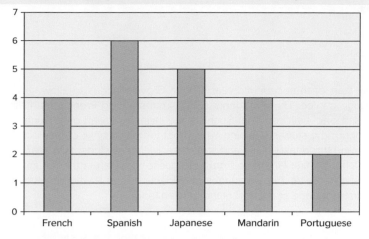

Second languages of students in Year 11 who study German

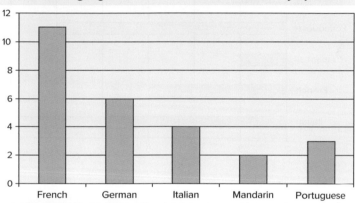

Second languages of students in Year 11 who study Spanish

1 What is the total number of students in Year 11?
   A 80
   B 101
   C 122
   D 143
   E Can't tell

2 The number of students who study Spanish as their only language is equal to the total number of students who study which two languages?
   A Mandarin and Portuguese
   B Italian and Mandarin
   C Italian and Japanese
   D Italian and Portuguese
   E Japanese and Portuguese

3 What percentage of students who study German also study Mandarin?
   A 4%
   B 11%
   C 19%
   D 26%
   E 43%

4 At the start of the academic year, Linden Grove decides to allow Italian as a first-language choice. Three students switch from studying French and Italian to Italian only, and one switches from Spanish and Italian to Italian only. During the autumn term: four new students joining Year 11 opt for Italian only; one selects French and Italian; and three take Italian and Japanese. Half of all students in Year 11 also decide to switch their first language from Portuguese to Italian in the autumn term. Which chart shows the second languages of students in Year 11 who are studying Italian as their first language at the end of the autumn term?

A

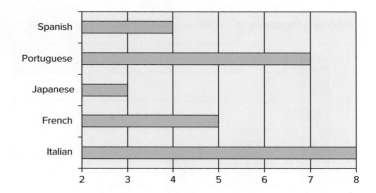

B

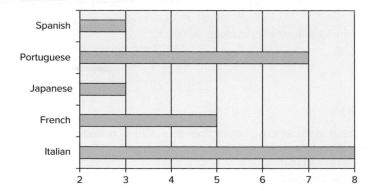

C

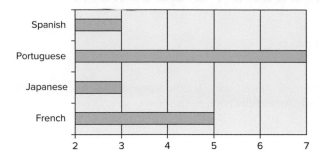

D

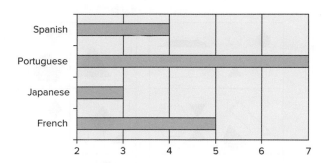

E

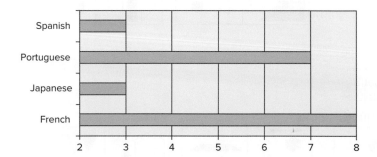

▌ UCAT section 3 questions

Time allowed 1 minute

Directions:

- Consider the pair of sets (which are the same for all five test shapes).
- For each test shape, select one answer only.

1. Test shape
   A   Set A
   B   Set B
   C   Neither

   Test shape   Set A   Set B

   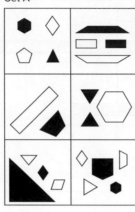
   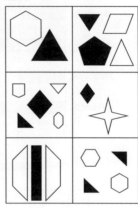

2. Test shape
   A   Set A
   B   Set B
   C   Neither

   Test shape   Set A   Set B

   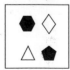
   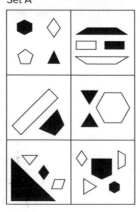
   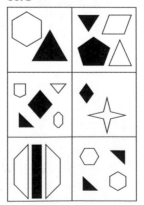

3. Test shape
   A Set A
   B Set B
   C Neither

   Test shape

   Set A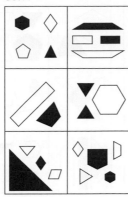

   Set B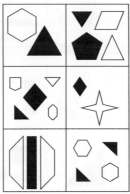

4. Test shape
   A Set A
   B Set B
   C Neither

   Test shape

   Set A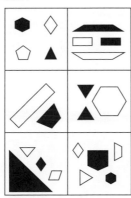

   Set B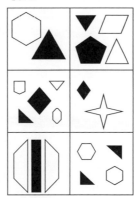

5. Test shape
   A Set A
   B Set B
   C Neither

Test shape

Set A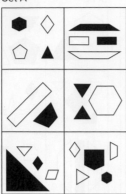

Set B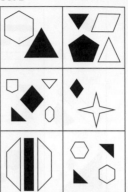

UCAT section 4 questions

Time allowed 7 minutes

Medieval tapestry code

Whilst cleaning a fourteenth-century tapestry, employees at the British Museum discover a previously undetected and rather elaborate code woven into its fabric. The code appears to consist of a series of letters and numbers (see 'Table of codes'), grouped together in sequences as coded messages that seem to tell a story. The employees call in an art historian, who hires you as his assistant to decipher these newfound codes.

On examining the tapestry, you determine that some of the information is strange or incomplete, but all of the messages contain some logic. Indeed, the code seems to follow certain patterns that indicate that an internal logic is built into its use. Thus you must make your assessments based on the codes rather than what seems the most predictable or literal translation.

UCAT section 4 questions

Every code has a best answer that makes the most sense based on all the information presented, but remember that this test requires you to make judgements rather than simply apply logic and rules.

1 What is the best interpretation of the coded message: C12, 1, 9, F(B3)?
   A Down from the castle, the noblewoman takes me as her equal.
   B The countess was my downfall.
   C I am taking the duchess into the castle.
   D I took the countess down from her castle.
   E The duchess and I found our downfall at the castle.

2 What is the best interpretation of the coded message: F(7,3), E8, 5, B(G6)?
   A The brave duke pulled the dangerous sword out of the tree.
   B The brave duke risked pushing the sword into the tree.
   C The duke bravely moved away from the treacherous tree with sword in hand.
   D The knight pulled the sword out of the tree.
   E The knight risked pulling the sword out of the tree.

3 What would be the best way to encode the following message: Many armies of knights came to the castle seeking the Holy Grail?
   A AF(7, 3), 8, G12, 14, H13
   B AF(7, 3), 8, D4, G12, 14, H13
   C ADF(7, 3), 8, G12, 14, H13
   D ADF(7, 3), 8, G12, 9(14, H13)
   E ADF(7, 3), 8, D4, G12, 14, H13

4 What is the best interpretation of the coded message: B(7, 3), 8, 10, (7, 3), 14, B10?
   A On his quest for peace, a fearful man sometimes moves against a brave one in battle.
   B A coward fights on, while a fearless man seeks peace.
   C A man who is not a knight went and fought one who was, on a search to end the war.

D A serf must go fight a knight in the name of peace.
E Peace is found when serfs and knights refuse to fight.

5 Which of the following would be the most useful and second most useful additions to the codes to convey the message accurately?
Message: The perilous woodland creatures alarmed my horse with their vulgar sounds.
A Peril
B Woodland
C Disturb
D Vulgar
E Noise

Table of codes

Operators and general rules	Specific information
	Basic codes
A = multiple	1 = I
B = opposite	2 = you
C = down	3 = man
D = group	4 = horse
E = danger	5 = sword
F = noble	6 = tree
G = into	7 = brave
H = special	8 = move
	9 = take
	10 = fight
	11 = creature
	12 = castle
	13 = goblet
	14 = search

▌ UCAT section 5 questions

Time allowed 7 minutes

Read the following scenario and answer the questions that follow.

> You are shadowing a Foundation Year 1 doctor in your local hospital for work experience. After just a morning of shadowing, you have noticed that the junior doctor appears inattentive, tired, and has not completed any of the jobs tasked to him on the morning ward round. He has also not responded to the last five bleeps he has received, and asks you to go and buy him a coffee while he 'recuperates' in the doctor's mess.

How appropriate are each of these responses by the medical student in this situation?

1. Ask the junior doctor why he appears to be neglecting his duties and putting his patient's safety at risk.
   - A very appropriate thing to do
   - Appropriate, but not ideal
   - Inappropriate, but not awful
   - A very inappropriate thing to do

2. Offer to buy him a coffee providing he responds to his pager.
   - A very appropriate thing to do
   - Appropriate, but not ideal
   - Inappropriate, but not awful
   - A very inappropriate thing to do

3. Report the junior doctor to your human resources point of contact at the end of the working day.
   - A very appropriate thing to do
   - Appropriate, but not ideal
   - Inappropriate, but not awful
   - A very inappropriate thing to do

4. Volunteer to answer his pager in the hope this will encourage the junior doctor to complete his professional duties.
   - A very appropriate thing to do
   - Appropriate, but not ideal
   - Inappropriate, but not awful
   - A very inappropriate thing to do

How important are these options in response to this scenario?

5. To ascertain, with certainty, whether the junior doctor is under the influence of alcohol.
   - Very important
   - Important
   - Of minor importance
   - Not important at all

6 Share your observations with the junior doctor's superiors, if you are concerned.
   - Very important
   - Important

- Of minor importance
- Not important at all

7 Identify if the pager is working and whether the junior doctor is currently responsible for answering his pager, before raising your concerns with anyone else.
- Very important
- Important
- Of minor importance
- Not important at all

8 Establish the junior doctor's medical school ranking in order to gain an impression of his clinical expertise.
- Very important
- Important
- Of minor importance
- Not important at all

▌ UCAT answers and commentary

UCAT section 1 answers

1. (A) True

This statement needs to be evaluated carefully. We're told in the first paragraph that Dumfries and Galloway was one of two local authority areas in which a majority of voters were not in favour of a Scottish Parliament having tax-varying powers. So the percentage of voters in favour of this question in Dumfries and Galloway must be 50% or less. We're also told that a majority of voters 'in every Scottish local authority area' were in favour of having a Scottish Parliament. Dumfries and Galloway is one of these areas, so a majority of voters, or more than 50%, were in favour of a Scottish Parliament. We don't know the exact number of voters in Dumfries and Galloway, but there must have been more in favour of a Scottish Parliament (at more than 50% of voters) than were in favour of tax-varying powers for that parliament (a number of voters at or below 50%). So the statement is 'True'.

2. (B) False

This statement is also rather challenging and requires you to read and think very carefully. The last sentence of the second paragraph tells us that the Scottish Parliament can 'set the basic rate of income tax, as high as three pence in the pound'. However, this statement says that Parliament 'can raise the basic rate of income tax by three pence in the pound'. Thus there must already be a basic rate of income tax, unspecified here, which is to be raised. Whatever the starting basic rate, raising it by three pence in the pound would result in a basic rate of income tax above three pence in the pound, which takes the rate beyond the level the Scottish Parliament may set it at. So the statement is 'False'.

3. (C) Can't tell

The text tells us very little about the National Assembly for Wales; its existence is merely noted, in brackets, as one of the regional bodies to which certain powers have been 'devolved', or transferred, from the UK Parliament at Westminster. We are told in the next sentence that 'Health (including NHS issues in Scotland)' are among the issues devolved to the Scottish Parliament, but we cannot infer from the text that similar issues in Wales are devolved to the Welsh National Assembly. We simply know nothing from the text about this Assembly, other than that it has some powers devolved to it. So the answer is 'Can't tell'.

4. (A) True

This statement requires you to do some maths, which shouldn't prove too difficult, so long as you don't misread the text! We're told that Scotland is divided into 73 local constituencies, each with one local MSP, and also into eight parliamentary regions, each with seven regional MSPs. So there are $73 \times 1 = 73$ local MSPs and $8 \times 7 = 56$ regional MSPs, making a total of $73 + 56 = 129$ MSPs in the Scottish Parliament. The statement is 'True'.

UCAT section 2 answers

1. (C) 122

We can eliminate one answer straight away: we seem to have enough data to calculate the total number of students in Year 11, so the answer can't be 'Can't tell'. Eliminate (E). The calculations, however, are not quite as straightforward as you might think, particularly if you did this question quickly, as it's not simply a matter of adding the number of students in the summary: $61 + 35 + 47 = 143$. These numbers include students who take a single language, as well as students who study two languages. Looking at the three charts, we see that students who study French and German, French and Spanish, or German and Spanish are counted twice. You must subtract them from the total of 143, so 143 − 11 − 4 − 6 = 122, and the correct answer is therefore **(C)** .

2. (E) Japanese and Portuguese

For this question, we need to read our charts carefully and do some basic sums—again, nothing terribly challenging, but it's very easy to make an error in the rush of trying to get through the question. First, we need the number of students studying Spanish as their only language. The first chart shows this as 21. We can then quickly count the number of students studying the other languages:

Italian: 7 + 0 + 4 = 11
Japanese: 2 + 5 + 0 = 7
Mandarin: 3 + 4 + 2 = 9
Portuguese: 9 + 2 + 3 = 14

Of those figures, we can only equal 21 by adding 7 and 14, the numbers of students studying Japanese and Portuguese, so the correct answer is **(E)** .

3. (B) 11%

Questions about percentages are very common on the UCAT and the key is to read carefully and make sure you don't make an error in your maths, as the common errors will likely be listed as wrong answer choices. This question asks for the percentage of students studying German who also study Mandarin. We see from the initial summary that 35 students study German. From the chart of second languages of students studying German, we see that four these students also study Mandarin. So our percentage is 4/35 × 100, or 11%. The answer is **(B)** .

4. (C)

Occasionally the UCAT will give you a question where the answers are new charts! These can be time-consuming. A good tip is to work backwards from the data in the answers and see if you can eliminate any of them straight away on this basis. In this instance, charts **(A)** and **(B)** include Italian as a second language. However, the question asks for a chart showing the second languages of students studying Italian. Thus, Italian can't be a second language choice, so we can eliminate **(A)** and **(B)**. We can then scan the remaining three charts for differences in the data. For instance, all three remaining charts list the number of students studying Japanese as three and students studying Portuguese as seven. So we cannot determine which is correct on the basis of these students. So let's try Spanish: we're told one student switches from Spanish and Italian to Italian only. There were four such students, so the number in our chart should be three. That eliminates **(D)**. Originally there were seven students studying French and Italian; we're told that three switch out of this group and one new student joins during the autumn term. Thus the total number of French and Italian students in our chart should be five and the answer is **(C)**.

UCAT section 3 answers

1. (A)

This set is all about colours and sides. In Set A, the total number of sides on the white shapes in each item is equal to the total number of sides on the black shapes. In Set B, the total number of sides on the white shapes is twice the total number of sides on the black shapes. The size, arrangement, or type of shapes is irrelevant. Our first test shape includes white shapes with a total of eight sides and black shapes with a total of eight sides, so it fits into Set A.

2. (C)

This test shape includes a black hexagon and pentagon, with a total of 11 sides, and a white diamond and triangle, with a total of seven sides. Thus it fits into neither set and the answer is **(C)** .

3. (C)

Counting the sides here, we find a total of eight sides on the black shapes and four sides on the white shape. This test shape fits into neither set, so again the answer is **(C)** .

4. (A)

This test shape contains two pentagons, one white, one black. As they have the same number of sides, the answer is **(A)** .

5. (B)

The final test shape in this set is the least like the rest of the lot, presenting two black triangles and four white triangles. The black shapes have a total of six sides and the white shapes a total of 12 sides. Therefore this test shape fits into Set B.

UCAT section 4 answers

1. (D)
Literal translation: down(castle), I, take, noble(opposite(man))

The basic approach with Decision Analysis is to write down the literal translation—taking care to group the elements of the code with commas or brackets, fitting the original. Then you can eliminate any answers that omit elements, or don't combine them correctly. Starting here with C12, or down(castle)—answers **(A)** and **(D)** keep these elements clearly together. Eliminate **(B)**, which omits the castle, and also **(C)**, which swaps 'down' for 'into' (which is a different letter in the code). Be very suspicious of **(E)**, which seems to separate 'down' and 'castle' (turning 'down' into 'downfall', a more elaborate concept than the code suggests). The three remaining answers contain 'I', but answer **(E)** drops out when we come to 'take', which is not included. The final element of the code could well become 'noblewoman', as in **(A)**, or 'countess', as in **(D)**. The elements of the code have been exhausted without accounting for the concept 'as her equal', which finishes **(A)**, so this cannot be correct. The correct answer is therefore **(D)**, which includes all the elements of the code and nothing more.

2. (E)
Literal translation: noble(brave, man), danger(move), sword, opposite(into(tree))

You don't need to take the code elements in order to eliminate answers. Here, the easiest might be the last element, which must mean something like 'out of the tree'. This matches answers **(A)** , **(D)**, and **(E)** and eliminates **(B)** and **(C)**. We might next consider the element 'danger', which is linked to 'move', which eliminates **(A)**, as this choice links 'danger' with 'sword'. The difference between **(D)** and **(E)** then is the difference between 'pulled' and 'risked pulling'—only the latter accounts for both 'danger' and 'move', so **(E)** is correct.

3. (C)

This question works in reverse, so we can go straight to the answers and see what elements they have in common; we can then make our judgements and eliminate as appropriate. For instance, the answers all start with 'AF(7, 3)' or 'ADF(7, 3)'—which best matches the start of our message, 'Many armies of knights'? The correct answer for question 2 rendered 'F(7, 3)' as 'knight'. In the code, A means 'multiple' and D means 'group', which would account for the 'many armies'. Eliminate answers **(A)** and **(B)**, as they omit the 'group' code (and would thus mean something like 'many knights'). All remaining answers include 8 ('move') and G12 ('into the castle'). They also include 14 ('search') and H13 ('special goblet'), which would fit 'Holy Grail' in the message. These elements, and nothing more, are found in answer **(C)**, which appears to be correct. Checking quickly, we can see that answer **(D)** groups 'search' and 'special goblet' with code 9 ('take'), which does not make sense with the message, and answer **(E)** adds in D4, or 'group of horses', also not in the message. This question also points up the value of using your correct responses from previous questions to help understand the patterns in the code, as these can recur again and again.

4. (B)
Literal translation: opposite(brave, man), move, fight, (brave, man), search, opposite(fight)
This coded message includes a 'brave man' and his opposite, so eliminate answers that don't: answers **(C)**, **(D)**, and **(E)** all render 'brave man' and the opposite as 'knight' and 'serf' (or 'not a knight'), but we've seen that the code requires F ('noble') to indicate that a brave man is in fact a knight. So that leaves **(A)** and **(B)**. Comparing these, it's quickly clear that answer **(B)** accounts for all the elements in the code and nothing more; answer **(A)** jumbles the order—moving the 'quest for peace' to the beginning and attributing it to the 'fearful man'; answer **(A)** also adds the element 'sometimes'. The better fit, and correct answer, is **(B)**.

5. (C) and (E)
This question is different from the rest, on two counts: we have to add something to the code, and we must find not one correct answer, but two. Once again, the quickest strategy is to eliminate the answers that are wrong. On this type of question, wrong answers most commonly fall into two categories: they are not part of the message, or they are already included in the code. All answers here are in the coded message—as 'disturb' means the same as 'alarm' in this context and 'noise' is the same as 'sound'. So eliminate those that are covered by the code: 'peril' means the same as 'danger', so eliminate answer (**A**). A 'group of trees', or D6, would be a 'woodland', so eliminate (**B**); and 'vulgar' also means 'common', which is the opposite of 'noble', or BF in the code. Eliminate (**D**), which leaves the correct answers as (**C**) and (**E**), as the code cannot cover the elements 'disturb' or 'noise'.

UCAT section 5 commentary

1. Appropriate, but not ideal
If you have concerns regarding the junior doctor's practice, it is appropriate to direct those concerns to the junior doctor in the first instance. This particular response is confrontational and more likely to antagonize the junior doctor than to successfully address the problem.

2. Inappropriate, but not awful
This attempt to cajole the junior doctor into completing his professional duties is inappropriate, and should not be necessary. You should not be expected to purchase coffee; the important point here is to address why the junior doctor is not responding to his pager.

3. Appropriate, but not ideal
It is reasonable to raise any concerns you have with your point of contact, but it would be more satisfactory to resolve your concerns more quickly with the junior doctor or, failing this, with his clinical superiors.

4. A very inappropriate thing to do
You are not qualified to be able to respond to the doctor's paged requests, and volunteering to answer his pages in an effort to encourage his fulfilment of clinical duties is unnecessary.

5. Not important at all

While the additional knowledge of the junior doctor being under the influence of alcohol would not be unhelpful, this is not something you need to ascertain with certainty, and you should not hesitate to raise any genuine concerns.

6. Very important

It is essential to share any concerns that you may have regarding patient safety with the responsible seniors.

7. Very important

There are various legitimate reasons why the junior doctor may not be responding to his pager, and the option offered enables you to gauge this in an appropriate fashion before escalating the matter further. Perhaps the pager messages were mistakenly sent without a return number, or were group messages or test calls unintended for the junior doctor and not requiring a response. Ascertaining this before accusing the junior doctor of shirking his responsibilities is important for the professional standing and reputation of the junior doctor, and yourself.

8. Not important at all

This should have no implication for the way you handle this situation, as all practicing doctors are considered competent and assumed clinically capable, and this would not be adequate justification for failing to perform one's clinical responsibilities.

▌ BMAT section 1 questions

Time allowed 7 minutes

1 A conductor of an orchestra makes the following remarks about the composers that her musicians adore:

All musicians in the orchestra adore Handel. Some cellists adore Schumann and some adore Bach. All flautists adore Mozart and some adore Rimsky-Korsakov. No percussionist adores Bach and all percussionists adore Rimsky-Korsakov.

Based on the conductor's remarks, which of the following statements must be true?

A Some cellists adore Handel, but not Schumann or Bach.

B Some cellists adore both Schumann and Bach.

C Some flautists adore Bach.

D Some flautists adore three composers.

E Some percussionists adore three composers.

2 A shop selling electrical goods lowers the price of a digital camera each day of a Bank Holiday weekend. On Saturday, the price of the camera is lowered by 10% from its price on Friday. On Sunday, the price is lowered 10% from its price on Saturday. On Monday, the price is lowered by 10% from its price on Sunday. The price of the camera on Monday is what percentage of its price on Friday?

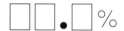

3 Media coverage of organ donation has increased as the Government considers making the donor registry 'opt-out', rather than 'opt-in'. Every week, newspapers and TV reports are filled with grim stories and statistics of waiting lists and deaths of those waiting for a transplant. Regardless of any changes to legislation, the media could do more to increase organ donation at present. For example, the frequent news reports on the need for more donated organs rarely mention how, exactly, members of the public can 'opt-in' to the donor registry. This practice stands in stark contrast to the presentation of such stories in other countries, such as the USA and Canada, where reports on the need for more organ donors almost always end with contact details for joining the donor registry. Providing viewers with a phone number or website for joining the registry is seen as a public service, part of the media's responsibility in calling attention to such a problem.

Which of the following best summarizes the main conclusion of the argument?

A It's easier to become an organ donor in the USA or Canada than in the UK.

B Sometimes the media can help to solve the problems it identifies.

C The Government wants to make organ donation compulsory.

D Many people die waiting for organs each year as there are too few donors opting-in to the registry.

E Everyone should be required to join the organ donor registry.

4 Shannon and Dave are hosting a dinner party for six friends. The dining table is circular, with chairs set out at equal distances around its circumference. Each chair is directly opposite one other chair (see diagram).

Dave prefers to sit directly opposite Shannon. Rachael and James are a couple and prefer to sit next to each other. Ben fancies Lola, and he's a bit shy, so he prefers to sit directly opposite her. Dave and Shannon can't stand Patrick, whom Cindy is seeing, so neither of them will sit next to him.

If the seating plan meets everyone's preferences, what is the probability that Cindy will be seated directly opposite Rachael?

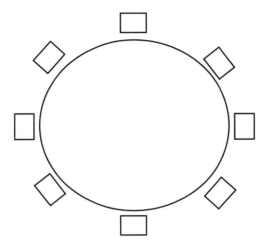

▎ BMAT section 2 questions

Time allowed 4 minutes

1 Haemophilia B (Christmas disease) is an X-linked recessive disorder. Both Jane's father and maternal grandfather suffer from haemophilia B. Which of Jane's relatives is neither a carrier of nor suffers from Christmas disease?

   A Her sister

   B Her father's monozygotic twin

   C Her maternal uncle

   D Her maternal aunt

   E Her paternal grandmother

2 Concerning acids:

   I   Citric acid ionizes partially in aqueous solution.

   II A 1 M solution of ethanoic acid has the same concentration of H+(aq) as a 1 M solution of nitric acid.

   III A 1 M solution of hydrochloric acid is a better conductor of electricity than a 1 M solution of lactic acid.

   Which of the following choices lists the statements that are correct?

   A I only

   B II only

   C III only

   D I and II only

   E I and III only

   F II and III only

   G I, II, and III

3 Three points in the (x, y) co-ordinate plane lie at: (a, b)

   $(a + 3 \sqrt{2}, b)$

   $(a + \sqrt{2}, b - 4\sqrt{2})$

   What is the area of the triangle described by these co-ordinates?

   A $\sqrt{2}$

   B 6

   C $5 \sqrt{2}$

   D 12

   E $12 \sqrt{2}$

4 A laser is shone through a small circular hole and the image is projected onto a screen. Which of the following choices represents the pattern shown on the screen?

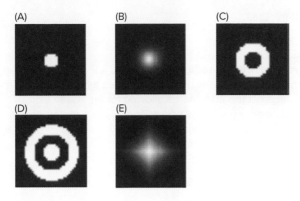

(A)

(B)

(C)

(D)

(E)

BMAT section 3 questions

Time allowed 30 minutes
Directions:

- Answer ONE question.
- Handwrite your answer on a single page of A4.
- You are permitted to make any preparatory notes as needed, but time spent on such notes counts against the 30 minutes allowed for the essay.
- Essays are assigned a numerical score. To achieve a top mark, you must address all aspects of the question and write compellingly with few errors in logic or in use of English.

BMAT section 3 questions

1 'A scientific man ought to have no wishes, no affections—a mere heart of stone.'

Charles Darwin

Write an essay in which you address the following points:

Why should those who practice science or medicine have 'no wishes, no affections'? What is the negative impact when scientists or doctors have 'hearts of stone'? How could a scientist or doctor best reconcile these competing concerns?

2 The self-inflicting diseases resulting from obesity should not be a burden for the National Health Service.

Explain the reasoning behind this statement and suggest arguments to the contrary. To what extent, if any, should the patient's responsibility of their disease shape clinical practice?

3 'The greatest enemy of knowledge is not ignorance; it is the illusion of knowledge.'

Stephen Hawking

Write an essay in which you address the following points:

In science, how is the 'illusion of knowledge' an 'enemy of knowledge'? Can you argue that ignorance is itself an 'enemy of knowledge'? By what criteria could you assess the comparative impact of these two, to determine which is the greater enemy of scientific knowledge?

4 'I observe the physician with the same diligence as the disease.'

John Donne, English poet (1572–1631)

Write an essay in which you address the following points:

Why would a patient observe his physician 'with the same diligence' as his disease? Under what circumstances might a patient be more concerned with his disease than with his physician? How would you advise a patient to best balance these two concerns?

▌BMAT answers and commentary

BMAT section 1 answers

1. (D) Some flautists adore three composers

This question is challenging as it hinges on the definition, in logic terms, of 'some', which simply means 'more than one'. The key, then, is in understanding what it means, and doesn't mean, to say that 'Some cellists adore Schumann and some adore Bach'. We know from the first sentence that all musicians adore Handel. Thus, we can divide cellists into at least two groups:

> Those who adore Handel and Schumann
> Those who adore Handel and Bach

However, answers **(A)** and **(B)** suggest two additional groups:

> Those who adore Handel, but neither Schumann nor Bach
> Those who adore Handel, Schumann, and Bach

In fact, either of these groups could exist without conflicting with the conductor's statements. She did not say that the 'some cellists' who adore Schumann and the 'some cellists' who adore Bach are mutually exclusive—nor did she say that they account for all the cellists in the orchestra. We can't infer beyond the logical meaning of her words, so the groups in **(A)** and **(B)** could exist, or they could not. However, the key is that they don't have to exist, on the basis of the conductor's words—they aren't definitely true, so these two answers are wrong.

Similarly, answer **(C)** says that 'Some flautists adore Bach'—this might or might not be true, as the conductor has not mentioned Bach in reference to the flautists. Since we don't know for certain, the answer is out.

Answer **(D)** says that 'Some flautists adore three composers'. How does this stack up to our statements? We know that all musicians adore Handel and all flautists adore Mozart. So all flautists must adore at least two composers—that's something that must be true, based on the conductor's remarks. We can go a step further and see that some flautists must adore at least three composers, as some adore Rimsky–Korsakov in addition to Handel and Mozart. So statement **(D)** must be true.

We cannot conclude the statement made in answer **(E)**, as we don't know for sure that any percussionists adore more than three composers. They all adore Handel and Rimsky–Korsakov, and none of them adores Bach, but we don't know about a third who any of them might adore. So this answer is out and our sole correct answer is **(D)**.

2. 72.9%

This question is tricky for two reasons: (1) we're not told the starting price of the camera; and (2) there are no answer choices. There's potentially a third twist, in that we're asked to give our answer as a percentage to one decimal place and do so without a calculator!

Kaplan has a helpful technique for percentage questions without a starting value for the original: always pick 100 for the original value. This makes the maths a lot simpler. Here, we can start with £100 for the price of the camera on Friday. It's marked down by 10% on Saturday, so the price on Saturday is £100 − £10 = £90, as £10 is 10% of £100. Then, on Sunday, the £90 is marked down another 10%: 10% of £90 is £9, so the price on Sunday is £90 − £9 = £81. Finally, on Monday, the price is marked down a further 10%: 10% of £81 is £8.10, so the final sale price on Monday is £81 − £8.10 = £72.90.

We calculate the percentage by dividing the price on Monday, £72.90, by the price on Friday, £100, and $\frac{72.90}{100} \times 100 = 72.9\%$.

You could do the problem without picking a number, using a variable such as p for the initial price of the camera on Friday. The price on Saturday would be 90% of the price on Friday, or 0.9p. The price on Sunday would be 90% of the price on Saturday, or 0.9(0.9p). Likewise, the price on Monday would be 90% of the price on Sunday, so the final sale price would be 0.9(0.9(0.9p)). This would multiply out as 0.729p, which is equal to 72.9%. If you have trouble conceptualizing that, then it's definitely quicker to pick a number for the starting value.

3. (B)

The conclusion of the argument is the author's main point. The rest of the argument as stated is evidence, backing up this main point in some way. Sometimes the conclusion comes as the final sentence of the argument; on the BMAT, this is not always the case. Here, the author's main point comes in the middle of the argument: 'Regardless of any changes to legislation, the media could do more to increase organ donation at present'. The rest of the argument is an example of how the media's current practice is deficient, as they rarely mention how readers or viewers can 'opt-in' to the organ donor registry. This shortcoming is contrasted with standard media practice in the USA and Canada, where viewers are routinely given contact details for the donor registry following stories on the need for more donated organs. The conclusion is nicely summarized in answer **(B)**, which admittedly abstracts things a bit but matches the author's main point directly.

All the other answers here touch on relatively minor points of the author's argument, or are not really part of it at all. For instance, one might infer that it is effectively easier to become an organ donor in the USA or Canada than in the UK, as answer **(A)** states, but this is hardly the author's main point, as the argument is focused on media coverage of the need for organ donors. Answers **(C)** and **(D)** are certainly true, on the basis of our argument, but neither is the author's main point. Finally, answer **(E)** makes a conclusion that is outside the scope of our argument. Our author never goes so far as to suggest that membership on the organ donor registry should be compulsory.

4. 50% probability

This question is a good example of a BMAT question that seems a lot trickier than it actually is. That's not to say that it's easy, but it's definitely doable—and without requiring terribly complicated maths.

The question is slightly odd in that the table is circular and we're told which people are meant to be seated next to each other, or directly opposite each other. From these rules, we will get enough information to determine the probability of Cindy sitting directly opposite Rachael. (This will be expressed as a fraction, with the number of such seating arrangements divided by the total number of possible seating arrangements.)

The good news: this question has a built-in shortcut, of sorts. One option is to consider all possible arrangements for sitting the full group of eight. The other, simpler option is to consider the pairs who can sit directly opposite each other. Our rules may well let us determine the probability of Cindy sitting opposite Rachael on this basis.

We know from our rules that Dave will sit opposite Shannon and Ben opposite Lola. That leaves four people with seating to be determined: Rachael, James, Patrick, and Cindy. We know that Rachael and James will sit next to each other, which means one of them will sit opposite Cindy and the other will sit opposite Patrick. That means there are two possible people who could sit opposite Rachael: either Cindy or Patrick. Cindy is one of those two possibilities, so the probability of Cindy sitting opposite Rachael is 50%.

BMAT section 2 answers

1. (C) Her maternal uncle
As Christmas disease is an X-linked recessive disorder, every carrier or sufferer has inherited a faulty gene on the X-chromosome. As Jane's paternal grandfather suffers from the disease, all of his female offspring must also be carriers. Therefore Jane's mother and maternal aunt must carry the faulty gene on one X-chromosome. As Jane's father suffers from the disease, he must have inherited the faulty gene on the X-chromosome from Jane's paternal grandmother. Jane's father's monozygotic twin will have an identical genotype to Jane's father himself. We know Jane's mother and father both carry copies of the faulty gene on their X-chromosomes. Therefore Jane and her sister must be either carriers or suffer from the disease. Therefore Jane's maternal uncle is the only possible relative in these answer choices who can be free from disease. The correct answer is **(C)**.

2. (E) I and III only
Weak acids are only partially ionized in aqueous solution, while strong acids are almost completely ionized in aqueous solution. Citric acid is a weak acid, so is only partially ionized in aqueous solution. Ethanoic acid is a weak acid, while nitric acid is a strong acid. So a 1 M solution of ethanoic acid will have a lower concentration of solvated protons than a 1 M solution of nitric acid. The electrical conductivity of a solution is greater when more ions are in solution. Hydrochloric acid is a strong acid and therefore will be almost completely ionized in aqueous solution, while lactic acid is a weak acid and will only be partially ionized in aqueous solution. So a 1 M solution of hydrochloric acid will be a better conductor of electricity than a 1 M solution of lactic acid, and the answer is **(E)**.

3. (D) 12
For a triangle, area = ½ × base × perpendicular height. The triangle in the question has one side parallel to the x-axis, as two of the points have an identical y-co-ordinate. This side is length $3\sqrt{2}$, the difference of the two x-co-ordinates. The perpendicular height of the third point is $4\sqrt{2}$. This is equivalent to its distance from b along the y-co-ordinate.

$$\text{Area} = \frac{3\sqrt{2} \times 4\sqrt{2}}{2} = \frac{3 \times 4\sqrt{2}}{2} = \frac{3 \times 4 \times 2}{2} = 12$$

or answer **(D)**.

4. (D)
The light passes through a circular hole, so the diffraction pattern will be circular. Light from the whole circumference of the circular hole will create a pattern of overlapping waves, causing circular rings of constructive interference (bright) and destructive interference (dim). The point of strongest constructive interference will be in the centre of the pattern. Laser light is of a single wavelength, so the size of the edges of the zones of interference will not be diffuse.

BMAT section 3 marking scheme

The essays will be marked by two examiners and, if the marks are similar, an average is taken; a third examiner is involved if there is a larger discrepancy. The content of the essay is scored out of a total of five, while the quality of English used is graded A to E. The markers are instructed to assess content based on the following:

- Have they answered the questions? Markers are asked to consider three specific categories, which often correspond to the three questions asked:
  - Explore the implications of the phrase.
  - Suggest counterarguments.

- Suggest ways to evaluate the different opinions.
- Clearly organized cogent arguments.
- Appropriate use of general knowledge and opinions.
- Breadth of arguments leading to a carefully considered conclusion.

Remember to consider each argument from multiple viewpoints in order to produce a balanced argument. If you are proposing a counterargument, consider what counterclaims could be made against each of your points and try to address them if appropriate.

Clear, concise, and fluent expression with the correct use of English spelling and grammar is scored from A (highest) to E (lowest). The composite mark of two scores is awarded (e.g. for an A and a C, a B would be awarded). If there is a larger discrepancy than two adjacent scores, the essay is marked for a third time by a senior assessor.

Key points

The full marking criteria for section 3 of the BMAT can be found at www.admissionstestingservice.org/bmat

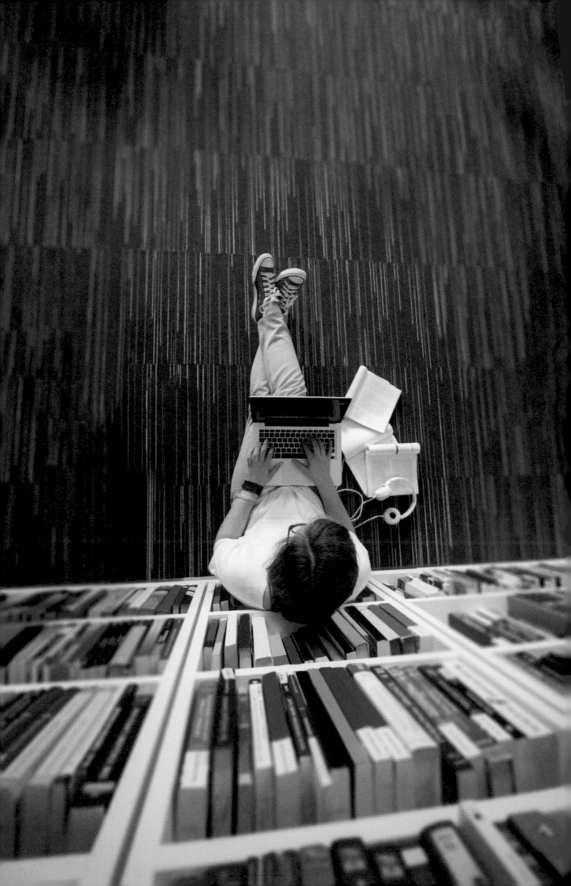

Appendix 2

Useful resources

Thinking about medicine

A deep insight into medicine comes from immersing yourself (as far as possible) in the culture of the profession you hope to join. Work experience (see p. 54) will help, but so will reading widely. Your understanding of how medicine works cannot help but pervade your personal statement and answers to interview questions.

Blogs

A number of doctors write blogs (i.e. online commentaries on their professional lives and issues affecting doctors). They are usually anonymous and so free to voice strong opinions on controversial topics. Take these for what they are and be cautious before reproducing the thoughts of these experienced (and often cynical) doctors at interview.

- **KevinMD** Insightful commentary on contemporary news and ideas, led by an American physician. www.kevinmd.com
- **Bad Science** Social commentary from self-styled 'evangelist for good science', Ben Goldacre. www.badscience.net

Books

Lots of books have been written about the process of becoming a doctor. They are usually written for a popular audience and inject comedy as well as insight into the profession. These are worth reading but beware—they often reflect the experiences of doctors training years ago when the system was very different, although many important themes persist in the NHS today.

- *Bedside Stories* A collection of short, humorous (yet insightful) anecdotes describing life as a doctor in the NHS. Bedside Stories: Confessions of a Junior Doctor. Michael Foxton. Atlantic Books.
- *Seven Signs of Life* A series of articles reflecting on life as an intensive care doctor. Seven Signs of Life. Aoife Abbey. Vintage.
- *In Stitches* A book in diary format, describing life as a doctor in Accident and Emergency. In Stitches: The Highs and Lows of Life as an A&E Doctor. Nick Edwards. The Friday Project Ltd.
- *This is Going to Hurt* The famous diary-entry book describing the career of an obstetrician from FY1 to pre-consultant training. *This is Going to Hurt: Secret Diaries of a Junior Doctor.* Adam Kay. Picador.

There are also more serious accounts of working within healthcare. These all raise issues that could come up in medical school interviews:

- *Complications* A collection of thoughtful essays on various issues that are raised in medicine. A very easy read. Complications: A Surgeon's Notes on an Imperfect Science. Atul Gawande. Profile Books.
- *Bad Science* This describes *how* we know treatments work. It is aimed at unravelling the debates around complementary medicine (e.g. homeopathy) but also explains the basis of clinical research. Bad Science. Ben Goldacre. HarperPerennial.
- *Do No Harm* A thought-provoking account of life as a neurosurgeon. Do No Harm: Stories of Life, Death and Brain Surgery. Henry Marsh. Weidenfeld & Nicolson.
- *Hippocratic Oaths* A collection of essays covering various aspects of healthcare. It is a challenging read because many concepts are complicated and hard to grasp.

However, if you enjoy reading and want to think hard about medicine, this book is worth the effort. Hippocratic Oaths: Medicine and its Discontents. Raymond Tallis. Atlantic Books.

Periodicals

It's worth subscribing to a good periodical. These lean towards either medicine (e.g. the *British Medical Journal*) or science (e.g. *New Scientist*). Keeping abreast of what's happening in medicine (and science) is better preparation before interviews that cramming for a week. Remember: if you subscribe, make a commitment to read every issue.

- *British Medical Journal (BMJ)* This is a weekly medical journal read by most doctors in the UK. Much of the content will be difficult to follow but letters, commentaries, and opinion articles highlight what doctors are thinking about now. www.bmj.com
- *New Scientist* A weekly international magazine covering recent advances in science. www.newscientist.com
- *Scientific American* Like the New Scientist, a popular science magazine. Worth a subscription if you want to learn about science beyond the A level curriculum. www.scientificamerican.com

TV shows

While most medical TV drama does not give an accurate representation of life in the NHS, one show does stand out:

- *Getting On* This BBC Four series, written by and starring Jo Brand, gives a cynical but extremely realistic portrayal of life on an NHS geriatric ward. Search the internet (and BBC iPlayer) to find episodes.

Application resources

The internet provides a wealth of resources for improving your application.

Online forums

Forums are great for keeping in touch with what's going on in the world of medical school selection. They are also good for letting off steam to people who know what you're talking about. Medical school admissions tutors have been known to prowl forums as well. However, be warned—forums are a mine of gossip and hearsay. Just because a poster articulates their views clearly, this doesn't mean their perceptions are correct or that things haven't changed since their experience. If there is doubt, call medical school admissions offices for clarification.

- **The Student Room** Probably the largest online resource for students, with over a million members. Although not specifically for medical applicants, it includes forums dedicated to every UK university, as well as medical applications. www.thestudentroom. co.uk

Learning about medical courses

- **The Medic Portal** A frequently updated resource providing lots of information about medical school applications. www.themedicportal.com/application-guide
- **UCAS** Database of all medical schools in the UK, with notes and entry requirements. www.ucas.com/students/coursesearch
- **Medical school websites** Web addresses for undergraduate and graduate courses.

Improving your personal statement

- **Studential** An online student community with a database of personal statements. Around 100 are for applications to medical school. Read these to gain an idea of how personal statements should look, but heed the plagiarism warning on p. 221. www. studential.com/personal-statements
- **The Student Room** Another database of over 100 medical personal statements. www.thestudentroom.co.uk/wiki/personal_statement_library

Admission tests

If you've exhausted the sample UCAT (see p. 82) and BMAT (see p. 86) questions, see the following website for additional resources:

- **Kaplan Test Prep and Admissions** Provides online and classroom-based preparation for the admissions tests; they supplied the test questions in this book. www. kaptest.com

Useful news outlets

Keeping abreast of the news is almost as important as knowing what is going on in healthcare. You need to come across to course selectors as someone who is interesting, broad-minded, and informed.

- **BBC** The BBC website provides up-to-date and impartial news through its website. Set it (or an equivalent site) as your internet home page and read stories that interest you. www.bbc.co.uk or www.bbc.co.uk/health
- *The Economist* This is an excellent way to keep up to date with current affairs; the articles are carefully researched and present thoughtful analyses of world events. www.economist.com

Social media

There is a thriving medical community on Twitter. The views expressed might not necessarily represent the medical profession as a whole but you can get a feel for what matters to doctors at any given time. This may help sway your views on pursuing medicine as a career and to stay informed as you approach interview time. The hashtag #medtwitter is popular and will help you choose who to 'follow'.

Money and careers

- **Royal Medical Benevolent Fund** A great resource to help you plan your finances and budget at medical school. Provides information on student loans, the NHS Bursary, and other sources of income available to medical students. https://rmbf.org/medical-students
- *So you want to be a brain surgeon?* The leading careers guide aimed at medical students. It is never too early to start thinking about your postgraduate career (see p. 6) and this is a good place to begin. So you want to be a brain surgeon? (4th edition). Edited by Lydia Spurr, Geoffrey Warwick, and Jessica Harris. Oxford University Press.

Index

Tables and figures are indicated by an italic *t* and *f* following the page number

F

failed applications 322–4
failed exams and resits 6, 8, 294, 323,
  325–7, 333
finance:
  debt 333, 340
  graduate entry students 16, 16t, 17,
    252, 253
  loans, grants and bursaries 14, 15–17, 239,
    252, 253, 340
  parental contributions 16, 17
  part-time jobs 16, 256
  Royal Medical Benevolent Fund 17, 383
  see also costs
fitness to practice 298–300, 318, 333
foreign students 101, 296
forums 76, 121, 260, 305, 322, 382
foundation courses 297
Foundation Programme 6, 9, 58
  application results, comparative data 114f
  graduate career destinations, comparative
    data 117f, 119f
Foundation Trusts 60
Freshers' Week 333, 334, 335, 341

G

GAMSAT (Graduate Medical School
  Admissions Test) 74, 254, 255
gap years:
  advantages and disadvantages 34, 38
  backpacking 39
  foreign travel 34, 36–7, 38–40, 43
  medical schools' perspective 35
  and personal statement 225
  practical arrangements 43
  sources of information 42–3
  volunteering 37, 38–9
  work experience placements 34, 36
gateway courses 297
gender reassignment 314
General Medical Council (GMC) 7, 90,
  200, 318
  fitness to practice 298–300, 318, 333
  international student registration 208, 210
  publications (Tomorrow's Doctors and
    Good Medical Practice) 221, 304, 318
general practitioners (GPs) 6, 7, 11, 58
Gillick case (capacity of children) 313
Glasgow 82, 92, 102, 297, 326
  comparative data 96, 98, 107, 109,
    112, 114–19
  profile 192–3
GMC see General Medical Council (GMC)
Good Medical Practice (GMC) 221, 304, 318
GPs (general practitioners) 6, 7, 11, 58
graduate entry 217, 252–3, 324, 327, 328–9
  applications

admission requirements 253–5, 260,
  261t, 266
  choosing a medical school 260–2
  extracurricular activities 256–7
  work experience 258–9
competitiveness of medical schools 252,
  253, 258, 261–2t, 328
costs of study 252, 290, 328
finance options 16, 16t, 17, 252, 253
GAMSAT (Graduate Medical School
  Admissions Test) 74, 254, 255
ScotGEM (Scottish Graduate Entry
  Medicine programme) 74, 261, 289f,
  290, 291t
see also non-traditional applications
grants, bursaries and loans 14, 15–17, 239,
  252, 253, 340
Grenada 209
gynaecology 12

H

health and wellbeing at university 340–1
healthcare, alternative careers in 324, 329
healthcare assistants 38, 57, 63, 67, 104
health concerns 298, 299, 340–1
heart attack 316
Herceptin (breast cancer drug) 314
Highers see A and AS levels
HIV/AIDS 38, 43, 299, 317
hobbies see extracurricular activities
honesty principle 310, 311
hospital porters 57, 67
Hull York 82, 92, 102, 297, 326
  comparative data 96, 99, 107, 110,
    112, 114–19
  profile 142–3
hypochondria 341

I

ill health 298, 299, 340–1
Imperial College, London 69, 86, 91,
  102, 326
  comparative data 96, 98, 107, 109,
    112, 114–19
  graduate entry 254
  profile 156–7
infectious diseases 299, 317
information resources 306–7, 318, 380–3
integrated courses 92, 100
integrity principle 310, 311
intensive care doctors 12
intercalated degree courses 90, 91, 103, 328
International Baccalaureate 22, 294
international students 101, 296
international study 208–9
interviews for medical school 19

chances of success (medical schools compared) 98–9t, 261–2t
ethical questions see ethics
format and marking criteria 304–5
information resources 306–7, 318, 380–1
'interview ammunition' 37, 62, 104 see also extracurricular activities; gap years; work experience
MMI (multi mini-interviews) 19
Oxbridge 104, 246–9, 316
predictable questions 308–9
preparing for interviews 103, 223, 305–7, 318–19
purposes 304
rejection at interview 323
scientific questions 316–17
see also applications to medical school
IVF (in vitro fertilization) 314

J

junior doctors see Foundation Programme
justice principle 310, 311, 314

K

Kaplan (preparatory course provider) 5, 74, 76, 382
Keele 82, 86, 92, 102, 326
    comparative data 96, 99, 107, 109, 112, 114–19
    graduate entry 74
    profile 144–5
Kent and Medway 82, 202
KevinMD (blog) 380
King's College, London 82, 102, 297
    comparative data 96, 98, 107, 111, 112, 114–19
    graduate entry 254, 255, 260, 261, 274
    profiles 158–9, 274

L

Lancaster 86, 102, 297, 326
    comparative data 96, 99, 107, 110, 112, 114–19
    profile 146–7
league tables of medical schools 106, 107–8t, 109–11t, 112–13t
learning at university 336–9
    course types 92–3t, 100, 102, 337
learning impairments 299
lectures 337
Leeds 86, 102, 326
    comparative data 96, 98, 107, 110, 112, 114–19
    profile 148–9
Leicester 82, 102, 297, 326

comparative data 96, 99, 107, 110, 112, 114–19
graduate entry 261, 266
profile 150–1
leisure see extracurricular activities
life-prolonging drugs 314
Lincoln 203, 297, 326
Liverpool 82, 92, 102, 104, 297, 326
    comparative data 96, 98, 107, 110, 113, 114–19
    graduate entry 74, 254, 255, 261, 262, 272
    profiles 152–3, 272
living costs 14–15t, 101
loans, grants and bursaries 14, 15–17, 239, 252, 253, 340
London:
    City and Islington College 296
    living costs 14, 101
    medical schools see Barts, London; Imperial College, London; King's College, London; St George's, London; University College London (UCL)

M

magistrates 257
maintenance loans and grants 15–16
Malta 208
mammograms 315
Manchester 82, 92, 102, 297, 326
    comparative data 96, 98, 107, 110, 112, 114–19
    profile 164–5
massive open online courses (MOOCs) 295
mature students 295, 296 see also graduate entry
MDT (multidisciplinary teams) 318–19
medical careers see career development
medical CVs 341, 345
medical ethics see ethics
medical press 225, 306, 309, 381
medical schools:
    admission requirements see admission requirements
    admission tests see admission tests
    applications see applications to medical school
    choosing a school see choosing a medical school
    comparative data
        graduate performance/ assessments 114–19f
        league tables 106, 107–8t, 109–11t, 112–13t
    costs of study 14–15t, 91, 101, 239, 340
        graduate entry 252, 290
        international students 296
    exams and assessments see exams and assessments

University College London (UCL) 86, 91,
    102, 326
    comparative data 97, 98, 107, 110, 112, 114–19
    profile 162–3
university experience *see* student experience
University of Central Lancashire *see* Central
    Lancashire
University of East Anglia *see* East Anglia (UEA)
university types 94*t*, 96–7*t*, 102

V

vaccinations 43
viral infections 317
visiting medical schools 18, 19, 94, 100,
    120–1, 305
volunteering:
    as extracurricular activity 49, 50, 51, 256
    in gap year 37, 38–9
    at university 256, 258
    see also work experience

W

Wales:
    medical schools *see* Cardiff; Swansea
    medical schools (maps) 197*f*, 285*f*
    Student Finance Wales 15
    tuition fees 14, 101

Warwick 102, 120
    comparative data 107, 111, 112, 114–19
    graduate entry 254, 255, 260, 261,
        262, 282–3
weblogs, medical 380
wellbeing and health at university 340–1
why do you want to be a doctor? 2–3, 224–6,
    308, 322
work experience 3, 4, 19
    advantages 54–5
    arranging placements 56–7
    combined with employment 66–7,
        104, 258–9
    in gap year 34, 36
    graduate entry applicants 258–9
    interview questions about 309
    medical schools' perspective 54
    and personal statement 225
    preparing for placements 58–60
    research-based 68–9, 257
    shadowing 57, 62–3, 66, 344
    at university 258
    unusual examples 70–1
    volunteering *see* volunteering
work-life balance 341
writing for publication/prizes 345

Y

York *see* Hull York